Molecular Description
of
Biological Membranes
by
Computer Aided Conformational Analysis

T0200596

Volume I

Editor

Robert Brasseur, Ph.D.

Laboratory for Interfacial Macromolecular Physical Chemistry
Free University of Brussels
Brussels, Belgium

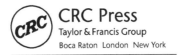

CRC Press
Taylor & Francis Group
Boca Raton London New York

CRC Press is an imprint of the
Taylor & Francis Group, an **informa** business

CRC Press
Taylor & Francis Group
6000 Broken Sound Parkway NW, Suite 300
Boca Raton, FL 33487-2742

Reissued 2019 by CRC Press

© 1990 by Taylor & Francis Group, LLC
CRC Press is an imprint of Taylor & Francis Group, an Informa business

No claim to original U.S. Government works

A Library of Congress record exists under LC control number:

Publisher's Note
The publisher has gone to great lengths to ensure the quality of this reprint but points out that some imperfections in the original copies may be apparent.

Disclaimer
The publisher has made every effort to trace copyright holders and welcomes correspondence from those they have been unable to contact.

ISBN 13: 978-0-367-26160-3 (hbk)
ISBN 13: 978-0-367-26161-0 (pbk)
ISBN 13: 978-0-429-29177-7 (ebk)

Visit the Taylor & Francis Web site at http://www.taylorandfrancis.com and the
CRC Press Web site at http://www.crcpress.com

PREFACE

The biological membrane represents a specific cellular domain as it constitutes a barrier between the inner and outer regions of the cell; it acts also as a crossing-point for all compounds which are either synthesized and released or absorbed by the cell. The assembly of amphiphilic molecules within the membrane results in the formation of a low dielectric constant medium in which hydrophilic compounds cannot easily dissolve. The hydrophobic character of this ultra-thin medium is stable enough to ensure an ionic concentration gradient across the membrane thickness.

The molecular description of the membrane constituents is difficult to achieve experimentally; therefore, one has to rely upon theoretical calculations to simulate the behavior of amphiphilic molecules, including both statistical and semi-empirical methods. Such approaches enable the unraveling of some of the mechanisms accounting for the membrane stability and for the function of compounds inserted in a lipid bilayer such as drugs, amphiphilic helices, and transmembrane peptides.

By all means, these theoretical models should be tested by comparison with all available experimental data. Such theoretical models can in turn give rise to new experimental approaches in order to validate the proposed mechanisms and structures.

Without the support of experimental evidence, conformational analysis would be like walking on the tightrope of science without a balancing pole.

Robert Brasseur

THE EDITOR

Robert Brasseur, Ph.D., is an established investigator of the Belgian National Fund for Scientific Research, working in the Laboratory for Interfacial Macromolecular Physical Chemistry, Free University of Brussels, Brussels, Belgium. Dr. Brasseur obtained his training at the Free University of Brussels, receiving the A.B. degree in 1974 and the Ph.D. degree in 1977 and the Aggregate in 1986. He served as an Assistant Professor and an Associate Professor at the Free University of Brussels between 1980 — 1984. He received a Research Fellowship of the World Health Organization (1984 — 86) and a permanent Research Associate of the Belgian National Fund for Scientific Research 1986.

Dr. Brasseur teaches a course on "Conformation of membrane components" at the Free University of Brussels and on "Statistical methods for the study of macromolecules" at the Agricultural University of Gembloux.

Dr. Brasseur is the author of 100 scientific papers. His current major research interests focus on theoretical approaches to study the conformation of lipid and protein components at interfaces.

CONTRIBUTORS

Volume I

Isak Bivas, Ph.D.
Research Fellow
Liquid Crystal Department
Institute of Solid State Physics
Bulgarian Academy of Sciences
Sofia, Bulgaria

P. Bothorel, Ph.D.
Professor
Centre de Recherche Paul Pascal
CNRS
Domaine Universitaire
Talence, France

Robert Brasseur, Ph.D.
Professeur
Laboratoire de Chimie Physique
  des Macromolecules aux Interfaces
Free University of Brussels
Brussels, Belgium

Michel Deleers, Ph.D., D.Sc.
Manager
Research Center
UCB Pharmaceutical Sector
Braine-L'Alleud, Belgium

E. Goormaghtigh, Ph.D.
Research Assistant
Laboratoire de Chimie Physique
  des Macromolecules aux Interfaces
Free University of Brussels
Brussels, Belgium

Helmut Hauser, Ph.D.
Professor
Biochemistry Department
ETH Zurich
Zurich, Switzerland

B. Lemaire, Ph.D.
Engineer
Centre de Recherche Paul Pascal
CNRS
Domaine Universitaire
Talence, France

Thomas J. McIntosh, Ph.D.
Professor
Department of Cell Biology
Duke University Medical Center
Durham, North Carolina

Ole G. Mouritsen, Ph.D., D.Sc.
Research Professor
Department of Structural Properties
  of Materials
Technical University of Denmark
Lyngby, Denmark

I. Pascher, Ph.D
Professor
Department of Structural Chemistry
Faculty of Medicine
University of Gothenburg
Gothenburg, Sweden

Richard W. Pastor, Ph.D.
Research Chemist
Biophysics Laboratory
CBER/FDA
Bethesda, Maryland

David A. Pink, Ph.D.
Professor of Physics
Physics Department
St. Francis Xavier University
Antigonish, Nova Scotia, Canada

J.-M. Ruysschaert, Ph.D.
Associate Professor
Chimie Physique des Macromolecules
  aux Interfaces
Free University of Brussels
Brussels, Belgium

H. L. Scott, Ph.D.
Professor of Physics
Physics Department
Oklahoma State University
Stillwater, Oklahoma

S. Sundell, Ph.D.
Professor
Department of Structural Chemistry
Faculty of Medicine
University of Gothenburg
Gothenburg, Sweden

Volume II

Robert Brasseur, Ph.D.
Professeur
Laboratoire de Chimie Physique aux
 Interfaces
Free University of Brussels
Brussels, Belgium

A. Burny, Ph.D.
Professor
Department of Molecular Biology
University of Brussels
Rhode-Saint-Genese, Belgium

Alan D. Cardin, Ph.D.
Research Associate
Department of Biochemical Sciences
Merrell Dow Research Institute
Cincinnati, Ohio

Pierre Chatelain, D.Sc.
Director
Sanofi Research Center
Brussels, Belgium

A.-M. Colson-Corbisier, Ph.D.
Department of Biology
University of Louvain
Louvain-La-Neuve, France

Bernard Cornet, Ph.D.
Laboratoire de Chimie Physique aux
 Interfaces
Free University of Brussels
Brussels, Belgium

Michel Deleers, Ph.D., D.Sc.
Manager
Research Center
UCB Pharmaceutical Sector
Braine-L'Alleud, Belgium

Hans De Loof, Ph.D.
Department of Clinical Biochemistry
A.Z. St.-Jan
Bruges, Belgium

David A. Demeter, Ph.D.
Chemist
Department of Chemical Sciences
Merrell Dow Research Institute
Cincinnati, Ohio

Joëlle De Meutter, Ph.D.
Laboratoire de Chimie Physique
 Macromolecules aux Interfaces
Free University of Brussels
Brussels, Belgium

E. Goormaghtigh, Ph.D.
Research Assistant
Laboratoire de Chimie Physique des
 Macromolecules aux Interfaces
Free University of Brussels
Brussels, Belgium

P. Huart, Ph.D.
Laboratoire de Chimie Physique des
 Macromolecules aux Interfaces
Free University of Brussels
Brussels, Belgium

Richard L. Jackson, Ph.D.
Director
Department of Biochemical Sciences
Merrell Dow Research Institute
Cincinnati, Ohio

Guy Laurent, M.B., Ph.D.
Research Associate
Institute of Cellular and Molecular
 Pathology
Catholic University of Louvain
Brussels, Belgium

Chi-Hao Luan, Ph.D.
Laboratory of Molecular Biophysics
University of Alabama
Birmingham, Alabama

P. Marichal, Ph.D.
Professor
Department of Comparative Biochemistry
Janssen Research Foundation
Beerse, Belgium

M. P. Mingeot-Leclerq, Ph.D.
Research Member
Laboratoire de Chimie Physiologique
Université Catholique de Louvain
Brussels, Belgium

H. Moereels, Ph.D.
Professor
Department of Comparative Biochemistry
Janssen Research Foundation
Beerse, Belgium

Michel Praet, Ph.D.
Laboratoire de Chimie Physique des
  Macromolecules aux Interfaces
Free University of Brussels
Brussels, Belgium

Alberte Pullman, Ph.D., D.Sc.
Doctor
Laboratoire de Biochimie Theorique
Institute de Biologie Physique Chimie
Paris, France

Maryvonne Rosseneu, Ph.D.
Researcher
Department of Clinical Chemistry
A.Z. St.-Jan
Bruges, Belgium

J.-M. Ruysschaert, Ph.D.
Associate Professor
Laboratoire de Chimie Physique des
  Macromolecules aux Interfaces
Free University of Brussels
Brussels, Belgium

Charles N. Serhan, Ph.D.
Assistant Professor of Medicine
Hematology Division
Brigham and Women's Hospital
Boston, Massachusetts

Bernard L. Trumpower, Ph.D.
Professor
Department of Biochemistry
Dartmouth Medical School
Hanover, New Hampshire

Paul M. Tulkens, M.D., Ph.D.
Senior Research Associate
Université Catholique de Louvain
Brussels, Belgium

Dan W. Urry, Ph.D.
Director
Laboratory of Molecular Biophysics
University of Alabama
Birmingham, Alabama

Hugo Vanden Bossche, Ph.D.
Professor
Department of Comparative Biochemistry
Janssen Research Foundation
Beerse, Belgium

M. Vandenbranden, Ph.D.
Senior Investigator
Faculty of Sciences
Free University of Brussels
Brussels, Belgium

B. Vanloo, Ph.D.
Department of Clinical Biochemistry
A.Z. St.-Jan
Bruges, Belgium

Herschel J. R. Weintraub, Ph.D.
Group Leader
Department of Chemical Sciences
Merrell Dow Research Institute
Cincinnati, Ohio

TABLE OF CONTENTS

Volume I

TABLE OF CONTENTS

Volume II

Part 1. Lipids Structures and Organizations

Part 1A. Computer Aided Description

Chapter 1.A.1

COMPUTER SIMULATION OF COOPERATIVE PHENOMENA IN LIPID MEMBRANES

Ole G. Mouritsen

TABLE OF CONTENTS

I. INTRODUCTION

A. COOPERATIVE PHENOMENA IN LIPID MEMBRANES

The number of lipid molecules in a typical prokaryotic cell membrane or in a giant lipid vesicle is typically of the order of 10.[11] Whereas it is the strong hydrophobic effect which leads to the formation of a thermodynamically stable bilayer aggregate[1,2] of such a large number of amphiphile molecules in water, it is the much weaker intralayer molecular interactions which are responsible for the very special dynamic and static physical properties of the lipid membrane. The pseudo-two-dimensional character of the bilayer, being only 50 to 80 Å thick, implies a condition of extreme mechanical anisotropy. Together with the physiological requirements for membranes of high fluidity and fast lateral molecular diffusion within the membrane, this condition presupposes that the molecular interactions support an unusually high degree of cohesion and mechanical strength.[3,4] The intramembrane interactions moreover govern the lateral organization of the membrane components and hence modulate the biological activity associated with the membranes,[5] e.g., lipid/protein-mediated enzymatic processes, cytosis, or passive and active transport.

The cooperative behavior of the ensemble of membrane molecules determines the thermodynamic phase of the membrane and hence its static physical properties, including average bulk macroscopic properties, such as specific heat, compressibility, and membrane thickness and area. The cooperative nature of the interactions also manifests itself in specific dynamic events involving large numbers of molecules, such as phase transitions, protein aggregation, and the formation of microscopic lipid domains and special interfacial regions in the membrane. The latter type of processes may be induced by thermal density fluctuations accompanying phase transitions and they lead to heterogeneous membrane structures and biologically differentiated regions of the membrane. These types of processes belong to a class of membrane cooperative phenomena which are of major importance for biological function. It is the computer modeling of this class of phenomena which is the main theme of the present review.

Fully hydrated lipid bilayers are the single most important class of model systems for biological membranes, experimentally as well as theoretically.[6,7] Another important class of model membranes is lipid monolayers spread on air/water interfaces.[8,9] In the present review, the term "lipid membranes" will be used to cover both lipid bilayers and monolayers. This is reasonable since the cooperative phenomena of the two classes of systems are very similar and there is a close relationship between the mechanical and thermodynamic properties of lipid monolayers and bilayers.[10] Consequently, the theoretical models used to describe the two classes of systems are very similar. Pure lipid membranes display phase transitions (for a recent review, e.g., see Reference 7) and have a very rich phase structure. We shall here mainly be concerned with the so-called main transition of the lipid membranes. The main transition takes the membrane from a low-temperature solid, chain-conformationally ordered phase to a high-temperature fluid, chain-conformationally disordered phase. Besides the transitions between lamellar and nonlamellar structures,[11] it is probably the main transition and the cooperative phenomena associated with this transition which have the potentially largest biological implications for membrane function. The main transition can be driven thermally or by electric fields, pH, lateral or hydrostatic pressures, or membrane composition. The phase transitions of a pure lipid membrane becomes smeared in the presence of other membrane components, such as other lipid species, cholesterol, proteins, or anesthetics. These other components often induce lateral phase separation in the membrane. In that case, it is the phase equilibria of the mixed system which govern the physical properties of the membrane.

From a physical-chemistry point of view, it is a challenge to describe and understand the phase transitions and phase equilibria of lipid membranes as systems in their own right. From the point of view of membrane biology, an understanding of membrane phase transitions is important due to two reasons: (1) the phase transitions and phase equilibria regulate many membrane functions,[5-7] and (2) the phase equilibria are very sensitive to the molecular interactions and may hence be used indirectly to assess aspects of the intramembrane forces, e.g., lipid-protein interactions.[12]

B. COMPUTER SIMULATION OF COOPERATIVE PHENOMENA

Coherent fluctuations and cooperative phenomena are restricted to systems with a large number of particles. Phase transitions occur in a strict sense only in the thermodynamic limit (i.e., for an infinite number of particles). The large number of molecules involved implies a principle difficulty for a theoretical description of such phenomena based on molecular microscopic interaction models. Only for very simplified models is it possible to perform any analytically exact calculations.[13] Such calculations are made possible at the expense of physical realism and detail of description. More complex and realistic models, which hold promise of a detailed and quantitative comparison with experimental data, do not lend themselves to an analytical approach. It is at this point that modern computer simulation techniques become useful and important for making further progress.[14] We shall in this review reserve the term "computer simulation" to exclusively comprehend the numerical techniques which are used to solve the statistical mechanical problems of systems consisting of many particles. These techniques include (1) Monte Carlo simulation methods which exploit various types of stochastics sampling methods, and (2) molecular dynamics simulation methods which solve the dynamical equations of motions in a way which is numerically exact.

When cooperative phenomena, and in particular phase transitions, are in focus,[14] numerical simulations on lipid membrane models are not without problems either. There are basically two different sources of difficulties. Firstly, the calculations have to be carried out on systems with a large number of particles. Secondly, the coherent fluctuations accompanying cooperative phenomena and phase transitions are characterized by large spatial correlation lengths, long time scales, and slow relaxation. The first difficulty is usually dealt with by employing finite-size scaling techniques by which the large-system behavior is extrapolated from calculations on a series of systems with different numbers of particles. The second difficulty is often circumvented by using a lattice approximation for the models and by imposing different types of stochastic dynamics in order to speed up the relaxation. Obviously, the use of stochastic dynamics in, for example, a Monte Carlo simulation[15] may prevent a study of the real dynamics of the system. A molecular dynamics calculation[15] will, on the other hand, simulate the real model dynamics, but for membrane systems, current computer capabilities only permit the study of a small number of molecules and very short time spans, typically up to 100 ps. Consequently, most of the current information on cooperative phenomena in lipid membrane models stems from Monte Carlo simulations on lattice models.

C. SCOPE

The current literature on computer simulation of cooperative phenomena in lipid membranes is rather sparse, the reason being the principal difficulties, mentioned in Section I.B, of a numerical approach to cooperative phenomena in many-particle systems. Most of the simulation results to be reviewed in this paper are consequently obtained from Monte Carlo calculations on lattice models. The discussion emphasizes the physical properties of lipid membranes and the central theme is that fundamental physical properties of membranes often provide simple and satisfactory explanations of many experimental observations of biomembrane phenomena. In particular, the review stresses the fact that many effects observed in membranes may be understood in terms of a cooperative phenomenon due to the interactions between a large number of molecules and that in many cases there is no basis or need for invoking more complicated and specific mechanisms.

The computer simulation approach to cooperative phenomenon in lipid membranes has previously been briefly reviewed in References 16 and 17 and somewhat more elaborately reviewed in Reference 18 (molecular dynamics simulations) and in Chapter 5 of Reference 14 (Monte Carlo simulations).

The present review article consists of four parts. Firstly, Section II gives some general aspects of computer simulation techniques applied to lipid membranes. This section also presents an overview of the literature in the field. Secondly, Section III describes the computer simulation techniques in some detail. Thirdly, Section IV contains a characterization of the statistical mechanical lattice models used to describe the lipid membrane main phase transition. Fourthly, Sections V to VII are devoted to the results on lipid membrane cooperative phenomena in bilayers as well as monolayers. Readers who are familiar with the computational techniques or who are only interested in the results may skip Sections II to IV and directly proceed to the sections with the results. The review is concluded in Section VIII.

II. COMPUTER SIMULATION OF LIPID MEMBRANES

A. GENERAL STRATEGY

Computer simulation methods have become indispensable tools in the statistical mechanical description of the physics and chemistry of many-particle systems. First having been developed and applied within the classical fields of fluids and liquids[19] and simultaneously within the lattice formalism of condensed matter statistical physics,[20,21] these methods have in recent years gained importance within biomolecular physics and chemistry. Undoubtedly, computer simulation methods will, along with the rapid development of computer hardware, have a dramatic impact on the advance of the molecular description of biological systems. Major steps forward[22] have already been seen in the fields of macromolecular dynamics, protein dynamics, dynamics of nucleic acids, and biological membranes. In particular, a tremendous effort is being presented in relation to protein dynamics, to a large extent stimulated and pushed by a strong commercial interest in rational design of drugs and enzymes. It is not surprising, therefore, that there is already a substantial literature on computer simulation of conformational properties and dynamics of water-soluble proteins.[22]

In contrast, much less work has been done within computer simulation of biological membranes,[14,18] and the major part of the work carried out so far is concerned with simple lipid monolayer and bilayer systems. Moreover, the simulation studies of membrane models with integral proteins are in most cases restricted to extremely simplified model proteins. This is particularly true of those studies which are concerned with cooperative phenomena in membranes. The main reason for this situation is that the quantitative experimental information on the structure and dynamics of membranes and membrane-bound proteins is much more limited than for water-soluble proteins. This implies that the membrane systems from a physical point of view are at the moment less well-defined and consequently more cumbersome to model theoretically.

The common strategy underlying the computer simulation studies on membrane systems to be described in this review involves basically two steps: (1) formulation of a microscopic interaction model which, in terms of a chosen set of variables (e.g., translational coordinates or conformational states), accounts for the forces between the constituents of the system and (2) numerical solution of the statistical mechanical problem posed by using either Monte Carlo or molecular dynamics methods. Step 1 always involves approximations of some type. These approximations are dictated by computational feasibility as well as by choice of properties to be calculated. No simulations have yet been performed which can describe the spontaneous formation of lipid membrane aggregates in water (although there is some interesting work on the stability of micellar amphiphile aggregates in water[24]). Most simulations, as a starting point, take the existence of the lipid membrane aggregate and model only the secondary effects of the lipid-water interactions.

B. ADVANTAGES AND DRAWBACKS OF A COMPUTER SIMULATION APPROACH TO COOPERATIVE PHENOMENA[14]

A computer simulation is in many ways like an experiment; it is built on as little bias as possible. The behavior of the model system is studied as it evolves in space and time subject to different external conditions. Only the fundamental physical laws governing the interaction between the microscopic constituents are invoked, and the nontrivial consequences for the macroscopic behavior are then derived using fully controlled numerical approximation schemes. This implies some general advantages such as simplicity, universal applicability, and susceptibility to systematic improvements. Contrary to a real experiment, the simulation is carried out on a well-defined system and there is full control over every "experimental parameter". Moreover, the simulation can be carried out under extreme physical conditions which may be difficult to realize in the laboratory. Of major importance is the fact that computer simulation, having all the microconfigurations at hand, provides information on the microscopic, molecular level. The availability of the microconfigurations allows a "close-up" picture to be formed of the static as well as the dynamic behavior of the system. This greatly enhances and guides our physical intuition of the phenomena under consideration. The outcome of a computer simulation study may be thought of both as "experimental data" for a model system as well as a theoretical result which can be used to asses the validity of assumptions underlying predictions of conventional theoretical approaches. Hence, computer simulation may serve as a valuable tool for design and development of models and for the identification of the variables relevant for a given phenomenon. This is of particular importance when modeling of such a complicated system as a lipid membrane is under consideration.

The general advantages and universal applicability of computer simulation methods to study cooperative phenomena is systems composed of many particles make such methods ideal for making advances in the theoretical description of lipid membrane phenomena. Computer simulation methods may readily be applied to the very complicated models of lipid membranes without essentially introducing further approximations. This is a very important point since only by working with fairly realistic (and hence complicated) membrane models is it possible to describe quantitatively and in sufficient detail the wealth of experimental data which has become available in recent years. Only in that case can the theorist have some hope of interacting fruitfully with the experimentalist and — in the light of the theoretical findings — interpret and propose interesting and relevant experiments. The direct access to the microstates of the model membrane systems presents a particular advantage in the study of coherent fluctuations, membrane heterogeneity, and lateral organization, as well as protein aggregation and segregation.

Undoubtedly, computer simulation is currently the most powerful and versatile theoretical tool for cross-fertilization of model theoretical and experimental approaches to cooperative phenomena in lipid membranes.

There is a rich and rapidly expanding literature on the applications of computer simulation techniques to cooperative phenomena and phase transitions in a great variety of physical systems.[4,19-21] This literature has convincingly demonstrated that it is indeed practicable to study quantitatively and in great detail systems displaying cooperative phenomena. The lessons learned from these studies are now becoming valuable for the study of biological systems. The general drawback of a computer simulation approach is that is involves a large amount of data processing and that it requires access to massive computer power. Furthermore, only a finite number of molecules can be simulated and for complicated intermolecular potentials, it is not possible to study a sufficiently large collection of molecules to reproduce a cooperative phenomenon. Hence, the art of computer simulation of lipid membrane phenomena is the balance of choosing a sufficiently interesting and realistic model which —

given the current computer resources — can be simulated to reproduce the phenomenon of interest.

C. GENERAL OVERVIEW

Some of the earliest computer simulation work related to lipid membranes dealt with enumeration of the conformational statistics of single hydrocarbon chains in confined geometries.[25,26] This type of work has later been extended by a number of authors.[27-35] The single chain approximation also forms the basis of the most celebrated model of the lipid membrane chain-melting transition due to Marčelja.[34,35] This model, so clearly inspired by liquid crystal work, was the first to take account of the chain conformer statistics and thereby revealed the chain internal entropy as the driving force for the main transition.

The computer simulation work on lipid membrane cooperative phenomena is conveniently classified according to the interaction potential and which degrees of freedom of the molecules the simulation models take into account. The main degrees of freedom include translation variables for the polar head groups, orientational variables for the long axes of the acyl chains, conformational variables of the chains, head group variables, and variables for water molecules.

The pioneering work in molecular dynamics simulation of cooperative phenomena in lipid membrane models is that of Cotterill,[36] who studied a two-dimensional dumbbell model governed by Lennard-Jones as well as Coulomb interactions. Another early study is that of Jacobs et al.,[37] who used the molecular dynamics calculation of the pressure for a hard disk system within a model which approximately accounted for the chain flexibility. Toxværd[38] studied by molecular dynamics methods the equation of state for a dense alcohol monolayer with rigid chains interacting via soft potentials. A number of Monte Carlo studies deal with two-dimensional, hard-object potentials and translational variables,[39,40] one of them[40] taking approximate account of the chain conformational degrees of freedom. A recent Monte Carlo study[41] deals with a monolayer of grafted hard rods with orientational and translational degrees of freedom.

A few Monte Carlo studies[42-44] have been reported on the hydrocarbon chain structure in small bilayer systems with both translational and conformational variables and with hard potentials. A large number of molecular dynamics studies have been devoted to lipid monolayer[45-47] and bilayer[48-52] models with translational and conformational variables and various types of polar head group interactions. The most detailed calculation to date of this type is that of Egberts and Berendsen[52] who simulated a sodium-decanoate/decanol/water system in full atomic detail except for the "united atom" approach used for the CH_2 and CH_3 groups.

Most of the studies referred to above provided only little insight into the cooperative phenomena in lipid membranes. The main reason for this is that the models studied did not include a sufficient large number of molecules. It is only with lattice model approach and Monte Carlo simulation of lipid monolayers[53-56] and bilayers[14,57-63] that substantial progress has been made regarding the lipid membrane main phase transition. Since this approach involves lattice models, the translational degrees of freedom are suppressed. However, the chain conformations are treated in detail and the potentials are soft. In some cases, the neglect of translational variables has been outbalanced by introducing certain crystalline variables.[54,56,60,61] Properties of mixtures of lipids and other membrane components have also been studied within lattice models, e.g., cooperative phenomena in lipid-cholesterol bilayers,[58,64] phase separation[65,66] and lateral organization[67-71] of lipid-protein (or polypeptide) bilayers, and protein diffusion[72-74] in lipid bilayers. Some Monte Carlo[75-79] and molecular dynamics[80-82] simulations have been reported on systems of cholesterol or proteins in lipid bilayers using off-lattice models, i.e., models which take account of the translational variables of the molecules. None of the off-lattice studies were performed on systems large enough to seriously deal with cooperative phenomena.

Of more sophisticated contributions, the following should be mentioned: Monte Carlo simulation on lattice models with vertical chain mobility leading to ripple phases,[83-86] Monte Carlo simulation on lattice models including hydrogen bonding,[87] molecular dynamics and Monte Carlo simulation on models incorporating interactions between lipid molecules and water,[52,88-91] and Monte Carlo simulation of pattern-formation processes and impurity-controlled solidification in lattice models of lipid monolayers.[92-95] Finally, it should be pointed out that there is a large amount of important computer simulation work being done on electrolyte systems in planar geometries[96-98] which is relevant to the charge distribution near membrane surfaces.

III. COMPUTER SIMULATION TECHNIQUES

This Section gives a brief introductory description of computer simulation techniques as they are currently being used to study cooperative phenomena in lipid membranes. The description is fairly general. The main emphasis is put on Monte Carlo importance sampling methods since these techniques have provided a major part of the results on cooperative phenomena. The subsection on molecular dynamics methods is included for completeness; it only deals with the basic principles, and its main virtue is that is presents the reader with references to the appropriate technical literature.

A. MONTE CARLO IMPORTANCE SAMPLING METHODS
1. Statistical Mechanics

The statistical mechanical description of systems which contain many molecules consider the macroscopic state of a system to be a weighted average over all the possible microstates which the system can possess. A microstate, or configuration, of a system is given by a set of specific values of the mechanical variables, $\vec{\Omega}$, which describe the molecules. $\vec{\Omega} = (\Omega_1, \Omega_2, \ldots, \Omega_N)$ includes all possible degrees of freedom for each of the N molecules.

The phase space of the system $\{\vec{\Omega}\}$, is the space spanned by all possible microstates. For a membrane molecule, $\vec{\Omega}_i$ would in general denote the specific values of the spatial coordinates, the impulses, the conformational state, the charges, etc. The properties of the system are governed by a Hamiltonian, $\mathcal{H}(\vec{\Omega})$, which couples the various mechanical variables of the molecules. Statistical mechanics now assigns a certain probability to each microstate. Within the canonical description, this probability is given by the Boltzmann probability distribution

$$\rho(\vec{\Omega}) = \frac{e^{-\mathcal{H}(\vec{\Omega})/k_B T}}{Z} \tag{1}$$

where Z is the partition function

$$Z = \sum_{\{\vec{\Omega}\}} e^{-\mathcal{H}(\vec{\Omega})/k_B T} \tag{2}$$

For convenience, we have in Equation 2 assumed that the phase space of the system is discrete. Having available the probability distribution, $\rho(\vec{\Omega})$ in Equation 1, of the microstates, the thermodynamic value of any physical quantity (macroscopic or microscopic), $f(\vec{\Omega})$, defined in terms of the mechanical variables, can be calculated:

$$\langle f \rangle = \sum_{\{\vec{\Omega}\}} f(\vec{\Omega}) \rho(\vec{\Omega}). \tag{3}$$

From Equations 1 and 3 follows a set of relationships between response functions and variances in the corresponding physical quantities. This is the so-called fluctuation-dissipation theorem which in the case of the specific heat, $C_P(T)$, and the isothermal lateral area compressibility, $\kappa(T)$, takes the following forms:

$$C_P(T) = \frac{\partial \langle \mathcal{H} \rangle}{\partial T} = \frac{1}{k_B T^2}(\langle \mathcal{H}^2 \rangle - \langle \mathcal{H} \rangle^2) \tag{4}$$

$$\kappa(T) = \frac{\chi(T)}{\langle A \rangle} = -\frac{1}{\langle A \rangle}\frac{\partial \langle A \rangle}{\partial \Pi} = \frac{1}{k_B T \langle A \rangle}(\langle A^2 \rangle - \langle A \rangle^2) \tag{5}$$

where A is the membrane area, $A = A(\vec{\Omega})$, and Π is the conjugate lateral pressure. The fluctuation-dissipation theorem formulas are particularly useful in relation to computer simulation calculations since they provide the response functions at single points without requiring a whole function as implied by the derivatives in the first parts of Equations 4 and 5.

2. Monte Carlo Importance Sampling[14]

Only in very few and extremely simplified situations, it is possible to calculate analytically exactly the partition function Z in Equation 2 and hence any thermal averages. Certainly, for realistic membrane models, the Hamiltonian is too complicated to allow an exact calculation of Z. It is now the basis of the Monte Carlo method first introduced into statistical mechanics by Metropolis et al.[99] to approximate Equation 3 by a sum over a finite subset

of $\{\vec{\Omega}\}$. This subset, $\{\vec{\Omega}_i\}_{i=1}^{M}$, includes a finite number of microstates which occur in the subset according to their Boltzmann probability and hence according to their importance for the thermal average so that

$$\langle f \rangle \simeq \sum_{i=1}^{M} f(\vec{\Omega}_i)\rho(\vec{\Omega}_i). \tag{6}$$

The subset $\{\vec{\Omega}_i\}_{i=1}^{M}$ is generated by introducing a stochastic principle (a Monte Carlo method) according to which a random walk is performed in phase space. By this random walk, in the limit of $M \to \infty$, microstates are visited with a frequency proportional to their Boltzmann factor, Equation 1. The correct limiting properties of the random walk are usually assured[14] by requiring that the transition probabilities, $p(\vec{\Omega}_k \to \vec{\Omega}_j)$, of going from state k to state j fulfill the detailed-balance condition:

$$\rho(\vec{\Omega}_j)p(\vec{\Omega}_j \to \vec{\Omega}_k) = \rho(\vec{\Omega}_k)p(\vec{\Omega}_k \to \vec{\Omega}_j) \tag{7}$$

as well as the steady-state condition

$$\rho(\vec{\Omega}_j) = \sum_{i=1}^{M} \rho(\vec{\Omega}_i)p(\vec{\Omega}_i \to \vec{\Omega}_j). \tag{8}$$

It is in principle always possible to set up such a random walk if the transition probabilities are ergodic,[14] i.e., assure that every microstate can be reached from any other state within the course of a finite number of transitions. The trick behind the Metropolis Monte Carlo method is to circumvent the difficulty of not knowing the partition function by choosing the transition probabilities in terms of conditional Boltzmann weights (i.e., ratios of Boltzmann factors where the partition function drops out), specifically:

$$p(\vec{\Omega}_j \rightarrow \vec{\Omega}_k) = p^*_{jk}; \qquad \rho(\vec{\Omega}_k)/\rho(\vec{\Omega}_i) \geq 1 \tag{9}$$

$$p(\vec{\Omega}_j \rightarrow \vec{\Omega}_k) = p^*_{jk}\rho(\Omega_k)/\rho(\Omega_j); \qquad \rho(\Omega_k)/\rho(\vec{\Omega}_j) < 1 \tag{10}$$

$$p(\vec{\Omega}_j \rightarrow \vec{\Omega}_j) = 1 - \sum_{k(\neq j)} p(\vec{\Omega}_j \rightarrow \vec{\Omega}_k). \tag{11}$$

p^*_{jk} is a set of transition probabilities which can be chosen arbitrarily as long as the ergodicity condition is obeyed. This other set of transition probabilities contains the flexibility of the Metropolis approach and the various options in particular realizations of the Monte Carlo method, cf. Section III.A.3, are collected in p^*_{jk}. In brief, the principle feasibility of the Metropolis Monte Carlo importance sampling method is demonstrated via Equations 9 to 11, whereas the practicability relies on clever choices of p^*_{jk}.

Before we proceed with a prescription of how to choose p^*_{jk}, it is instructive to point out that the random walk in phase space described above may be considered a dynamical process, a so-called Markov process,[14] by which a time sequence of microconfigurations is visited. The discrete index for the set $\{\vec{\Omega}_i\}^M_{i=1}$ corresponds to a time parameter, the Markov time t. The random walk is then seen to be governed by the master equation:

$$\frac{d\rho(\vec{\Omega}_j,t)}{dt} = -\sum_k p(\vec{\Omega}_j \rightarrow \vec{\Omega}_k)\rho(\vec{\Omega}_j,t) + \sum_k p(\vec{\Omega}_k \rightarrow \vec{\Omega}_j)\rho(\vec{\Omega}_k,t). \tag{12}$$

In thermal equilibrium, $d\rho(\vec{\Omega}_j,t)/dt = 0$ and $\lim_{t \rightarrow \infty} \rho(\vec{\Omega}_j t) = \rho(\vec{\Omega}_j)$. The characteristic time scale r of this dynamics is determined as $\tau^{-1} \sim p^*_{jk}$. It is obvious, however, that there may be several different time scales in a given realization depending on the choice of p^*_{jk}. The standard unit for the time parameter is Monte Carlo steps per particle (or per site for a lattice model), MCS/S.

Usually, the dynamics implied by the master equation in Equation 12 is not the true physical dynamics of the system since the correct equations of motion have not been invoked. However, in cases where either the Hamiltonian does not have a dynamics of its own or a real physical time can be assigned to each of the transitions, an interpretation of the Monte Carlo calculation in terms of a dynamical process may be possible. However, great care should be exercised in defining the time scales of p^*_{jk} in order to be able to calculate, e.g., diffusion constants,[100]

$$D = \lim_{t \rightarrow \infty} \langle r^2(t) \rangle / 6t, \tag{13}$$

where $r(t)$ is a spatial coordinate.

The number, M, of microstates needed to make Equation 6 a good approximation to the true thermodynamic average depends on the system as well as the phenomenon under consideration. It also depends on the specific values of the thermodynamic parameters, such as temperature, pressure, and composition. In principle, the approximation can be made as good as desired, provided the values of the system size, N, and the statistical ensemble size, M, are chosen appropriately. Ultimately, this is a question of available computer resources. Part of the finite-size effects may be suppressed by using appropriately chosen periodic boundary conditions. In the case of cooperative phenomena and phase transitions, it becomes very demanding to make Equation 6 a good approximation, in particular close to critical points. The reasons for this are twofold: (1) cooperative phenomena and phase transitions require large values of N to establish themselves, and (2) close to a cooperative phenomenon, a large part of phase space contributes to the thermal averages, thus demanding large values of the ensemble size M.

3. Realization of the Monte Carlo Method[14]

The Monte Carlo importance sampling method as described above is extremely general and can in principle be used for any statistical mechanical system. However, the method will be practicable to study cooperative phenomena only when the energy of the microstates,

$E_i = \mathcal{H}(\vec{\Omega}_i)$, is easy to calculate. This will be the case for most nonquantum systems. The precise realization of the method, i.e., the choice of the transition probabilities p^*_{jk} of Equations 9 to 11, depends in a detailed manner on the type of model under consideration. Nevertheless, it is quite straightforward to visualize the construction of p^*_{jk} going from one type of model to the other. Without loss of generality, we shall therefore here focus attention on a particular realization used for lattice models of lipid membranes.[14]

Let us consider a system of N molecules positioned on a lattice (e.g., a two-dimensional triangular lattice) and let us assume for simplicity (and again without loss of generality) that

the state of each molecule is characterized by a single number, α, i.e., $\vec{\Omega} = (\alpha_1, \alpha_2, \ldots, \alpha_N)$; α could, as an example, be a label of an acyl chain conformation of a lipid molecule or a label which distinguishes different molecular species. In the general case, the state α can carry a multiplicity, D_α, which for an acyl chain would be the degeneracy, or the single-chain density of states. The canonical density function, Equation 1, would then read:

$$\rho(\vec{\Omega}) = Z^{-1}(\Pi_{j=1}^{N} D_{\alpha_j})e^{-\mathcal{H}(\vec{\Omega})/k_\mathbf{B}T}. \qquad (14)$$

p^*_{jk} is usually chosen to correspond to rather localized events, e.g., one-particle excitations (Glauber dynamics[14]), exchange of molecules on neighboring sites (Kawasaki dynamics[14]), or combinations of these two events, i.e., $\alpha_n \rightarrow \alpha'_n$ and/or $\alpha_n \leftrightarrow \alpha_m$ (m and n are neighbor sites). Whatever these changes are, they will imply a certain change in energy:

$$\Delta E = \mathcal{H}(\vec{\Omega}_k) - \mathcal{H}(\vec{\Omega}_j) \qquad (15)$$

and change in the internal entropy, Δs, which is related to appropriate ratios of degeneracies. For example, in the case of a single-chain conformational excitation, the internal entropy change takes the form:

$$\Delta s = k_B \ln(D_{\alpha'_n}/D_{\alpha_n}). \qquad (16)$$

In terms of the above quantities, a possible realization of the Markov chain of microstates may then be described by the following simple algorithm:

1.   Choose an arbitrary initial configuration, $\vec{\Omega}_1$.

2. Pick a trial state, $\vec{\Omega}'_2$, according to the transition probability, p^*_{12}.

3. If $\Delta E - T\Delta s \leq 0$, the transition to the trial state is accepted, i.e., $\vec{\Omega}_2 = \vec{\Omega}'_2$.

4. If $\Delta E - T\Delta s > 0$, a random number, $\xi \in [0,1]$ is drawn. If $\exp[-(\Delta E - T\Delta s)/k_B T]$
   $> \xi$, the transition to the trial state is accepted, i.e., $\vec{\Omega}_2 = \vec{\Omega}'_2$. If $\exp[-(\Delta E -$
   $T\Delta s)/k_B T] \leq \xi$, the transition is not performed and $\vec{\Omega}_2 = \vec{\Omega}_1$.

5. A new trial state, $\vec{\Omega}'_3$, is considered, etc.

If p^*_{jk} is ergodic, this algorithm will in the limit of a large number of attempted transitions, so-called Monte Carlo steps, lead to a sequence of microstates which are distributed according to the equilibrium Boltzmann distribution at the prescribed temperature. Step 4 of the above algorithm involves the use of random numbers and this step constitutes the core of the stochastic Monte Carlo approach to calculation of statistical mechanical properties.

The remaining options in the choice of p^*_{jk} are used to optimize the rate of convergence to equilibrium. Often, p^*_{jk} is subject to certain conditions formulated in terms of conservation laws. For example, in the canonical description, the total number of molecules of each species is a conserved quantity. It is straightforward to modify the canonical Monte Carlo importance sampling technique to simulate grand canonical sampling where the molecular densities fluctuate and are controlled by appropriate chemical potentials.

Since the canonical Monte Carlo importance sampling techniques described above operate directly on the level on the microconfigurations, $\vec{\Omega}$, it is obvious that such techniques are extremely powerful to elucidate aspects of membrane lateral organization, heterogeneity, and coherent fluctuations, as well as they permit a detailed conformational analysis of the lipid molecules to the finest level of the underlying microscopic interaction model.

B. MOLECULAR DYNAMICS METHODS

In contrast to the Monte Carlo simulation methods described in Section III.A which are built on stochastic principles, the molecular dynamics simulation methods[15,19] are fully deterministic (although such methods can also simulate stochastic dynamics). As an input, a molecular dynamics calculation needs a potential function (a Hamiltonian or Lagrangian) $V(r_2, r_j)$, which couples the degrees of freedom for all the molecules of the system. The calculation then simply consists of a numerical solution to Newton's equations for the coupled many-particle problem

$$m_i \frac{d^2 r_i(t)}{dt^2} = -\sum_j \nabla_{ij} V(r_i, r_j), \tag{17}$$

where $V(v_2, v_j)$ is a pair potential function defined on the spatial coordinates, r_i, and m_i is the mass of the ith particle. The potential function for a membrane model may, for example, contain atom-atom Lennard-Jones potentials, bond-bending potentials, torsional potentials, and Coulomb potentials for charged sites. Often the potentials used for flexible hydrocarbon chains are those developed by Ryckaert and Bellemans.[101]

The molecular dynamics approach hence implies the determination of a true dynamical trajectory in phase space, often subject to the conservation of the total energy, i.e., microcanonical sampling. (However, also other ensembles may be simulated.[15]) Ensemble averages are then obtained by averaging over several of such trajectories, using different initial configurations. The practicability of a simulation according to the molecular dynamics method relies on the availability of effective and numerically accurate integration algorithms.

For membrane simulations,[18,45-49,51,52] it is common for this purpose to use the Verlet third-order predictor algorithm[19] (or the mathematically equivalent but computationally more efficient leap-frog algorithm):

$$m_i[r_i(t + dt) - 2r_i(t) + r_i(t - dt)] = -\sum_j \nabla_{i,j} V(r_i, r_j) dt^2. \qquad (18)$$

The Verlet method requires an approximation for the initial velocities. For lipid systems, the equations of motion are often solved under the constraint of fixed bond lengths.[102,103] The temperature is derived from the velocity distribution using the equipartition theorem.

From the trajectories sampled by the molecular dynamics simulation, static thermodynamic averages may be obtained (exploiting the ergodic nature of the system) as well as dynamic correlation functions. Hence, a molecular dynamics simulation provides the full information about the structural as well as dynamical details of the model system under consideration. In this respect, the molecular dynamics approach is potentially much more powerful than the stochastic Monte Carlo approach. However, the faithful reproduction of the dynamical modes is made possible at the expense of computer time. This implies that, for such complicated systems as lipid membranes, only rather small systems may be simulated and the accessible time span is short (typically less than 200 ps). Until now, only limited information about cooperative phenomenon in lipid membranes has therefore been gained by the use of molecular dynamics methods.

IV. STATISTICAL MECHANICAL LATTICE MODELS OF THE LIPID MEMBRANE MAIN TRANSITION

We shall mainly be concerned with the cooperative phenomena in lipid membranes near their main transition, the so-called gel-to-fluid chain melting transition. Over the last couple of decades, physicists and physical chemists have found it a real challenge to model this transition and to reveal its underlying physical mechanisms. Many of the early theoretical models have been reviewed critically by Nagle.[13]

A proper theoretical modeling of the main transition must seriously deal with the following aspects of the system:

1. The rotational isomerism of the acyl chains
2. The anisotropic van der Waals' forces between the hydrophobic parts of the lipids
3. The polar forces between the head groups
4. The excluded volume interactions in a dense aggregate
5. The interaction with water

Any model that attempts to include all these considerations as realistically as possible is going to be computationally intractable. Consequently, different degrees of realism are built into the theoretical models used in practice. The particular choice and design of a model of the main transition is, at the present stage of development of a theory, usually dictated by what type of experimental information one wants to compare with. Since the experimental activities in biomembrane physics have by now reached a quantitatively rather detailed and sophisticated level, there is a call for models which both are reasonably realistic and at the same time computationally tractable.

Due to the particular difficulties in dealing with cooperative phenomena, the work on theoretical modeling, aided by computer simulation techniques, of the lipid membrane main transition is almost exclusively performed using lattice models in which the excluded volume interactions automatically are taken into account. A particularly useful class of lattice models includes the so-called multistate models, being first proposed by Doniach,[104] refined by Caillé et al.,[105] extended by Pink et al.,[106,107] and further developed by Mouritsen and Zuckermann[60,61] to account for effects of crystallization. The lattice formulation suppresses the translational coordinates of the lipid molecules and confines the glycerol backbones of the lipids to a plane. On the other hand, the lattice models account in a detailed manner for the statistics of the rotational isomerism. The use of lattice models makes it possible to treat by Monte Carlo simulation techniques a sufficiently large number of molecules to be able to reproduce cooperative phenomena.

We shall below describe the multistate lattice models of the bilayer main transition and the various results which have been obtained from these models. These models are, via their construction, equally good models for the liquid-condensed/liquid-expanded phase transition of lipid monolayers spread on air/water interfaces. Hence, the description of the models in Sections IV.A and B also serves as a description of the models which are used to derive the results reviewed in Section VI on monolayer cooperative phenomena. The prototype system to be considered is a one-component lipid membrane of DPPC (dipalmitoyl phosphatidylcholine). With appropriate scaling, the results presented will be equally applicable to other phosphatidylcholine membranes. Moreover, some of the general phenomena described will have qualitative relevance for a much larger class of phospholipids.

A. MULTISTATE MODELS WITH CONFORMATIONAL DEGREES OF FREEDOM

Within this class of models, the lipid bilayer is considered as two noninteracting independent monolayers. Each monolayer is represented by a two-dimensional triangular lattice, cf. Figure 1A, where each site can be occupied by an acyl chain. The two chains of the diacyl lipid molecule are considered as independent and the carbonyl groups of the chains (or the glycerol backbone) are restricted to lie in the plane of lattice, cf. Figure 1B. The multistate models are characterized by certain single-chain properties as well as by the form of interaction between the chains.

The single-chain description builds on the rotational isomeric model[108] by which the rotations around each saturated C–C bond of the acyl chain can only be performed corresponding to three discrete angles, leading to a *trans* and two energetically degenerate *gauche* angles. The *trans* and the *gauche* levels are separated by an energy of 0.45×10^{-13} erg. The rotational isomeric model reduces the number of chain conformations to $3^{n_s - 1}$ where n_s is the number of CH_2-monomers. This is a very large number of conformations of which only a modest number will occur and pack reasonably well in a condensed membrane. The central idea of the multistate models is then to select a small number, q, of the more important conformations and use these as the accessible single-chain states. Each of these q states, α, is described by an internal conformational energy, ϵ_α (which is proportional to the number of *gauche* rotations of the conformation), a cross-sectional area, A_α (which is the cross-section of the effective cylindric volume occupied by the chain), and finally a degeneracy (or multiplicity), D_α (which is a number denoting how many chain states are characterized by the same values of ϵ_α and A_α). D_α is the single-chain density of states. Two states[104] which always occur in a multistate model are the all-*trans* conformation ($\alpha = 1$) and a hypothetical conformationally disordered or fluid state ($\alpha = q$) which is characteristic of the fluid phase. Roughly, it is the entropy difference between these two states, $\Delta s = k_B \ln(D_q/D_1)$, which provides the driving force for the chain melting transition. A set of eight gel-like intermediate states was chosen by Pink[106] as the lowest-lying excitations of the all-*trans* conformation subject to conditions of low conformational energy and optical packing. These intermediate states are all approximated as conformations which can be mapped onto a triangular lattice, i.e., with C–C–C bond angles of only 120°, cf. Figure 1B. By this construction, and by assuming that the first C–C–C segment is all-*trans* and parallel to the

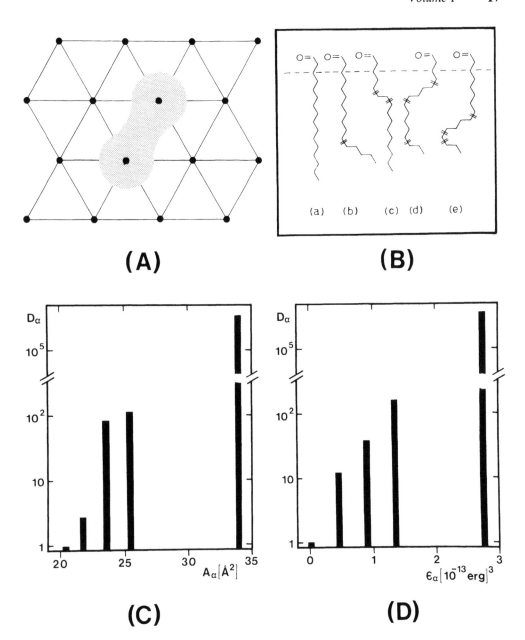

FIGURE 1. Pseudo-two-dimensional lattice model of the main lipid membrane transition. (A) Top view of a triangular lattice with sites which can be occupied by lipid molecules. The positioning of a diacyl lipid molecule is indicated schematically; (B) some acyl chain conformations of the multistate Pink model for saturated lipids with 16 C-monomers (e.g., DPPC): (a) all-*trans* state; (b) intermediate state with a single jog; (c) intermediate state with two *gauche* rotations (kink); (d) and (e) intermediate states with three *gauche* rotations. (From Caillé, A., Pink, D., de Verteuil, F., and Zuckermann, M. J., *Can. J. Phys.*, 58, 581, 1980. With permission.) (C) Single chain degeneracy, D_α, vs. cross-sectional area, A_α, per acyl chain; (D) single-chain degeneracy, D_α, vs. conformational energy per chain, ϵ_α. Note that the plots of D_α are semilogarithmic.

TABLE 1

Single-Chain Parameter with the Ten-State Pink Model for Chains with 16 Monomers (DPPC)

State	α	Cross-sectional area, $A_\alpha [\text{Å}^2]$	Conformational energy, $\epsilon_\alpha [10^{-13}\text{erg}]$	Degeneracy D_α
All-*trans*	1	20.4	0	1
Jog	2	21.86	0.45	4
	3	23.54	0.45	4
	4	25.5	0.45	4
Kink	5	21.86	0.9	20
	6	23.54	0.9	16
	7	25.5	0.9	12
	8	23.54	1.35	64
	9	25.5	1.35	96
Fluid	10	34.0	2.78	354,294

bilayer normal (cf. Figure 1B), there is a simple relationship between the chain state and the hydrophobic length, d_α, of that state; d_α is measured from the carbonyl group to the terminal CH_3-group. The cross-sectional area of the various states is determined from an assumption about the hydrophobic membrane volume being approximately constant.[34,109]

$$A_\alpha = \frac{d_1 A_1}{d_\alpha},$$

(19)

where $A_1 = 20.4 \text{Å}^2$ for DPPC.[110] The cross-sectional area of the fluid chain state is taken to be[106] $A_q = 34 \text{Å}^2$. The degeneracies are finally determined by simple combinatoric arguments.[107] A compilation of the single-chain properties for the ten-state Pink model of DPPC bilayers is given in Table 1. The single-chain contribution to the model Hamiltonian of a membrane with N acyl chains is now written:

$$\mathcal{H}_1 = \sum_{i=1}^{N} \sum_{\alpha=1}^{q} \epsilon_\alpha \mathcal{L}_{\alpha i},$$

(20)

where $\mathcal{L}_{\alpha i} = 0,1$ is a quantity which specifies the state of the chain at site i. The average of this quantity, $\langle \mathcal{L}_{\alpha i} \rangle$, is an occupation number and hence $\Sigma_\alpha^q \langle \mathcal{L}_{\alpha i} \rangle = 1$.

Turning now to the interaction between the lipid molecules, it is anticipated that this interaction for a lattice model has to be written in terms of the area variables. Combining Wolf's[111] theory for the orientational energy between anisotropic molecules in liquid crystals with Salem's[112] approximation for the distance dependence for the van der Waals' interaction between two long cylindrical rods, the anisotropic van der Waals' interaction Hamiltonian is written[107]

$$\mathcal{H}_2 = -\frac{J_0}{2} \sum_{i,j}^{N} \sum_{\alpha,\beta=1}^{q} V_{\alpha\beta} S_\alpha S_\beta \mathcal{L}_{\alpha i} \mathcal{L}_{\beta j}.$$

(21)

The summation in Equation 21 is over nearest neighbors only. J_0 is an interaction constant and the nematic shape factor, S_α, or the acyl chain order parameter, is given by

$$S_\alpha = \frac{1}{2(n_s - 1)} \sum_{n=2}^{n_s} (3 \cos^2 \Theta_{\alpha n} - 1),$$

(22)

where the summation extends over the segments of the acyl chain and Θ_{an} is the angle between the bilayer normal and the normal to the plane spanned by the nth CH_2-group of the chain. By geometrical reasons it is then found that

$$S_\alpha = aA_1A_\alpha^{-1} + b \tag{23}$$

where $a = 1.8$ and $b = -0.8$ are geometrical factors. Hence, within the multistate Pink models, the acyl chain orientational order parameter is linearly related to the hydrophobic thickness.[113] In the all-*trans* state, $S_1 = 1$. The distance dependence of the interaction is determined by the approximation:[107]

$$V_{\alpha\beta} = V_\alpha V_\beta = \left(\frac{A_\alpha}{A_1}\right)^{5/4}\left(\frac{A_\beta}{A_1}\right)^{5/4} \tag{24}$$

The form of the interaction, Equation 21, with Equations 22 and 24 is not expected to hold strictly for the fluid chain state, $\alpha = q$. Hence, for that state, a "weakening factor", w_q, is introduced[58] so that $V_q \to w_q V_q$. It has been found[58] that $w_q = 0.4$.

It should be noted at this point that the concept of a lattice model of the present type is a rather subtle one since the acyl chains interact with a distance-dependent potential, Equation 24. The distance between two chains is related to the areas of these chains, specifically, $r_{\alpha\beta} \simeq (A_\alpha/\pi)^{1/2} + (A_\beta/\pi)^{1/2}$. In the present context, the lattice is merely a topological structure which assures that each chain interacts with six neighbors corresponding to a close-packed arrangement. The chains are, however, assigned different amounts of space depending on their conformational state. The model may therefore be termed a pseudo-two-dimensional model since the three-dimensional character of the chains and their interactions is mapped onto a two-dimensional representation.

The interaction between the polar parts of the lipid molecules may, as first suggested by Marčelja,[34] be expressed in terms of an intrinsic lateral pressure, Π:

$$\mathcal{H}_3 = \Pi \sum_{i=1}^N \sum_{\alpha=1}^q A_\alpha \mathcal{L}_{\alpha i} \tag{25}$$

which assures bilayer stability. It is through Equation 25 that a close relationship between bilayer and monolayer thermodynamics is made possible.[63] The interaction between the polar heads can be modeled more explicitly by

$$\mathcal{H}_4 = -\frac{K_o}{2}\sum_{i,j}^N \sum_{\alpha,\beta}^q Y_{\alpha\beta}\mathcal{L}_{\alpha i}\mathcal{L}_{\beta j}, \tag{26}$$

where

$$Y_{\alpha\beta} = Y_\alpha Y_\beta = \left(\frac{A_1}{A_\alpha}\right)^\nu\left(\frac{A_1}{A_\beta}\right)^\nu \tag{27}$$

and ν is the exponent of the central force between the polar heads. It has been shown[14,58] that the more accurate form, Equation 26 (with $\nu = 1$ corresponding to Coulomb forces), is effectively accounted for by Equation 25 which therefore will be considered in the following.

The multistate models defined above do not account for direct interaction with water. Furthermore, they disregard the properties of the $P_{\beta'}$-phase. Modification of the models to include effects due to translational variables will be described below. Other modifications include vertical mobility of the acyl chains[85] and hydrogen bonding between amide groups.[87]

B. MULTISTATE MODELS WITH CRYSTALLINE DEGREES OF FREEDOM

The multistate model formalism described above focuses at the acyl chain conformational degrees of freedom as those of single importance for the lipid membrane main transition in equilibrium. Certainly, the acyl chain disordering is responsible for the main contribution to the large transition enthalpy, $\Delta S \simeq 8.7$ kcal/mol for hydrated DPPC multilayer systems. Still, the translational variables will lead to two-dimensional crystallization at low temperatures, although the corresponding entropy contribution is estimated[104] to be only about 1 kcal/mol. For bilayers, the crystallization and chain ordering processes are believed to be coupled.[61] However, in nonequilibrium, the effects of the crystallization process are expected to have a dramatic influence on the transition properties.

In order to model, within the simplest possible approximation, the effects of the crystallization process on the main transition, Mouritsen and Zuckermann[60,61] have recently proposed an extension to the multistate Pink model. This extension seeks to model the crystallization process on a lattice by introducing a new set of lattice site variables, so-called Potts variables, $p, p = 1,2, \ldots ,Q$, which for each site label the orientation of the crystalline domain in which the molecule at that site prefers to participate. Molecules in the same crystalline arrangement have the same value of p. Molecules with different values of p repel each other according to the Potts interaction

$$\mathcal{H}_5 = J_P \sum_{i,j}^{N} \sum_{\alpha,\beta}^{q-1} \sum_{p,p'}^{Q} (1 - \delta_{pp'}) \mathcal{L}_{\alpha p i} \mathcal{L}_{\beta p' j}, \tag{28}$$

where $\delta_{pp'}$ is the Kronecker delta function and $\mathcal{L}_{\alpha p i}$ is a variable which is 1 if the ith chain in the αth conformational state assumes the pth Potts state, and zero otherwise. J_P is a positive interaction constant. Note that only chains which are in gel-like conformations interact via their Potts variables since only in that case can they enter a crystalline matrix. The interaction in Equation 28 may hence be said to model the interaction due to crystalline misfit and packing defects. The constant J_P can be interpreted as a grain boundary energy. In order to model the large (in principle infinite) number of possible crystalline orientations, the number of Potts states, Q, has to be chosen as a large number. General work on polycrystalline aggregates[114] indicates that Q = 30 is sufficient to approximate the large Q limit. As it will turn out, cf. Section VII.A, the usefulness of the multistate model modified to account for crystalline degrees of freedom is most clearly revealed through the modeling of the effects of intrinsic molecules (such as cholesterol) on the lipid membrane cooperative phenomena.

V. LIPID BILAYER COOPERATIVE PHENOMENA

A. STATIC PROPERTIES NEAR THE MAIN TRANSITION

1. Nature of the Main Transition. Membrane Area and Free Energy

In Figure 2 are shown the results[58] for the average cross-sectional area per lipid molecule;

$$\langle A(T) \rangle = \sum_{\alpha=1}^{q} A_\alpha \langle \mathcal{L}_{\alpha i} \rangle \tag{29}$$

as obtained from Monte Carlo simulations on the ten-state Pink model with parameter values $J_o = 0.70985 \times 10^{-13}$erg and $\Pi = 30$ dyn/cm, i.e., for the Hamiltonian, $\mathcal{H} = \mathcal{H}_1 + \mathcal{H}_2 + \mathcal{H}_3$, cf. Equations 20, 21 and 25. Figure 2 demonstrates how the temperature dependence of $\langle A(T) \rangle$ depends on the size of the lattice used for the simulation. It is noted that for systems with more than 1800 molecules, the results for $\langle A(T) \rangle$ are fairly insensitive to the system size and hence represent the thermodynamic limit. Systematic analyses of the type

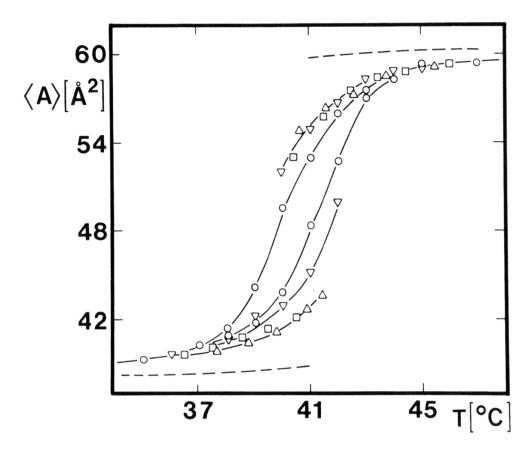

FIGURE 2.   Temperature dependence of the average cross-sectional area per lipid molecule, $\langle A(T) \rangle$, as obtained from Monte Carlo simulations on the ten-state Pink model of a DPPC bilayer system. Systems with different numbers, N, of molecules are considered: N = 450 (○), N = 800 (▽), N = 1800 (□), and N = 4050 (△). The dashed lines denote the mean-field result. (Adapted from Reference 58.)

shown in Figure 2 have to be carried out for each individual quantity considered. In the following, we shall assume that such analyses have been performed and only present data which closely reproduce the thermodynamic limit.

There are several important pieces of information in the data set of Figure 2. Firstly, the transition region is seen to be strongly influenced by thermal fluctuations. This becomes clear by comparing with the mean-field results which are known to suppress the fluctuations. Hence, we conclude that fairly large systems are required to reproduce the true transition behavior of the model. Secondly, the transition is associated with a rather pronounced hysteresis of 1 to 2°. The width of the hysteresis, however, depends on the equilibration time, i.e., the number of configurations included in the ensemble after a change of temperature. The data in Figure 2 correspond to an equilibration time of 1000 MCS/S. Only for such short times is it possible to trap the system into metastable states. The finding of metastable states indicates that the transition is of the first order.

The first-order nature of the main transition is more clearly demonstrated via a calculation of the free energy, F(T). It is notoriously difficult to calculate F(T) directly by computer simulation techniques,[21] but it may be obtained indirectly from numerical investigation,[14,58] provided that good data are available for the internal energy, $E = \langle \mathcal{H} \rangle$,

$$F(T) = \frac{T}{T_o}F(T_o) + T \int_{T_o^{-1}}^{T^{-1}} E(x)dx. \tag{30}$$

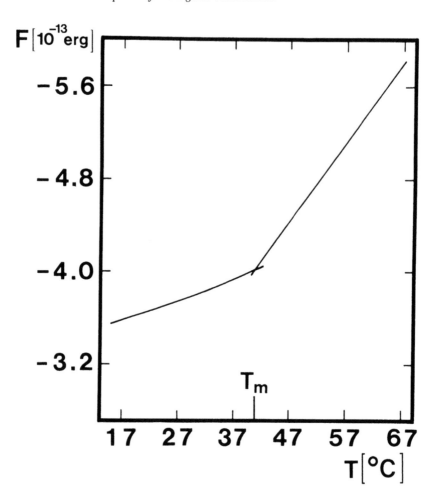

FIGURE 3.   Free energy per lipid molecule F(T), Equation 30, vs. temperature as obtained from Monte Carlo simulations on the ten-state Pink model of a DPPC bilayer. The transition temperature is $T_m = 41°C$. (Adapted from Reference 58.)

In Equation 30, T_o is a temperature at which $F(T_o)$ is known. By choosing appropriate values of T_o deep into, respectively, the high- and low temperature phases where the mean-field theory is exact, a branch of F(T) is obtained in each of the two phases as shown in Figure 3. By integrating along the metastable branches, it is then possible to locate the point of intersection which is the transition point, $T_m \simeq 41°C$. A difference in the slope of the two F(T) branches at this point shows unequivocally that the main transition is of first order. The transition entropy and enthalpy may then be obtained as follows

$$\Delta S/T_m = \Delta H = \Delta \left(\frac{\partial F(T)}{\partial T} \right)_{T_m} \tag{31}$$

This leads to $\Delta H \simeq 7$ kcal/mol for DPPC bilayers.

Turning now to the membrane area again, it has been found[57] that longer relaxation times in the transition region lead to a smearing of the transition and eventually to a smooth and continuous variation of $\langle A(T) \rangle$ through the transition. Details of the simulation suggest that the transition proceeds via a series or cascade of long-lived metastable states (see also Section V.C.1) and that the continuous appearance of the first-order transition is caused by an intrinsic molecular property of the bilayer system. To shed some further light on this problem, Mouritsen[57] conducted a systematic study of the transition in a series of q-state Pink models. These models were constructed by deleting an appropriate number of the intermediate chain states of the ten-state model, keeping the total number of states (i.e., $\Sigma_\alpha D_\alpha$) a constant. The results of this study are shown in Figure 4A which shows that for models with $q \leq 5$, a clear first-order discontinuity is found, whereas for more intermediate states, the transition appears as continuous. These findings suggest that the continuous appearance of the main transition may be explained as a result of kinetically caused metastability of intermediate lipid chain conformations. The microscopic phenomena underlying this effect are described in Section V.B.2 in terms of soft interfaces formed between different lipid domains in the transition region.

The theoretical finding of a "continuous" main transition is in agreement with experimental measurements on unchanged lipid bilayers using a variety of techniques, including NMR,[115,116] micromechanics,[117] and calorimetry.[118] In fact, no experiment has been reported of discontinuous behavior in any bilayer property at the main transition. The computer simulation work removes a puzzle in interpreting these experiments as consistent with a first-order transition by pointing out that the apparent continuous behavior is caused by molecular properties of the lipid systems. There is no need to ascribe the effect to the presence of impurities or as due to experimental inadequacies. The smearing of the first-order transition, on the other hand, makes it difficult to compare quantitatively experimental and theoretical values of transition enthalpy and change in cross-sectional area.

It is difficult to measure experimentally the absolute membrane cross-sectional area. It is, however, possible by micropipette aspiration techniques[117] for single giant vesicles to determine the fractional change in area as a function of temperature. Data obtained by these techniques have been reported for DMPC vesicles,[117] but we are not aware of any measurements for DPPC. As will be described in Section V.A.3 below, it is possible to indirectly derive an approximation for the membrane area from deuterium NMR measurements[119] of the average acyl chain orientation order, $\langle S \rangle$, cf, Equation 33. Results obtained in this way are shown in Figure 4B. Considering the approximations underlying this derivation, the agreement between the experimental $\langle A \rangle$ and the computer simulation result from the ten-state Pink model (Figure 4A) is satisfactory. It should be noted that the experimental data in Figure 4B below the main transition exhibit effects due to the $P_{\beta'}$-phase and the pretransition not accounted for in the theoretical model.

2. Lipid Chain Statistics

Having all the microscopic variables available, the Monte Carlo computer simulation allows a detailed description of the relative occurrence of the various chain states via the occupation variables, $\langle \mathscr{L}_{\alpha i} \rangle$, $\alpha = 1,2 \ldots ,10$. In Figure 5 are shown the temperature variations of the occurrence of the all-*trans* ($\langle \mathscr{L}_{1i} \rangle$), the fluid ($\langle \mathscr{L}_{10i} \rangle$), and the intermediate chain states, ($\Sigma_{\alpha=2}^9 \langle \mathscr{L}_{\alpha i} \rangle$). It is seen that the intermediate states have a very high probability in a fairly large region around the transition.

3. Membrane Hydrophobic Thickness and Acyl Chain Orientational Order Parameters

Due to the assumption underlying the multistate Pink models that only chain conformations which have C–C–C bond angles of 120°, the membrane hydrophobic thickness $\langle d \rangle$ is by geometrical reasons linearly related to the average chain orientational order parameter $\langle S \rangle$:

$$\langle d \rangle = (\langle S \rangle - b) a^{-1} d_1, \qquad (32)$$

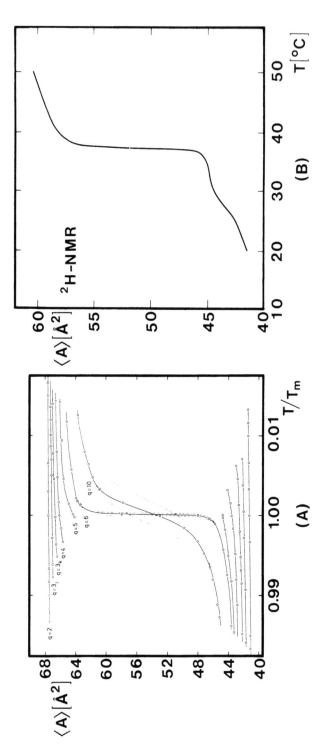

FIGURE 4.   (A) Average cross-sectional area per lipid molecule, $\langle A(T)\rangle$, as a function of reduced temperature, T/T_m, for a series of q-state Pink models. The data ($\circ$) are obtained from Monte Carlo simulations on DPPC bilayer systems with 1800 molecules. In the case of $q = 3$, the subscript refers to models with only the kink (k) or jog (j) intermediate state (cf. Table 1). The dashed loops specify for the $q = $ six and $q = $ ten-state models, the range over which metastable states have been detected. (Adapted from Reference 57.) (B) Average cross-sectional area per lipid molecule as derived from ^{2}H-NMR data for d_{62}-DPPC using Equations 19 and 32 to 34. (Adapted from Reference 113.) The experimental data are those of Vist. (From Vist, M. R., *Partial Phase Behavior of Perdeuterated Dipalmitoyl-phosphatidylcholine/Cholesterol Model Membranes*, M.Sci. Thesis, University of Guelph, Ontario, 1984. With permission.) Note that the main transition temperature of d_{62}-DPPC bilayers is $T_m = 37^\circ$C.

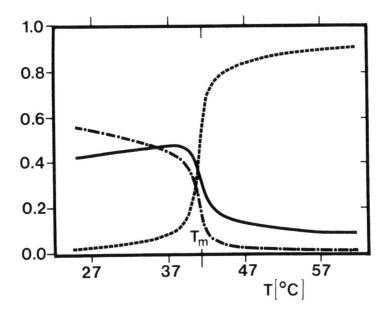

FIGURE 5.   Temperature dependence of chain state occupation variables as obtained from Monte Carlo simulations on the ten-state Pink model of a DPPC bilayer: (·—·—·), all-*trans* state $\langle \mathcal{L}_{1i} \rangle$, (------), fluid state $\langle \mathcal{L}_{10i} \rangle$; and (——), intermediate states $\Sigma_{\alpha = 2}^{9} \langle \mathcal{L}_{\alpha i} \rangle$. The data are derived from a system with 5000 molecules.

where a and b are the constants of Equation 23. $\langle S \rangle$ in turn is calculated as

$$\langle S \rangle = \sum_{\alpha=1}^{q} S_\alpha \langle \mathcal{L}_{\alpha i} \rangle. \tag{33}$$

The hydrophobic length of the all-*trans* state is taken to be $d_1 = 19.7$ Å for DPPC.[34] The Monte Carlo simulation data for $\langle S \rangle$ are shown in Figure 6A. Since $\langle S \rangle$ is a measure of the average segmental order of the acyl chains, cf. Equation 22, Figure 6A shows how the chains disorder during the main transition.

The acyl chain orientational order parameter is an important quantity since it can be measured directly in ^{2}H-NMR experiments on perdeuterated lipid samples.[119,120] The deuterated lipid membranes lead to a quadrupolar spectrum whose first moment, M_1 is related to the C–D bond order parameter $\langle S_{CD} \rangle$:

$$M_1 = \frac{2\pi}{3\sqrt{3}} \Delta\nu_Q \langle | S_{CD} | \rangle, \tag{34}$$

where $\Delta\nu_Q$ is the maximum quadrupolar splitting for a deuteron on a CD bond.[113,115] Since $\langle S \rangle = 2\langle | S_{CD} | \rangle$ for axially symmetric averaging[120] (which will be the case in the fluid phase), the moment M_1 can in certain cases be used as a way of measuring membrane thickness without relying on complicated diffraction methods.[113] The numerical data of Figure 6A for $\langle S \rangle$ is in good agreement with the experimental data[119] in Figure 6B provided these data are appropriately renormalized in the low-temperature phase. Such a renormalization is required since the experimental system contains information from low-temperature structures not accounted for by the ten-state Pink model.

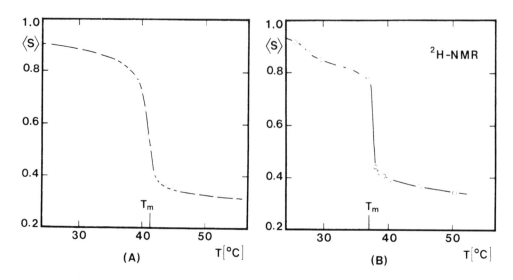

FIGURE 6.   (A) Acyl chain orientational order parameter, $\langle S(T) \rangle$ in Equation 33, as obtained from Monte Carlo simulations on the ten-state Pink model of a DPPC bilayer with 5000 molecules; (B) $\langle S(T) \rangle$ as derived from the first moment M_1 of the quadrupolar NMR spectrum of d_{62}-DPPC membranes using Equation 34. The experimental data, which are renormalized by requiring that $\langle S \rangle = 1$ at $T = 10°C$ are those of Vist. (From Vist, M. R., Partial Phase Behavior of Perdeuterated Dipalmitoylphosphatidylcholine/Cholesterol Model Membranes, M.Sci. thesis, University of Guelph, Ontario, 1984. With permission.) Note that the main transition temperature of d_{62}-DPPC bilayers is $T_m = 37°C$.

4. Specific Heat and Lateral Compressibility. Pseudocritical Phenomena in Lipid Bilayers

Figure 7A gives the Monte Carlo simulation data for the specific heat, $C_p(T)$, of the ten-state Pink model. It is seen that the specific heat has a dramatic peak at the transition and that there are pronounced wings at both sides of the transition signaling strong thermal fluctuations. Such a behavior is reminiscent of critical behavior. A similar behavior in the specific heat has been found in DSC[118,121,122] (cf. Figure 7B) and AC calorimetric[123-126] investigations of a variety of phospholipid bilayer membranes. In a sharp first-order phase transition, C_p has a δ-function singularity superimposed on the background specific heat. The area of this anomaly corresponds to the transition enthalpy, ΔH. In an experiment as well as in a computer simulation, the Δ-function will appear as a broadened peak of finite intensity. The background specific heat has been shown by AC calorimetry,[123-126] in accordance with the data of Figure 7A, to have a sharp divergence at T_m as well as intense wings on both sides of T_m. In contrast to DSC, steady-state AC calorimetry does not measure the latent heat of the transition and is only sensitive to thermal fluctuations. A recent careful analysis of the wings in C_p measured by DSC has also revealed fluctuation-induced wings.[127]

The lateral area compressibility, $\chi(T)$, as calculated from the fluctuation-dissipation theorem, Equation 5, is shown in Figure 8A for the ten-state Pink model. Similar to the specific heat, $\chi(T)$ has a dramatic peak at the phase transition with wide wings extending into both phases. This behavior is the macroscopic signal of strong thermal density (area) fluctuations and a pronounced softening[59] of the bilayer in the transition region.

It is experimentally extremely difficult to measure the lateral area compressibility of bilayer membranes. Basically two types of experiments have been performed, osmometry on multilayer dispersions[128] and micromechanical measurements on single vesicles.[4,117,129] Data obtained from these different techniques are not consistent and the whole subject is very controversial at the moment. We are not aware of any data which systematically show the temperature dependence of the compressibility for DPPC bilayers in the transition region. However, in Figure 8B, the corresponding results for DMPC vesicles obtained by micro-

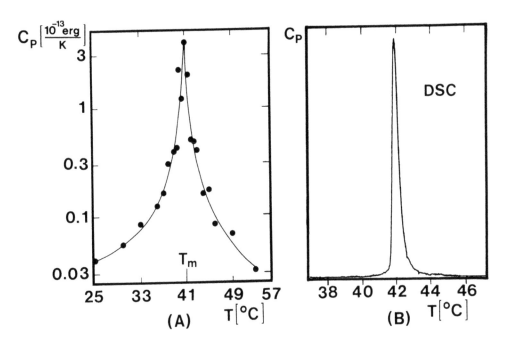

FIGURE 7. (A) Specific heat per lipid molecule, $C_P(T)$ in Equation 4, as obtained from Monte Carlo simulations on the ten-state Pink model of DPPC bilayers with 5000 molecules. Note that the vertical axis is logarithmic. (B) Specific heat, $C_P(T)$ (in arbitrary units on a linear scale), as measured experimentally by DSC techniques. The scan rate is 10°C/h. (From Mouritsen, O. G., unpublished data, 1983.)

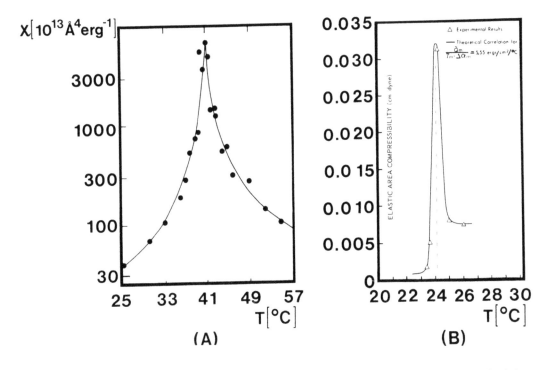

FIGURE 8. (A) Isothermal lateral area compressibility, $\chi(T)$ in Equation 5, as obtained from Monte Carlo simulations on the 10-state Pink model of DPPC bilayers with 5000 molecules. Note that the vertical axis is logarithmic. (Adapted from Reference 64.) (B) Elastic area compressibility of DMPC vesicles. (From Evans, E. and Kwok, R., *Biochemistry*, 21, 4874, 1982. With permission.)

mechanical measurements[117] are reproduced. The data are rather sparse, but a peak is seen at the phase transition temperature. It is not possible to conduct a quantitative comparison between theoretical and experimental results, Figures 8A and B, with respect to the wings in $\chi(T)$. The experimental data are too limited and there are subtleties with respect to the interpretation of the experimental data in the gel phase due to the compliance of the ripples of the $P_{\beta'}$-phase.[4]

The pronounced peaks in the response functions, $C_P(T)$ and $\chi(T)$, suggest that the bilayer system may exhibit pseudocritical behavior at the main transition. Pseudocritical behavior implies that the first-order transition is subject to strong precursor effects and that the spinodal points are close to the transition temperature. Mouritsen and Zuckermann[59] analyzed and their Monte Carlo simulation data for the lateral compressibility of the six-state Pink model in terms of an effective power-law singularity:

$$\chi(T) \sim A_{\pm} \mid \tau \mid^{-\gamma\pm}, \qquad \tau = (T - T_m)/T_m \rightarrow \pm 0, \tag{35}$$

where $\gamma_{\pm}$ are the pseudocritical exponents. (For the six-state model, the pseudospinodal temperatures[59] are within 0.1% of T_m and hence the reduced temperature τ in Equation 35 can to a good approximation be defined uniquely in terms of T_m.) The results of this analysis are shown in Figure 9 which demonstrates that Equation 35 accurately describes the data and moreover that the scaling relation, $\gamma_+ = \gamma_-$, is fulfilled, and $A_+/A_- \simeq 1$. The values of $\gamma_{\pm}$ are found to depend on the number of states, q, included in the multistate model.[59] Hence, there is no apparent universality in the pseudocritical behavior of the multistate bilayer models.

A softening of lipid bilayers and the description of the bilayer response functions near T_m in terms of pseudocritical phenomena have been reported in a number of experimental studies. In addition to the specific heat measurements,[123-126] pseudocritical behavior has been observed for ultrasonic relaxation,[130,131] dynamic fluorescence,[132] motional narrowing of NMR spectra,[133] and fluorescence lifetime heterogeneity.[134] Moreover, studies of passive transmembrane permeability, e.g., of small cations[135] show similarly strong and related anomalies at the main transition. We shall return to this point in Section V.B.3.

5. Interaction Between the Two Sheets of the Bilayer

The multistate lattice models of the lipid bilayer assume that the interaction between the two monolayers is negligible. There is some experimental evidence in support of this assumption.[136] Georgallas et al.[63] have studied a model of coupled monolayer lattices in order to determine the effect of the strength of this coupling on the phase transition within each monolayer. The two monolayers are each described by a generalized two-state model where the lower state has specific temperature-dependent properties to approximately account for intermediate states.[17] Georgallas et al.[63] observed that the problem of two coupled triangular lattices can be mapped onto a honeycomb lattice with nearest and next-nearest neighbor interactions. By combining results from series expansion techniques with those from Monte Carlo simulation, it was found that it is possible to match lipid bilayer and lipid monolayer thermodynamic data for the phase transition in accordance with experiment, provided that the interlayer coupling is about 2% of the intralayer van der Waals' coupling, J_o. Hence, the interaction between the two sheets of the lipid bilayer is rather weak, but has to be considered in order to account for the difference between lipid monolayer and bilayer thermodynamic behavior.

6. Cooperative Models of Chain Tilting

In order to allow simulations in the transition region, the multistate lattice models of the lipid bilayer do not include translational variables and they are not solved using the true

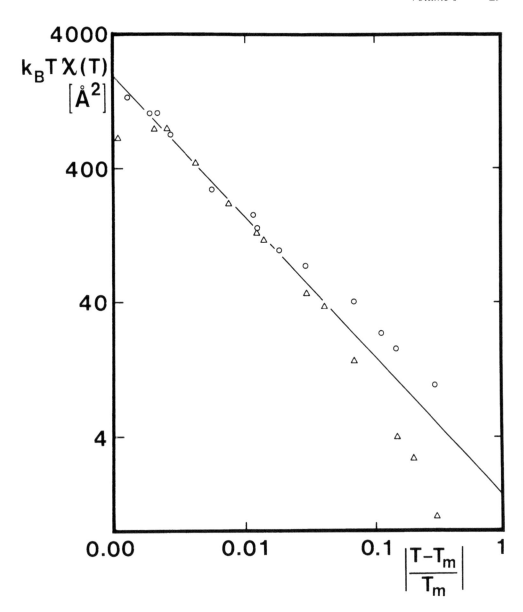

FIGURE 9.   Double-logarithmic plot of the reduced lateral area compressibility, $k_BT\chi(T)$, per lipid molecule, vs. reduced temperature, $|T - T_m|/T_m$, for the six-state Pink model. The data are obtained from Monte Carlo simulations on a system with 1800 molecules of a DPPC bilayer $\circ$, $T > T_m$; $\triangle$, $T < T_m$. The solid line denotes the power law $k_BT\chi(T) \sim |(T - T_m)/T_m|^{-\gamma}$, in Equation 35, with $\gamma \simeq 1.05$. (Adapted from Reference 59.)

equations of motion. The true dynamics of a lipid bilayer model with translational variables was considered by van der Ploeg and Berendsen.[48,49] These authors studied by molecular dynamics simulation a bilayer membrane model with interactions, including Lennard-Jones, dihedral, and bond angle potentials subject to a bond-length constraint. The interaction with water was represented by a harmonic restoring force for the head groups. Moreover, an external pressure was exerted on the head groups in order to assure bilayer stability. Model simulations were performed for bilayers of 2×16 and 2×64 decanoate molecules at temperatures in the fluid phase. Although it is not possible to study the main transition with systems of this size, the molecular dynamics simulations[48,49] revealed a very exciting co-operative effect in terms of a slowly fluctuating cooperative tilt mode of the chains. The

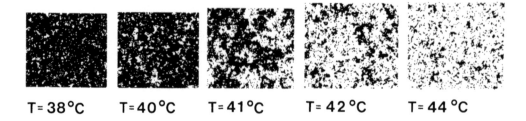

T= 38°C   T= 40°C   T= 41°C   T= 42°C   T= 44 °C

FIGURE 10.   Snapshots of microconfigurations typical of a series of temperatures in the neighborhood of the main transition T_m = 41°C of the ten-state Pink model of DPPC bilayers. The configurations are obtained from Monte Carlo simulations on a system with 10,000 acyl chains on a triangular lattice. The lattice parameter has been scaled with the square root of the membrane area so as to display the lateral expansion of the membrane. Black dots denote chains in gel conformations (all-*trans* and intermediate states) and blank areas denote chains in the fluid conformational state. (Adapted from Reference 62.)

correlation time of the fluctuations was found to be around 10 to 20 ps with an extended spatial correlation length of 10 Å. The molecular alignment was strongly correlated with the tilt angle, van der Ploeg and Berendsen[48] used their results to explain the characteristic experimentally observed orientational order parameter profile (observed by NMR[120]) as due to an average tilting of the acyl chains.

B. FORMATION OF LIPID DOMAINS AND INTERFACIAL REGIONS

The strength of a computer simulation approach to cooperative phenomena in lipid membranes becomes evident in the search for the microscopic phenomena which accompany and support the strong thermal density fluctuations observed in the macroscopic membrane properties, cf. Figures 6 to 9 , in the region of the main transition. Not only do the simulation results reveal the microscopic lateral organization and heterogeneous structure of the membrane, but they may also stimulate the development of theories and models for particular membrane functions associated with differentiated regions of the membrane. As an example, the lipid domain boundary formation to be described below has inspired modeling of passive ion permeability and facilitated an understanding of the function of interfacially active membrane-bound enzymes such as phospholipase.

1. Lateral Density Fluctuations, Lipid Domains, and Clusters. Cooperativity of the Main Transition

In Figure 10 are shown snapshots of microconfigurations typical of different temperatures in the transition region of the ten-state Pink model. The figure distinguishes between lipid chains in gel-like states and chains in the fluid state. It is seen that the thermal fluctuations manifest themselves in the formation of lipid domains or clusters.[57,59,62] Below T_m, domains of the fluid phase are formed in the gel matrix; above T_m, clusters of the gel phase are formed in the fluid matrix. Hence, heterogeneous membrane structures prevail in the transition region. The size of the domains increases as T_m is approached from either side. The domains are dynamic entities of finite lifetime. They fluctuate persistently in position and size. At the very transition temperature, the bilayer fluctuates strongly between the two phases in a sort of dynamic coexistence.

It is important to realize that the domain formation process discovered by the simulations is a highly nontrivial phenomenon which is a consequence of a cooperative phenomenon, i.e., due to the buildup of long-range correlations in a many-particle system. It is here derived from first principles via the computer simulation which takes the Hamiltonian of the interacting system as its only input. This is in contrast to other theoretical approaches to the problem which into the theory built the presence of lipid domains.[137-140]

Despite their dynamic and fluctuating nature, the domains in Figure 10 are described by a temperature-dependent equilibrium size-distribution function[59,62] $n_\ell^i(T)$, i = gel or fluid, where $n_\ell^i(T)$ denotes the number of i-domains with ℓ lipid molecules. The domains are defined via a nearest-neighbor correctivity criterion in accordance with the nearest-neighbor interaction range. The distribution function has a maximum at $\ell = 0$ and a tail toward the large domains. The tail rises in intensity as T_m is approached from either side.[59] The average domain size is calculated as

$$\bar{\ell}(T) = \sum_\ell \ell n_\ell^i(T) / \sum_\ell n_\ell^i(T), \tag{36}$$

where the summation is restricted by a lower cut-off in the value of ℓ in order to avoid small clusters in the average. This lower cut-off determines the width of the average domain size function shown in Figure 11 for a cut-off corresponding to three acyl chains. The figure shows that $\bar{\ell}$ has a sharp peak at T_m. Freire and Biltonen[122] have analyzed DSC data for the lipid bilayer main transition in terms of a bilayer partition function which allows a calculation of a cluster distribution function without assuming any particular model of the transition. The results obtained in this way for $\bar{\ell}$ are strikingly similar to the Monte Carlo data presented in Figure 11.

The experimental observations of a continuous behavior of the lipid bilayer main transition have often been rationalized in terms of "lack of cooperativity"[9,118,141,142] and the size of the cooperative unit has been estimated indirectly by a simple Van't Hoff analysis. It is interesting to note that the sizes found in this way[9,122,143-146] are of the same order of magnitude as the average lipid domain sizes found near the transition in the computer simulations. A piece of direct experimental evidence for the formation of lipid domains during the main transition comes from an electron microscopy study of isolated phosphatidylcholine vesicles.[146] In Section V.C.1, we shall return to a description of the kinetics of the lipid domain formation process and how this influences the appearance of the main transition.

2. Soft Domain Interfaces and Their Biological Significance

We now proceed one step deeper into the spatial analysis of the lipid domain pattern and the membrane heterogeneity discovered in the computer simulation of the lipid bilayer main transition, cf. Figure 10. The membrane plane is now divided into three regions:[62] the background phase (the bulk, b), the domains or clusters (c), and the interface (i) between the clusters and the bulk. In order to exclude very localized random events caused by the stochastic Monte Carlo dynamics (cf. Section III.A.3), only clusters with more than seven molecules are taken into account. The cluster-bulk interface is probed via a series of molecular layers. The first layer is defined as those acyl chains which are connected by nearest-neighbor bonds to the cluster boundary; the second layer is defined as those chains which are nearest neighbors to the first layer, etc. By these definitions, the membrane heterogeneity may be described by the relative amounts, a_b, a_c, and a_i, of the membrane area found in the three regions. In Figure 12 are shown the Monte Carlo simulation results for these quantities obtained from the ten-state Pink model.[62] The interfacial and cluster areas display pronounced peaks at the transition.

The very nature of the interfacial region between the bulk and the lipid clusters is revealed by examination of the occurrence of the various acyl chain states in the interface and comparing it with that in the bulk. In Figure 13 is shown the relative occurrence as a function of temperature of the all-*trans*, the intermediate, and the fluid acyl chain conformational states in the first (A) and second (B) interfacial layer compared to that of the bulk (C). These figures demonstrate very clearly the special nature of the first interfacial layer as being strongly dominated by chains in intermediate conformational states. Conversely,

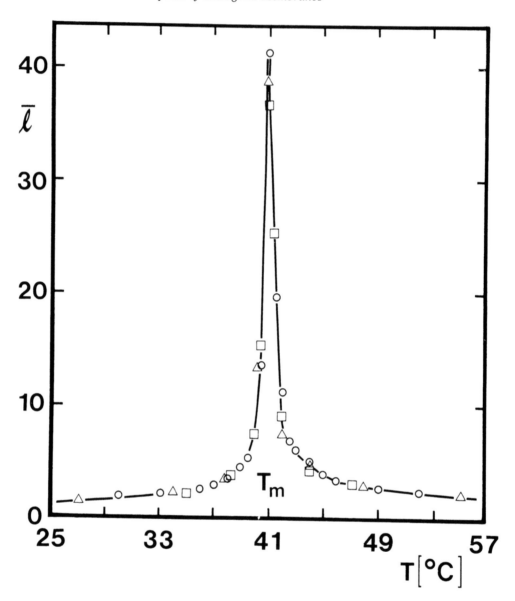

FIGURE 11.   Average domain size (number of molecules), $\bar{\ell}(T)$ in Equation 36, as a function of temperature as obtained from Monte Carlo simulations on the ten-state Pink model of a DPPC bilayer with 200 ($\triangle$), 800 ($\square$), and 5000 ($\bigcirc$) molecules. The lower cut-off cluster size was chosen to be one and a half molecules (three acyl chains) for this figure. (Adapted from Reference 62.)

the states in the second interfacial layer occur with the same probability as in the bulk. Hence the interface is soft and well localized in space. The interface attracts excited gel-like acyl chain conformations.

The softness of the domain-bulk interfaces leads to a lowering of the interfacial free energy and hence a weakening of the driving force for growth and shrinking of the domains. This has important consequences for the kinetics of the main transition (cf. Section V.C.1) as well as for the lateral distribution and physiological function of interfacially active membrane-bound molecules, such as cholesterol (cf. Section V.II.A.3) and certain enzymes. The soft interface will act as a sink for foreign molecules and facilitate the insertion of newly synthesized proteins and lipids.[147] Moreover, the interface may by its particular structure

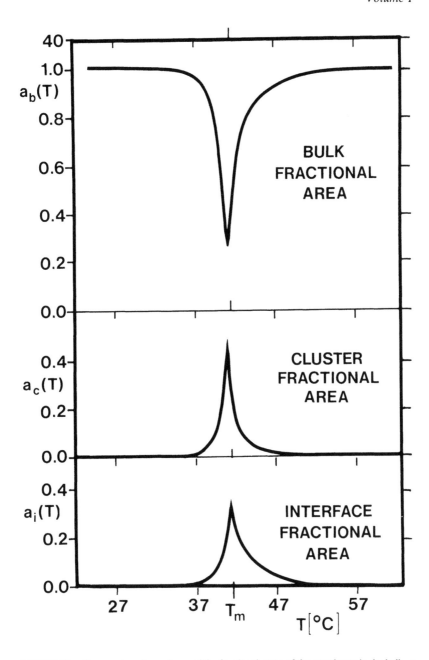

FIGURE 12.   Temperature dependence of the fractional areas of the membrane in the bulk, a_b, in the clusters, a_c, and in the interfaces, a_i. The interface is defined as the first interfacial layer of lipid chains. The data are obtained from Monte Carlo simulations on the 10-state Pink model of a DPPC bilayer with 5000 molecules. (Adapted from Reference 62.)

facilitate or inhibit certain enzymatic functions. A particularly striking example is that of pancreatic phospholipase for which it is known that hydrolysis only occurs in the transition region.[148,149] The rate of activation of this enzyme varies strongly with temperature and it changes two orders of magnitude within 1°C of the phase transition.[150] It has been shown[150] that this dramatic dependence on temperature can be related to the lipid domain formation and it has been proposed that the interfacial region of the membrane may facilitate certain conformational changes in the enzyme which enhances its activity. As will be pointed out

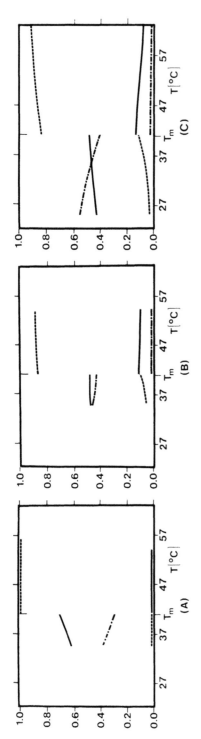

FIGURE 13. Relative occurrence of all-*trans* (·——·), intermediate (——), and fluid (------) acyl chain conformational states of (A) the first interfacial layer of chains; (B) the second interfacial layer of chains; and (C) the bulk. The data derive from Monte Carlo simulations on the ten-state Pink model of a DPPC bilayer with 5000 molecules. (Adapted from Reference 62.)

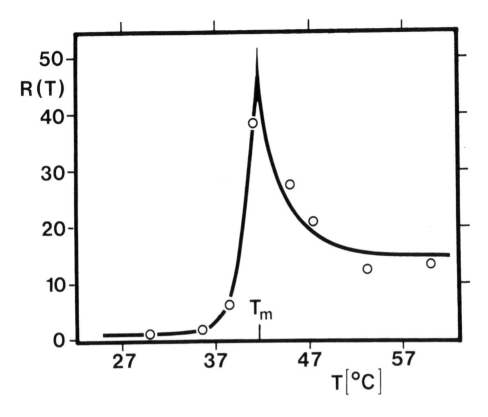

FIGURE 14.   Relative permeability, R(T) in Equation 38 of Na$^+$ ions in liposomes as measured experimentally[147] by radioactive ^{22}Na techniques (O) and as calculated theoretically (———) via Equation 37 using Monte Carlo simulation data for the interfacial area (cf. Figure 12). The scale of R(T) is relative to the experimental value at T = 25°C. The Monte Carlo data are obtained from the ten-state Pink model of a DPPC bilayer with 5000 molecules. (Adapted from Reference 62.)

in Section V.II.A.4, other interface active membrane-bound molecules, such as cholesterol or cholate, may then couple to the enzymatic activity by altering the interfacial area.

3. Relationship Between Lipid-Domain Interfaces and Passive Transmembrane Permeability

Lipid bilayers are generally characterized by very low passive permeability to small ions such as Na$^+$ and K$^+$. An anomalous behavior in the permeability of Na$^+$ ion was first observed by Papahadjopoulos et al.[135] who at the phase transition of liposomes discovered a sharp enhancement in the permeability, cf. Figure 14. Papahadjopoulos et al.[135] explained this striking phenomena as caused by the formation of specially leaky interfaces in the membrane due to coexisting gel and fluid domains. This explanation was questioned by others,[151,152] who argued that such interfaces could not exist on thermodynamic grounds. Still others[104,153] proposed that the peak is a result of enhanced density fluctuations.

Cruzeiro-Hansson and Mouritsen[82] used their finding from Monte Carlo computer simulation of an enhanced interfacial area, cf. Figure 12, at the main bilayer phase transition to propose a simple minimal model for passive ion diffusion through membranes. This model assigns a high relative permeation rate to the domain interfaces and identifies the interfacial area as the membrane property which has the proper temperature variation to account for the conspicuous peak in the experimental data. By writing the probability for an ion of crossing the lipid membrane once it has hit it as:

$$P(T) = a_b(T)p_b + a_c(T)p_c + a_i(T)p_i, \tag{37}$$

Cruzeiro-Hansson and Mouritsen[62] arrived at an expression for the relative permeability:

$$R(T) = C\langle A(T)\rangle^{-1/2}T^{1/2}P(T), \tag{38}$$

where C is a constant which gives a point of reference for R(T). In Equation 37, p_b, p_c, and p_i are temperature-independent regional probabilities of ion transfer, $p_i > p_b, p_c$. The results of the model calculation are also shown in Figure 14. It is seen that the proposed minimal model can quantitatively account for the experimental data.

The results of the computer simulation study of cooperative phenomena in lipid bilayers reported above lend strong support to the general idea[140,143] that it is the special nature of interfacial regions of the membrane, e.g., structural defects and mismatch in molecular packing, which is responsible for leakiness and enhanced permeation of ions near the main transition. This idea not only applies to Na^+ ions, but also to other cations (K^+, Rb^+, Ca^+)[153] and larger molecular species. This is supported by the observation of permeability peaks for such different molecules as TEMPO (2,2,6,6,-tetra-methylpiperidinyl-1-oxy)choline,[143] ANS (8-anilino-1-napthalinesulfonate),[140] and water.[154] In this context, it is interesting to note that the width of the permeability peak predicted on the basis of the computer simulation results will be smaller the larger the lower cut-off in Equation 36 is for the domain size. Since the permeation process of larger molecules presumably will require larger sizes of the defects, i.e., larger cut-off values, it is reassuring to find that the permeability peak for the large ANS molecules is very sharp.[140]

C. NONEQUILIBRIUM PROPERTIES AT THE MAIN TRANSITION
1. Kinetics of the Main Transition

The computer simulation results reported in Section V.A and B for the ten-state Pink model have already forecast that the main transition is associated with some interesting and unusual kinetics. Since the Monte Carlo simulation approach exploits a scheme of stochastic dynamics, it is in principle not possible from such calculations to obtain quantitative information about time-dependent processes. Still, by relying on physically motivated excitation mechanisms (e.g., Glauber dynamics) and by referring to the master equation interpretation of the Monte Carlo process, Equation 12, it is possible to gain some information on the kinetics of the ordering processes and the phase transitions in the membrane models.

Clearly, the simulations have shown that the first-order main transition, cf. Figures 2 to 6, is accompanied by metastabilities (leading to hysteresis) and complicated relaxation behavior which produces a "continuous" melting behavior. The relaxation toward equilibrium is slowed down by the intermediate chain conformational states which are found to have a tendency to appear on the surface of the lipid domains formed near the transition, cf. Figures 10 and 13. This so-called softening of the interfaces decreases the ratio between the domain surface free energy and the bulk free energy and hence lowers the driving for the growth or shrinking of the domains. This furthermore implies that the interaction between the domains is screened which effectively slows down the tendency for the domains to fuse and form a new phase. The overall kinetics of the main transition is therefore slow. These observations from the computer simulation studies can be recast[14] into the language used for the kinetics of phase transitions: the main transition involves three steps:

1. A rapid *nucleation* mediated by the creation of intermediate states which decrease the surface tension of the nucleating domains
2. A fast *growth* of the nucleation centers due to the gain in internal conformational entropy

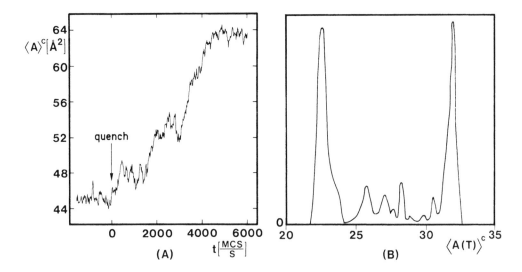

FIGURE 15. (A) Coarse-grained average, $\langle A(T) \rangle^c$, of the cross-sectional area per lipid molecule as it evolves in time (in units of MCS/S) subsequent to a thermal quench from immediately below to immediately above the transition temperature. The data are obtained from Monte Carlo simulations on the six-state Pink model of a DPPC bilayer with 1800 molecules. The time parameter, t, is in units of Monte Carlo steps per site (MCS/S). (Adapted from Reference 14.) (B) Distribution for the cross-sectional area per lipid chain for the time-evolution seen in (A). The vertical scale is in arbitrary units.

3.   A slow *coarsening* of the nucleated domains due to the screening mentioned above

Hence, Step 3 becomes the rate-limiting one. This step implies a kinetic stabilization of metastable domain distributions. The macroscopic consequence is a "continuous" variation of the system properties through the transition region.

Mouritsen[14] has performed a temperature-quenching Monte Carlo simulation on the multistate Pink model which shows that the metastabilities and the relaxation phenomena associated with the main transition are considerably more involved than those accompanying standard first-order phase transitions.[20] In Figure 15A is shown the variation with time (in units of MCS/S) of the coarse-grained cross-sectional area, $\langle A(T) \rangle^c$, of the six-state Pink model (cf. Figure 4A) for which the temperature is quenched from 0.3°C below the transition to 0.3°C above the transition. The coarse-grained average is an average taken over a small number of consecutive configurations in the ensemble generated by the Markov process (cf. Section III.A.2). Use of coarse-grained averages permits a time-resolved picture to be formed of the variation of a quantity. The conspicuous finding from the data presented in Figure 15 is that the relaxation through the transition into the new phase proceeds as a cascade with a number of well-defined steps corresponding to a set of similarly well-resolved peaks in the distribution function for $\langle A(T) \rangle^c$, cf. Figure 15B. This distribution function[14] measures the relative occurrence of microconfigurations with a specific value of the membrane area. The peak positions are not simply related to the discrete set of single-chain cross-sectional areas in Table 1. Each peak in Figure 15B corresponds to a plateau in Figure 15A. From direct inspection of the microconfigurations along the quench, it is found that each plateau is characterized by a specific metastable domain configuration. Cascade relaxation is found only in models with a large number of intermediate states.[14] Hence, cascade kinetics seems to be related to the smearing of first-order transitions. The precise shape of the cascade and the number of resolved intermediate steps depends on the details of the quench, such as initial state and the change in temperature. However, since cascading is always seen in simulated quenches through the transition, cascade kinetics is established as a genuine

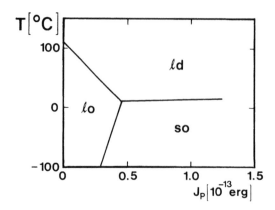

FIGURE 16.   Mean-field phase diagram of the ten-state Pink model with crystalline degrees of freedom for a DPPC lipid bilayer. The transition temperature is plotted vs. grain boundary energy, J_P, for van der Waals' energy parameter $J_o = 1.32 \times 10^{-13}$ erg. Three first-order phase boundaries are shown which divide the diagram into a solid-ordered (so) phase, a liquid-disordered (ℓd) phase, and a liquid-ordered (ℓo) phase. The three phase boundaries meet in a triple point. (Adapted from Reference 61.)

property of the multistate models. Since it is not possible to relate the Markov time of the computer simulation directly to real time, it is not possible to derive the relaxation time for the various steps in Figure 15A.

There has recently been a strong interest in experimental studies of the kinetics of lipid membrane phase transitions, not only of the main transition,[132,155-164] but also of the pretransition[165,166] and the subtransition.[167] The field has greatly advanced with the use of modern time-resolved synchrotron X-ray diffraction techniques.[160,162,163,167] A general finding from the various temperature-jump,[132] pressure-jump,[157] and volume-perturbation[164] techniques (the latter two taking advantage of the small volume expansion during the main transition[109]) has been that the main transition is characterized by several relaxation times (up to five[132]) in the range from 10^{-9} to 10^{-3} s. The processes in the time regime 3×10^{-4} to 3×10^{-3} s have been suggested as being cooperative processes involving a large number of molecules via cluster formation and cluster melting.[132] The finding of a cascading relaxation process in the computer simulation,[14] cf. Figure 15, is in overall accordance with the interpretation of the experimental kinetic data and suggests that a more careful and quantitative analysis of the computer simulation data may be rewarding.

2. Effects of Crystallization and Interfacial Melting

The results described so far on the main bilayer phase transition were predominantly obtained from Monte Carlo simulations of the multistate lattice models of Section IV.A. These models incorporate only the acyl chain conformational degrees of freedom and are believed to provide an accurate description of equilibrium properties. Outside the thermodynamic equilibrium, however, the translational variables and the effects of two-dimensional crystallization will be important for characterizing the kinetic processes and the approach to equilibrium.

Mouritsen and Zuckermann[60,61] have investigated the ten-state Pink model with crystalline variables (Potts variables) in order to study within the simplest possible setting the coupling between the acyl chain ordering process and the crystallization. The Hamiltonian of this model study is $\mathcal{H} = \mathcal{H}_1 + \mathcal{H}_2 + \mathcal{H}_3 + \mathcal{H}_5$, cf. Equations 20, 21, 25, and 28. The added feature of crystalline variables in the Hamiltonian leads to a richer phase behavior. In Figure 16 is shown the mean-field phase diagram spanned by temperature and grain

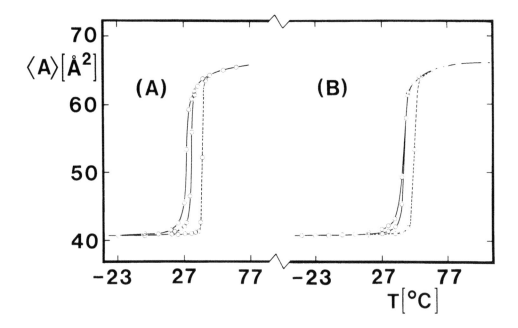

FIGURE 17. Temperature dependence of the average cross-sectional area per lipid molecule, $\langle A(T) \rangle$ in Equation 29, for the ten-state Pink model with crystalline variables for a DPPC bilayer. Data as obtained from Monte Carlo simulations on a system with 5000 molecules are shown for two different values of the grain-boundary energy, J_P. (A) $J_P = 0.55 \times 10^{-13}$ erg; (B) $J_P = 0.525 \times 10^{-13}$ erg. The system has been equilibrated at each temperature value for a time corresponding to 4000 MCS/S. (Adapted from Reference 61.)

boundary energy, J_P. The diagram contains three phases separated by first-order phase boundaries: an so phase (solid-ordered), an ℓd phase (liquid-disordered), and an ℓo phase (liquid-ordered). The phases are labeled by two indices. The first index refers to the bulk two-dimensional thermodynamic phase characterized by the crystalline variables (Potts variables), i.e., the solid is a crystalline solid. The second index refers to the average state of the acyl chains, i.e., ordered means gel and disordered means fluid (liquid-crystalline). The three phase lines meet in a triple point, J_P^*. Above the triple point, the acyl chain, ordering process and the crystallization are coupled and there is a single transition. Below the triple point, acyl chain ordering and crystallization are decoupled processes and there are two thermal transitions. This gives way to a new intermediate phase, the ℓo phase. The ℓo phase is a structurally disordered phase which is a gel and at the same time a liquid with fast in-plane lateral mobility. The parameters of the model are determined by requiring that the coupled so-ℓd transition (the main transition) occurs at $T_m = 41°C$ for DPPC. This leads to $J_o = 1.32 \times 10^{-13}$ erg. The triple point from the Monte Carlo simulations is then found to occur at $J_P^* \simeq 0.535 \times 10^{-13}$ erg (which is smaller than the mean-field value). There is at present no way of estimating the value of J_P in terms of molecular properties[61] and it is therefore left as an undetermined model parameter.

Mouritsen and Zuckermann[60,61] conducted a series of Monte Carlo simulations of the model in the neighborhood of the triple point. In Figure 17 are shown some data for the cross-sectional area, $\langle A(T) \rangle$, as the model is thermally cycled through the transition immediately above (Figure 17A) and immediately below (Figure 17B) the triple point. The thermal cycle, initiated in the equilibrium so phase — heated through the transition region, cooled back again, and finally reheated — has three branches. The extent of the associated

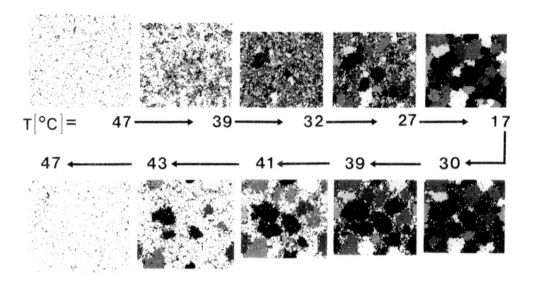

$$T\left[°C\right] = \quad 47 \longrightarrow \quad 39 \longrightarrow \quad 32 \longrightarrow \quad 27 \longrightarrow \quad 17$$

$$47 \longleftarrow \quad 43 \longleftarrow \quad 41 \longleftarrow \quad 39 \longleftarrow \quad 30 \longleftarrow$$

FIGURE 18.   Snapshots of microconfigurations illustrating the nonequilibrium process of grain-boundary formation and subsequent interfacial melting (Figure 17A) for a lipid bilayer with 10,000 acyl chains. White areas indicate fluid domains and symbols indicate lipid chains in gel conformations, with each symbol labeling the crystalline variable (Potts state) of the chain. The lattice parameter has been scaled so as to display the thermally induced area contraction and expansion of the lipid bilayer during the nonequilibrium thermal cycle. The data derive from Monte Carlo simulations on the 10-state Pink model with crystalline variables for a DPPC bilayer with 5000 molecules. The equilibration time at each temperature corresponds to 4000 MCS/S. (Adapted from Reference 61.)

hysteresis loops obviously depends on the equilibration time which for the sake of comparison is chosen to be the same at each successive temperature in both Figures 17A and B. Figure 17 shows that the hysteresis behavior is more pronounced in the case of coupled transitions.

The nonequilibrium microscopic phenomena underlying the thermal cycles of Figure 17 are illustrated in the case of coupled transitions in Figure 18. This figure gives selected snapshots of typical microconfigurations obtained along the lower thermal loop of Figure 17A. It is seen that the bilayer model, being initiated in the ℓd phase and then taken below the main transition temperature, firstly gels and that the structure being formed has a low coherence in the crystalline variables. The domains of the resulting granualar structure or polycrystalline aggregate grow only slowly. If this nonequilibrium configuration is heated before the solid has fully annealed, the phenomenon of interfacial melting[60] is observed: the system melts uniformly from the grain boundaries rather than in the bulk. This phenomenon is similar to grain-boundary melting in metals and alloys.[60,168] The interfacial melting process, being a nonequilibrium phenomenon, occurs at temperatures below the bulk equilibrium transition temperature due to the tension in the grain boundaries. In the case of a larger value of J_p, the interfacial melting process becomes more pronounced.[61] For values of J_p below the triple point, an equally interesting phenomenon is discovered[61] which could be termed interfacial "glassification." During a heating process of a granular structure, the acyl chains at the interfaces remain in gel-like states rather than fluidizing and the crystalline structure changes into that of an amorphous or glassy system. Only at higher temperatures do the chains undergo the disordering process, cf. Figure 16.

It has been suggested[60,92] that lipid membranes are exceptional candidates for experimental observation of interfacial melting phenomena because the melting in these systems proceeds via an internal degree of freedom. Since in general the cooperativity in the chain conformational degrees of freedom is much faster to manifest itself than the cooperativity in the crystalline (translational variables), it is possible to manipulate the system so that chain melting can proceed before the grain-growth process is completed. For conventional materials, such as simple metals, the time scales of the two processes are such that either the annealing is completed before melting takes place or the grain-boundary region is too small to be monitored experimentally.[169]

For phospholipid bilayers, the chain ordering and crystallization processes are found by time-resolved X-ray synchrotron diffraction to be coupled in equilibrium,[160,162] but decoupled out of equilibrium.[163] The question remains whether long-range crystalline order actually is obtained in the low-temperature phase of lipid bilayers. From DSC[170] and static X-ray studies[171] of quickly frozen lipid multibilayers, it was argued that the lipid phase is either a glass or a polycrystal composed of very small grains. The low-angle synchrotron X-ray work by Caffrey[162] on DHPE could be interpreted as showing that a substantial part of the sample is in an amorphous phase. Since this work concentrates on the three-dimensional nature of a multibilayer sample via the lamellar repeat distance, none of these experimental studies are capable of directly studying the phenomenon of interfacial melting. Finally, it should be pointed out that for phosphatidylcholine bilayers, the presence of the ripple $P_{\beta'}$-phase complicates the grain structure of the solid phase[172] and a three-dimensional representation has to be used. Hence, the phenomenon of interfacial melting predicted by the Monte Carlo computer simulation work[61] is most likely to be observed in bilayers, e.g., of DPPE which do not support a ripple phase.

D. COOPERATIVE PHENOMENA IN THE CONDENSED BILAYER PHASES

The results of the lipid bilayer cooperative phenomena reported in Section V.A to C above were predominantly derived from models which were specially designed to describe the main phase transition in terms of the acyl chain conformational degrees of freedom. These models do not claim to account for the detailed properties of the condensed $P_{\beta'}$ or L_{β} low temperature phases of lipid bilayers. In this brief section we shall review some of the few computer simulation studies which have been performed on models which illuminate some aspects of the structure and cooperative phenomena in the condensed phases. There are basically two types of approaches. One,[36,40] which models the liquid crystalline properties of the glycerol backbone (or the anisotropic molecular cross-section) of diacyl lipids, and another,[83-86] which accounts for the vertical motion of the acyl chains in the gel phase. Either of these approaches may or may not simultaneously incorporate acyl chain flexibility and hence the coupling to the main transition. A third type of approach,[87,173] which we shall not be concerned with, deals with the thermodynamic effects of hydrogen bonding on the gel phase properties of hydrated cerebroside membranes.

1. Effects Due to the Anisotropic Shape of the Glycerol Backbone

Most theoretical modeling of lipid membranes disregards the fact that the molecules which make up membranes of diacyl lipids include a tight glycerol backbone coupling between pairs of acyl chains. This produces an extra degree of freedom being the glycerol backbone orientation or the asymmetric shape of the lipid molecule, cf. Figure 1A.

In Cotterill's[36] pioneering work on molecular dynamics simulation of model membrane dynamics, a model was studied which assumes the individual lipid molecules to be in the form of rigid cylinders with a dumbbell cross section, the two ends of the dumbbell corresponding to the two hydrocarbon chains. This model does not account for the conformational degrees of freedom of the chains. The individual chains are assumed to interact via a Lennard-Jones potential and the intermolecular polar head group interactions are modeled by a Coulomb potential. Since the dumbbells in this two-dimensional model have translational as well as orientational degrees of freedom, their dynamics are described by the Newton-Euler equations.[36] By molecular dynamics simulation, the model was found to exhibit an interesting dislocation-mediated two-dimensional melting transition at a temperature which is sensitive to the electrostatic screening (i.e., the pH). These results may have some interesting implications for the structural properties of bilayer condensed phases. The experimental picture of the backbone orientational ordering is at the moment rather unclear. On the basis of freeze-fracture investigations, Hatta et al.[174] suggested a parallel ordering of the backbones similar to that seen in Cotterill's simulations, with defect lines which were suggested as being related to the texture seen in the ripple phase.[172]

In a recent Monte Carlo simulation study, Fraser et al.[40] focused on the two-dimensional liquid-crystalline structural properties of a membrane model. In this model, which is a sort of hybrid between the model studied by Werge and Binder[39] and that proposed by Scott,[175] the lipid molecules are modeled by hard triatomic particles of varying length corresponding to the long axis of the cross section of the lipid molecule. In Scott's[175] model (being similar to the Pink models[107]), the cross sections reflect the conformational states of the acyl chains and a statistical weight is assigned to each state in order to account for the degeneracy. Hence, the simulations carried out by Fraser et al.[40] are very interesting in that they incorporate translational as well as conformational degrees of freedom. The Monte Carlo simulations were performed in both the constant NVT and NPT ensembles. The main results of this study, which were carried out on systems including up to 900 molecules, are that there appears to be no long-range orientational order established before the system freezes and that the short-range orientational order increases with area density. It is unclear, however, whether the simulations have actually reached the state of equilibrium at low temperatures. Furthermore, the absence of a clear first-order main transition in this model may be caused by the small system size and possibly by the neglect of attractive forces.[40]

2. Vertical Motion of Chains, Steric Effects, and the Ripple Phase

There is strong experimental evidence[176] that the phospholipid acyl chains in bilayer undergo vertical fluctuations. The time scale of these fluctuations (10^{-8} to 10^{-9}) is in between that of *trans-gauche* isomerization and that of chain melting. The vertical modes are therefore expected to be relevant for an understanding of the condensed phases of the bilayers.

Pearce and Scott[177] have proposed a model for the condensed bilayer phases which includes the vertical motion of the lipid molecules, but suppresses the acyl chain conformational degrees of freedom. The model is arrayed on a square lattice with "Γ"-shaped molecules which have two coupled discrete degrees of freedom: one being the direction of the bar of the "Γ" along a preferred axis of the square lattice and the other being the molecular displacement perpendicular to the plane of the membrane. The asymmetric "Γ"-shape of the molecule reflects the mismatch between head group and acyl chain cross-sectional areas for phosphatidylcholine bilayers. Obviously, the construction of this model is inspired by general work on magnetic systems with competing interactions for which it is known that modulated structures can arise.[178] From Monte Carlo simulations on this model, Scott[83] found that there is a region of the parameter space where the model has three phases: a low-temperature chain-tilted phase, and intermediate ripple phase, and a high-temperature disordered phase. The mechanism responsible for the spontaneous formation of the spatially modulated ripple phase is the competition in the packing conditions for the polar heads and the acyl chains. Scott's simulations furthermore showed that the kinetics of formation of the ripple phase from the tilted phase is extremely slow. Obvious drawbacks of the model by Pearce and Scott[177] are that it is formulated on a square lattice (whereas acyl chain packing is known to be hexagonally close-packed) and that the modulation is undirectional in contrast to the experimental observation of three preferred ripple propagators.[172] A more sophisticated model has recently been proposed and simulated by Scott[86] in which the vertical molecular displacement degree of freedom is described by a continuous variable. Also this model has a ripple phase.

The model proposed by Georgallas and Zuckermann[85] contains vertical mobility of the chains as well as conformational degrees of freedom. Furthermore, this model is arrayed on a triangular lattice. On the other hand, in contrast to Pearce and Scott's model,[177] it does not include the competitive element in the packing conditions for the head group and the chains. Hence, Georgallas and Zuckermann's[85] model is not capable of describing condensed lipid bilayer phases with tilted chains. In this model, the chains are free to move vertically under a harmonic restoring potential due to the neighboring chains. The force constant of this potential is related to the internal bilayer pressure. The new feature of this model is that it includes explicitly steric effects by allowing chains to twist into the free volume created by a vertical displacement of neighboring chains. Monte Carlo simulations on a one-dimensional version of the model lend some evidence to the idea that the interplay between the twist and the vertical motion can lead to coherent ripple modes. Whether these will survive as a ripple phase in a two-dimensional model remains to be demonstrated.

VI. LIPID MONOLAYER COOPERATIVE PHENOMENA

Condensed phases of lipid monolayers spread on an air/water interface[179] constitute an important class of model systems for biological membranes. In particular, they provide an ideal assay for studying interactions with other membrane-bound molecules, such as proteins,[180,181] cholesterol,[182,183] and anesthetics.[184] Moreover, lipid monolayers have an interesting physics and physical chemistry of their own, encompassing such diverse phenomena as the hydrophobic effect, interfacial tension, phase transition, and pattern formation. In particular, the cooperative phenomena displayed by lipid monolayers as functions of lateral pressure have attracted considerable attention and the nature of the various phase transitions has been a central issue of investigation. Despite the considerable efforts which have been presented, these are still two basic questions which have not yet been fully answered. One is the question of the very nature of the liquid-condensed/liquid-expanded phase transition (the chain melting transition equivalent to the main transition in lipid bilayers) and an explanation of the experimentally observed nonhorizontal isotherms. The other is the question of the in-plane lateral structure of the low-temperature solid phases. Some important progress has been made in recent years toward answering these questions. Firstly, Pallas and Pethica[185] have performed thermodynamic monolayer studies on ultrahigh purity lipid monolayers subject to high standards of humidity control. These authors found horizontal isotherms and consequently argued that the chain melting transition is of first order. Some theoretical support for this conclusion was subsequently provided by Nagle.[186] Secondly, recent use of fluorescence microscopy[187-192] and X-ray synchrotron radiation[193-197] has provided new information on the monolayer lateral structure. The fluorescence work has revealed the formation of different patterns of solid domains during the transition[194] and the anisotropy of the fluorescence emission has indicated that the solid domains have long-range orientational order.[191,192] The X-ray synchroton work[197] supported classical work[9] suggesting two pressure-induced phase transitions, but showed also that the liquid-condensed phase of DMPA and DMPE is a crystalline solid only at very high pressures and that the coherence length of the crystal is small. At lower pressures, there is an intermediate solid phase with long-range orientational order and short-range positional order. The nature of this intermediate phase is, however, subject to some uncertainty and a number of different theoretical interpretations have been suggested.[49,54,194]

Many of the computer simulation model studies on lipid monolayers to be reported below are closely related to the lipid bilayer studies described in Section V. In fact, the microscopic interaction models underlying the theoretical monolayer studies are in many cases formally equivalent to the bilayer models.

A. STATIC PHASE BEHAVIOR OF LIPID MONOLAYERS

The main part of the computer simulation results on lipid monolayer cooperative phenomena and phase transitions derives from Monte Carlo work on multistate lattice models.[53-56] The early molecular dynamics simulations by Kox et al.[45] and Northrup and Curvin[46] dealt with less than 100 acyl chains and provided more structural and dynamic information within the phases than quantitatively reliable information on the transitions themselves. Kox et al.[45] found evidence of a first-order gas-liquid transition and Northrup and Curvin[46] discovered that chain-tilting disorder may be a precursor for the onset of the chain melting transition. The Monte Carlo study by Chen et al.[41] on a system of grafted rods with orientational variables, but without chain degrees of freedom, showed that this model system does not undergo an orientational ordering transition in the liquid condensed phase. Hence these authors concluded that the two transitions inferred from the X-ray work[193] must be induced by the coupling between chain flexibility and the orientational degrees of freedom.[41] The molecular dynamics study by Bareman et al.[47] on the structure of the intermediate phase will be discussed in Section VI.B.1. None of the multistate lattice model simulations reviewed below allow for chain tilting which should be kept in mind when comparisons with experimental data are performed.

1. Isotherms and the Nature of the Liquid-Expanded/Liquid-Condensed Transition

The first Monte Carlo simulation on a multistate lattice model of lipid monolayer phase behavior is that of Georgallas and Pink,[53] who studied a special two-state model with certain temperature-dependent properties of the lower acyl chain state mimicking average properties of the intermediate states. The statistics of Georgallas and Pink's simulations are insufficient and the systems simulated are too small to give a detailed picture of the liquid-expanded/liquid-extended monolayer transition region. One important result of these simulations is that they show how the isotherms depend on impurity concentration. Since it was found that unrealistically large impurity concentrations (~4%) are required to produce isotherms with a shape similar to that of experimental observations, it must be concluded that a two-state model is not adequate to faithfully model monolayer phase behavior.

The Monte Carlo simulation study of the ten-state Pink model of a lipid monolayer by Mouritsen et al.[55] is the first one to give detailed insight into the fluctuation effects with accompany the chain melting transitions. In Figure 19 is shown a selection of equilibrium isotherms derived from this model. At low temperatures, the isotherms have a horizontal section and they are highly asymmetric with a low-pressure kink and a high-pressure rounded shoulder. The horizontal section as well as the asymmetry get progressively less pronounced as the temperature is increased. Below 34.1°C, there are clear signs of a first-order transition, whereas for higher temperatures, the change of phase is rather smooth. In the first-order region, thermal cycles with incomplete equilibration give rise to hysteresis phenomena, cf. Figure 20. At the highest temperatures in the first-order region, e.g., at 30°C, the simulated isotherm has a finite slope and the transition appears as "continuous". No discontinuity may be resolved. This is similar to the finding for the thermally induced chain melting transition in lipid bilayers, cf. Figure 4A, and is caused by the same mechanism: the diversity of acyl chain conformations results in a cascade of metastable states and a slow relaxation in the transition region reminiscent of critical slowing down.

A comparison with the experimental isotherm at 30°C for DPPC is provided in Figure 21. This comparison should not be taken too far into the liquid-expanded phase since the lattice model used for the simulations is not a proper model of this phase due to the neglect of free volume.[198] The difference between the data from the two different experimental groups[9,187] is due to difficulties in controlling the absolute amount of lipid applied. Both experimental and theoretical isotherms are nonhorizontal in the transition region. This shows that it is not necessary to invoke complications such as impurity effects,[53] polar-head group

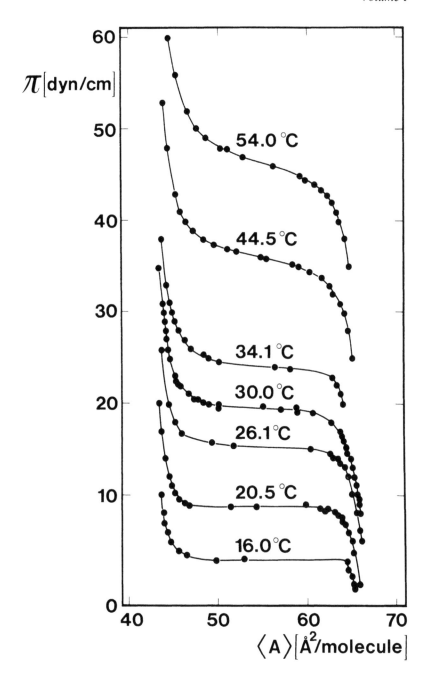

FIGURE 19.   Isotherms for the 10-state Pink model of a DPPC monolayer as obtained from Monte Carlo simulations on a system with 5000 molecules. (Adapted from Reference 55.)

interactions,[199] or interphase strain[186] to explain the experimental nonhorizontal isotherms, although impurities can also lead to a smearing of the transition.[185] The round high-pressure shoulder is also common for the experimental and simulated isotherms in Figure 21, although the experimental isotherms are smooth over a larger pressure range. However, even the set of experimental isotherms has some deviations at this point. These differences have been interpreted[55] as being due to a nonequilibrium crystallization and grain-growth process[54] which we shall return to in Section VI.B.1.

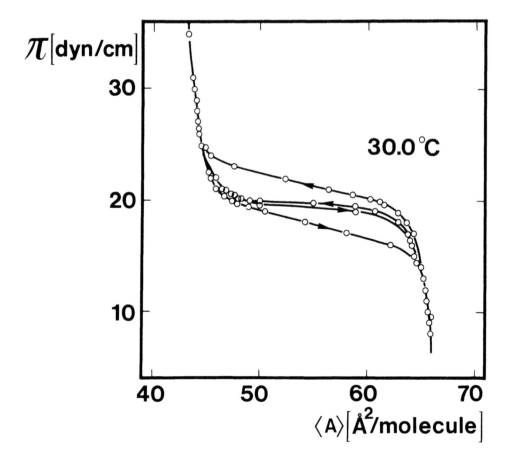

FIGURE 20.   Isotherm at 30°C for the ten-state Pink model of a DPPC monolayer as obtained from Monte Carlo simulations on a system with 5000 molecules. The outer and inner hysteresis loops correspond to equilibration times of 100 and 1000 MCS/S, respectively. (Adapted from Reference 55.)

Figure 22 provides a comparison between experimental and theoretical results for the transition pressure $\Pi_m(T)$ as a function of T for a DPPC monolayer. The theoretical results are shown from computer simulations on different models and from an analytical theory.[200] Each set of data is described approximately by a linear relationship, $\Pi_m(T) \sim T$. It should be pointed out that the determination of the transition pressure becomes progressively less precise as the temperature is raised. The correlation between the experimental data and the computer simulation results from the ten-state Pink model is satisfactory considering that the parameters of the model have not been fine-tuned to be material specific.[55]

2. Cluster Formation and Cluster Statistics

The microscopic phenomena accompanying the chain melting transition in the ten-state Pink model of a monolayer are illustrated in Figure 23 which gives a series of typical microconfigurations along different isotherms. The manifestations of lateral density fluctuations in terms of lipid domain formation are similar to those of the bilayer, cf. Figure 10. In the region of clear first-order transitions, $T < T_c$, where $T_c \simeq 35$ to 45°C, the lipid domains increase in size as the temperature is raised toward T_c. The domains or clusters are compact but ramify as T_c is approached. Above T_c, the signals of a phase transition are absent and there is smooth change of phase, cf. Figure 23 at 54°C.

A quantitative formulation of the statements above is made possible by an analysis of the cluster statistics. In Figure 24 are shown for different temperatures the average domain

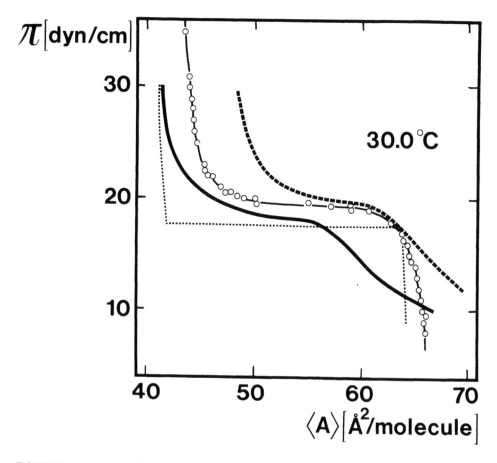

FIGURE 21. Isotherm at 30°C for a DPPC monolayer. Results are shown as obtained from the experimental work by Albrecht et al.[9] (------) and von Tcharner et al.[187] (———) and from Monte Carlo simulations (○) on the 10-state Pink model with 5000 molecules. For comparison is shown the mean-field prediction for the ten-state Pink model (······). (Adapted from Reference 55.)

size, $\bar{\ell}(\Pi)$, cf. Equation 36, as a function lateral pressure around the inflection points of the isotherms. For all temperatures, $\bar{\ell}(\Pi)$ has a sharp peak. The intensity of the peak increases and the width decreases as T_c is approached from either side. These observations are strong indications of the presence of a critical point (rather than a tricritical point) at T_c.

3. Nature of the Solid Phase: Decoupling of Chain Ordering and Crystallization

By including the crystalline variables in the ten-state Pink model, cf. Section IV.B, it is possible to study aspects of the structural properties of the liquid-condensed monolayer phase.[54,56] In the plane spanned by lateral pressure and grain-boundary energy, J_P, cf. Equation 28, the phase diagram of the ten-state Pink model with crystalline variables as derived from Monte Carlo simulations[54] is as shown in Figure 25. In analogy with the corresponding bilayer phase diagram, cf. Figure 16, the model is seen to have three phases separated by three first-order lines which meet in a triple point, J_P^*. Above the triple point, the acyl chain ordering transition is coupled with the crystallization and a single phase transition separates the solid-ordered (so) phase from the liquid-disordered (ℓd) phase. Below the triple point, the liquid-ordered (ℓo) phase intervenes and there are two pressure-driven phase transitions. The phase line between the ℓo and so phases is extremely steep reflecting the fact that once the acyl chains are ordered, very high pressures are required to produce crystallization. Hence, from this phase diagram it is anticipated that the ℓo-so transition may

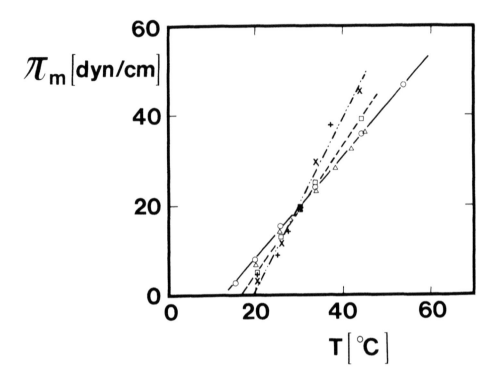

FIGURE 22.   Pressure Π_m of the chain melting transition for a DPPC monolayer. Results are shown as obtained from the experimental studies by Albrecht et al.[9] (+) and von Tscharner et al.[187] (+) and from theoretical model calculations: Monte Carlo simulations on the ten-state Pink model (o), Monte Carlo simulations on the two-state model of Georgallas and Pink[53] ($\triangle$), and the analytical theory due to Georgallas and Pink[200] ($\square$); (·····) is used as a guide for the eye for both sets of experimental data (——) is used for both sets of computer simulation data, and (·—·—·—·) is used for the analytical theory. (Adapted from Reference 55.)

be associated with slow kinetics related to that of grain growth in polycrystalline aggregates.[114] In summary, the model predicts two possible senarios: (1) coupled chain ordering and crystallization above the triple point and (2) decoupled chain ordering and crystallization below the triple point. The value of J_p valid for phospholipids is at present unknown. In the light of the experimental findings of uncoupled transitions,[193,197] it is obviously of interest to investigate the model below the triple point.[56]

In Figure 26 are shown the computer simulation results for the model in the case of decoupled acyl chain ordering and crystallization immediately below the triple point, cf. Figure 25. (Note that the van der Waals' interaction constant has not been adjusted to accurately fit the DPPC monolayer isotherm.) The main branch of the isotherm (the solid line) is obtained from a series of increasing lateral pressures starting from the ℓd phase. For an equilibration time corresponding to 4000 MCS/S, the isotherm is almost reversible in the ℓo and ℓd phase with a modest hysteresis in the transition region. The relaxation in the ℓd-ℓo transition is extremely slow, causing the isotherm to be nonhorizontal. The ordering kinetics of the ℓo-so transition is even slower and only for a small system is it possible, by the Monte Carlo calculations, to make the system enter the uniformly ordered crystalline phase, so (Potts ordered phase), within a reasonable time. Hence it is difficult to accurately locate the high-pressure transition. The area discontinuity associated with this transition is estimated to be about 0.8 Å² from Figure 26, which is in good agreement with that derived from the synchrotron X-ray data for a change in the molecular nearest-neighbor distance parameter.[194]

Typical snapshots of microconfigurations taken along the 30°C-isotherm in Figure 26

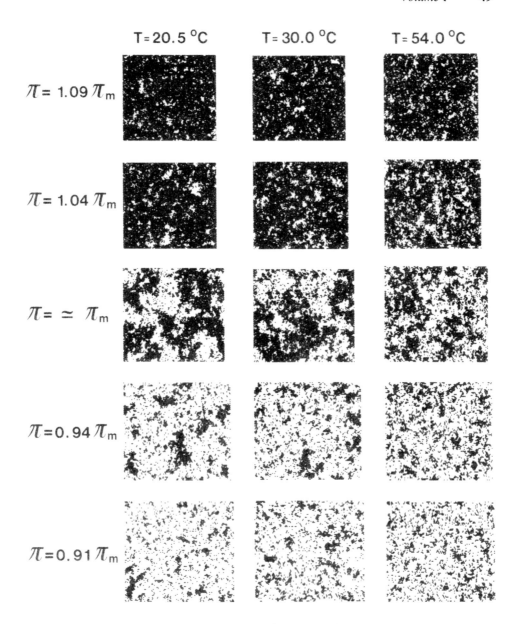

FIGURE 23.   Snapshots of microconfigurations typical of equilibrium for a DPPC monolayer near the chain melting transition at Π_m. These configurations are obtained from Monte Carlo simulations on the 10-state Pink model with 5000 lipid molecules. The gel state acyl chains are denoted by black dots and the fluid chains are indicated by white regions. The lattice parameter has been scaled so as to display the lateral expansion and compression of the monolayer. (Adapted from Reference 55.)

are displayed in Figure 27. The configurations illustrate the structure of the monolayer as it is being compressed laterally. For pressures below the ℓo-so transition, these snapshots (a to e) are typical of equilibrium, whereas at higher pressures equilibrium has not been attained. The figure shows that during the ℓd-ℓo (liquid-expanded/liquid-condensed) transition the monolayer is transformed into a condensed glassy phase. The approach to the so phase is then signalled by the appearance of clusters of chains in the same Potts state (Figures 27d and e). These clusters are akin to density fluctuations. We shall return to a description of the nonequilibrium properties of the so phase and the ℓo-so phase transition in Sections VI.B.1 and 2.

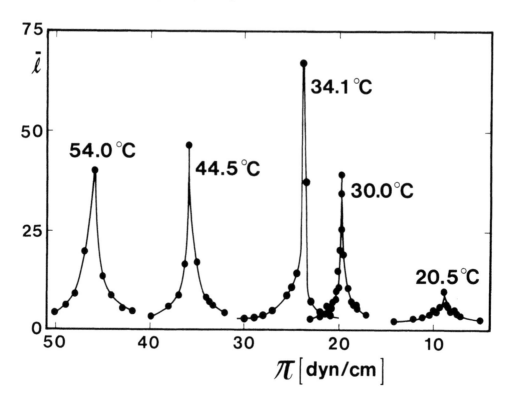

FIGURE 24. Average cluster size $\bar{\ell}(\Pi)$ in units of number of molecules as a function of lateral pressure Π near the chain melting transition. Results as obtained from Monte Carlo simulations on the 10-state Pink model of a DPPC monolayer with 5000 molecules are shown for 5 different isotherms of Figure 19. The cluster formation phenomena underlying the peaks in $\bar{\ell}(\Pi)$ are illustrated in Figure 23. (Adapted from Reference 55.)

4. Lateral Compressibility and Specific Heat

The lateral monolayer compressibility $\kappa(A)$, along the 30°C isotherm is shown in Figure 28. It is seen to have two distinct features. Firstly, the ℓo-so transition is signaled by a shoulder in $\kappa(A)$. Secondly, the compressibility of the uniformly ordered Potts phase is considerably lower than that of the softer metastable grain structure, cf. Figure 27g and h. This difference is consistent with the experimentally found difference[194] between the "macroscopic" lateral compressibility (obtained from the slope of the isotherm) and the "microscopic" compressibility (obtained from the pressure variation of the crystal lattice parameters determined from the X-ray scattering). Helm et al.[194] suggested that this difference is due to a possible influence on the macroscopic compressibility of defect annealing as well as merging and deformation of solid domains. This is in excellent accordance with the computer simulation results.[56] Furthermore, the shape of $\kappa(A)$ in the transition, cf. Figure 28, is rather similar to that reported in the experimental study on DPPC monolayers by Albrecht et al.[9] Some deviations are expected, however, due to the neglect in the model of the tilting mode.

The specific heat, C_Π, along the 30°C isotherm is shown in Figure 29. C_Π has a sharp peak at the ℓd-ℓo transition and a second peak at the ℓo-so transition. The signaling of the latter transition is much stronger in C_Π than in $\kappa(\Pi)$.[54] The reason for this is that the area fluctuations are only slightly influenced by the Potts ordering (crystallization) process. The specific heat data in Figure 29 above the ℓo-so transition are subject to large nonequilibrium fluctuations caused by a grain growth process. It is not possible to measure C_Π experimentally for a single monolayer.

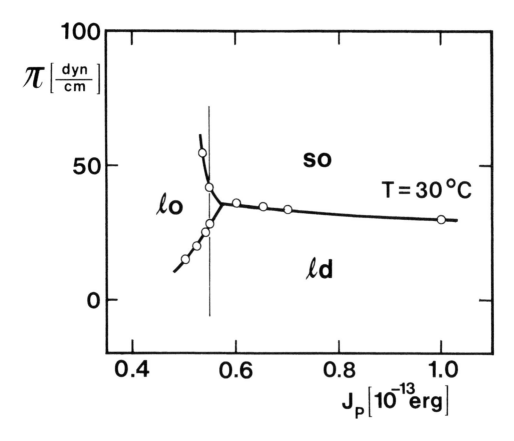

FIGURE 25. Phase diagram of the ten-state Pink model with crystalline variables for a DPPC monolayer as derived from Monte Carlo simulations. The transition lateral pressure is shown vs. the grain boundary energy, J_P. Three first-order phase boundaries are shown which divide the diagram into a solid-ordered (so) phase, a liquid-disordered (ℓd) phase, and a liquid-ordered (ℓo) phase. The three phase boundaries meet in a triple point. The horizontal line denotes a scan through the phase diagram at $J_P = 0.55 \times 10^{-13}$ erg which leads to results as given in Figures 26 to 30. (Adapted from Reference 56.)

B. NONEQUILIBRIUM PROPERTIES OF LIPID MONOLAYERS
1. Nonequilibrium Isotherms and Growth of the Solid Phase

The part of the isotherm (solid line) in Figure 26 in the neighborhood and above the ℓo-so transition corresponds to a nonequilibrium situation. This leads of a rounded shoulder similar to that observed experimentally,[9,187] cf. Figure 21. This shoulder is much more pronounced than that obtained from a model with acyl chain conformational degrees of freedom only, cf. Figure 21. The shoulder is caused by the nonequilibrium growth of crystalline domains which form a polycrystalline aggregate as seen in Figure 27h. The polycrystalline aggregate is characterized by a random network of grain boundaries separating the competing crystalline domains. The domain pattern anneals extremely slowly in time, as illustrated in Figure 30. The reason for this is that the lateral pressure only couples to the Potts ordering via the fluid chain states which are almost absent in the highly condensed ℓo and so phases. Figure 30 shows that there are even domains of the disordered ℓo phase intercalated in the grain boundaries. This element of a disordered interface between the grains tends to screen the interaction between the ordered domains; it lowers the driving force for grain growth and consequently slows down the kinetics of the growth. In other words, it may be said that in the case of decoupled transitions, the lateral pressure becomes a "weak" thermodynamic variable[56] for inducing order.

The finding of low crystalline coherence in the so phase is consistent with the interpre-

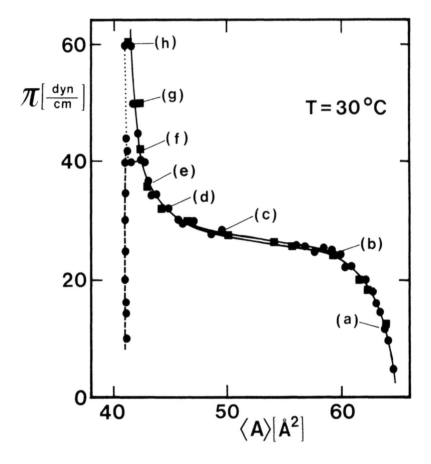

FIGURE 26.   Isotherm at 30°C for the ten-state Pink model with crystalline variables of a DPPC monolayer in the case of decoupled crystallization and acyl chain ordering, cf. Figure 26 at $J_p = 0.55 \times 10^{-13}$ erg. The data are obtained from Monte Carlo simulations on systems with 5000 (solid squares) and 450 (solid circles) lipid molecules: (——) denotes an isotherm which at high lateral pressures corresponds to a nonequilibrium monolayer with a domain structure; (······) refers to an equilibrium expansion at high pressures which continues at lower pressures into a nonequilibrium state (------) of a metastable monolayer with a single crystalline domain. Points (a) to (h) on the isotherm refer to the microconfigurations in Figure 27. (Adapted from Reference 56.)

tation of the synchrotron X-ray work on DMPA and DMPE lipid monolayers.[197] In these experiments, it was found that only crystalline regions were formed with a coherence length of less than 100 Å. Due to the neglect of true translational variables in the ten-state Pink model with crystalline variables, it is of course not possible to produce a hexatic phase[201] with bond orientational order. Therefore the computer simulation studies of the multistate models are not capable of revealing the possibly more subtle details of the intermediate phase.

In contrast, the molecular dynamics simulation by Bareman et al.[47] is performed on a monolayer model with chain flexibility as well as translational coordinates for the head groups being confined to the membrane plane. The most striking finding from this study is that the system in the intermediate phase breaks up into regions ($\sim$ 20 Å) of ordered and disordered chains. The ordered regions have a distinct tilt of the chains. The breaking up in domains leads to a dramatic decrease in the density profile normal to the monolayer as the surface area is increased. The resulting density distributions are very similar to those observed experimentally.[197] Bareman et al.[47] concluded from their molecular dynamics study

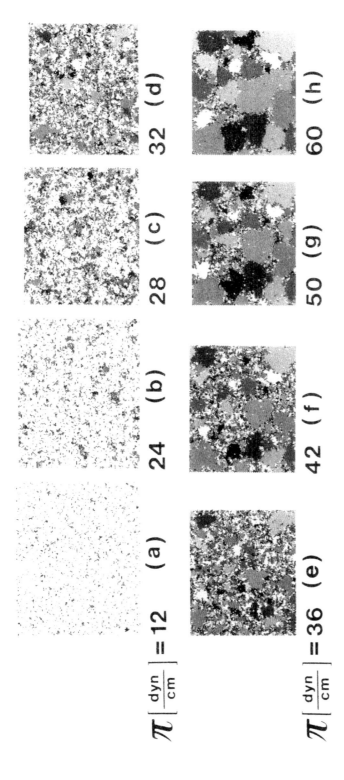

FIGURE 27.   Snapshots of microconfigurations typical for points along the 30°C isotherm of a lipid monolayer. The data are obtained from Monte Carlo simulations on the ten-state Pink model with crystalline variables in the case of decoupled crystallization and acyl chain ordering, cf. Figure 26 at $J_P = 0.55 \times 10^{-13}$ erg. The monolayer lattice contains 5000 DPPC molecules. White areas indicate fluid domains and symbols indicate acyl chain in gel-like conformations, with each symbol labeling the crystalline variable (Potts state) of the acyl chain. The lattice parameters has been scaled so as to display the lateral compression of the monolayer as the lateral pressure is increased from (a) to (h). Each configuration is typical for an equilibration time corresponding to 4000 MCS/S. (Adapted from Reference 56.)

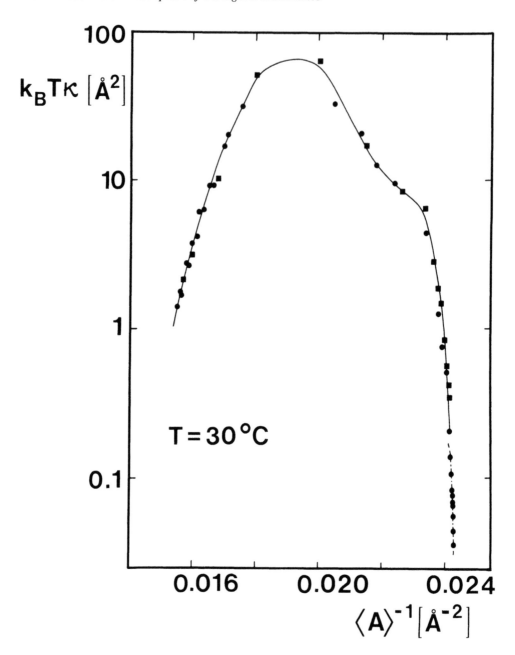

FIGURE 28.   Isothermal area compressibility, $\kappa(A)$ in Equation 5, vs. inverse average cross-sectional area per lipid molecule along the DPPC monolayer isotherm of Figure 26. The data are obtained from Monte Carlo simulations on the ten-state Pink model with crystalline variables for systems with 5000 (solid squares) and 450 (solid circles) lipid molecules. The solid and dashed lines refer to the corresponding branches of the isotherm in Figure 26. (Adapted from Reference 56.)

that the driving force for the observed structural and conformational changes in the monolayer may be related to the tendency for close-packing of the CH_3 groups of the lipid chains.

2. Fractal Pattern Formation and Impurity-Controlled Solidification

A particularly striking manifestation of a nonequilibrium cooperative phenomenon in lipid monolayers has been observed by Miller et al.,[202,203] who studied the growth of solid

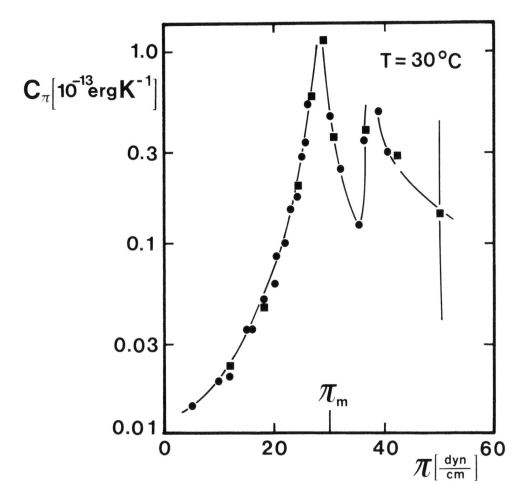

FIGURE 29. Specific heat per lipid molecule, $C_P(T)$ in Equation 4, vs. lateral pressure, Π, along the DPPC monolayer isotherm of Figure 26. The data are obtained from Monte Carlo simulations on the ten-state Pink model with crystalline variables for systems with 5000 (solid squares) and 450 (solid circles) lipid molecules. (Adapted from Reference 54.)

domains in DMPE monolayers on the air/water interface by fluorescence microscopy. Subsequent to a rapid compression in the coexistence region, these monolayers, which contain a dye impurity, form solid domains with a variety of morphologies ranging from compact to very tenuous, depending on the temperature, the size of the pressure jump, and the dye concentration.[203] The tenuous domains, of which an example is displayed in Figure 31A, are characterized by a tip-splitting fractal morphology.[204,205] A similar type of fractal pattern formation process has recently been observed in monolayers of myristic acid.[206] Miller et al.[202] explained their finding of fractal growth in monolayers as caused by a diffusion-limited aggregation mechanism which becomes operative by a constitutional supercooling effect due to the low miscibility of the dye impurity in the solid phase.

Sørensen et al.[92-95] have reported in a series of papers the results of computer simulation studies on a model designed to study the influence of mobile impurities on a two-dimensional solidification process in lipid monolayers. Within this model, the solidification process is controlled by two mechanisms: one being the gel ↔ fluid isomerization of the acyl chains which occurs on the time scale τ_S and the other being the diffusion of impurities in the fluid phase which occurs on the time scale τ_D. The model is implemented on a square lattice. The nature of the lattice and in fact the lattice approximation as such is irrelevant for the

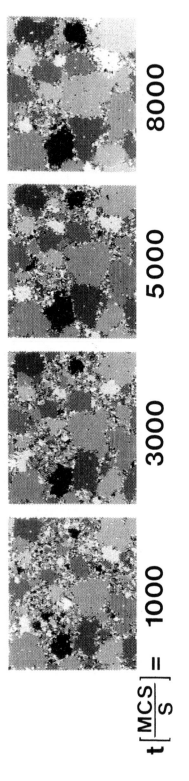

FIGURE 30. Snapshots of the time evolution of microconfigurations of the DPPC monolayer isotherm of Figure 26 for $\Pi = 50$ dyn/cm. The configurations are obtained from Monte Carlo simulations on the ten-state Pink model with crystalline variables in the case of decoupled crystallization and acyl chain ordering. The monolayer lattice contains 5000 lipid molecules. White areas indicate fluid domains and symbols indicate acyl chains in gel-like conformations, with each symbol labeling the crystalline variable (Potts variable) of the acyl chain. (Adapted from Reference 56.)

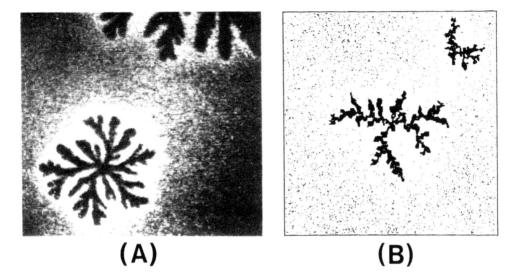

(A)   **(B)**

FIGURE 31.   Fractal growth patterns in lipid monolayers. (A) Fluorescence microscopic picture of a DMPA monolayer doped with a fluorescent dye impurity. The monolayer has been rapidly compressed to a lateral pressure of 0.5 dyn/cm above the transition pressure. The dark fractal patters are solid domains being formed in the fluorescing fluid phase. The radius of the solid is about 50 μm. (From Miller, A., Knoll, W., and Möhwald, H., Fractal growth of crystalline phospholipid domains in monomolecular layers, *Phys. Rev. Lett.*, 56, 2633, 1986. With permission.) (B) Fractal domain of solid as obtained from a Monte Carlo simulation of the growth model described in Sec. VI.B.2. The dark dots in the white background denote lipid chains in the fluid state. (Courtesy of H. C. Fogedby.)

results obtained. The diffusion of the latent heat away from the solidification front is not taken into account since the water subphase is effectively thermocoupled with the lipid molecules. The model is described by a Hamiltonian which Sørensen et al.[94,95] chose to be a simple version of the two-state Doniach model[104] of the acyl chain melting transition. The impurities are modeled by an annealed dilution of vacancies. The relationship between the concentration of site vacancies and the potency of the actual dye impurity to dissolve the solid is unclear. However, it is anticipated that the effective potency of the actual dye impurity to dissolve the solid is unclear. However, it is anticipated that the effective potency is not restricted to a single site. The time evolution of the model subsequent to a sudden temperature quench was studied by a Monte Carlo technique which used Glauber dynamics for the acyl chain conformational transitions and Kawasaki nearest neighbor pair exchange between vacancies and chains in the fluid state to simulate translational diffusion of the impurities (cf. Section III.A.3). It is expected that the solidification process during a temperature quench will be similar to that observed after a pressure jump. The model is related to the standard models used to study diffusion-limited aggregation,[207] but it is the first model which uses a Hamiltonian formalism. This makes it possible to study not only early time irreversible aggregation and solidification phenomena, but also the crossover in both time and temperature to the equilibrium growth conditions.

In Figure 32 are shown typical solid domains grown by the model of Sørensen et al.[93] in the low-temperature regime for various values of the time scale ratio, τ_S/τ_D. It is seen that the faster the diffusion is, the more compact do the solid domains grow. The very fractal-forming mechanism is revealed by studying the radically averaged impurity distribution, P(R), cf. Figure 33, as it evolves in time. The data in Figure 33 show that there is an elevated level of impurities in the active growth zone. This leads to an interface instability which in turn causes the interface to develop fingers. Obviously, the slower the diffusion is, the more impurities are piled up at the solidification front and the more ramified the

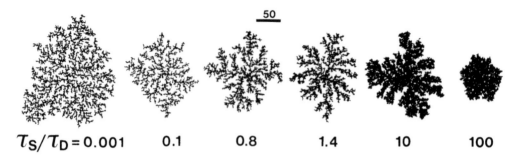

FIGURE 32. Typical lipid monolayer solid domains grown from the impurity-controlled solidification model of Section VI.B.2 at low temperatures for different time scale ratios, τ_S/τ_D, for lipid chain solidification and dye impurity lateral diffusion. The impurity concentration is 70%. The solids consist of about 10,000, 500, 6000, 7000, 13,000, and 5000 acyl chains, respectively. The solid bar indicates 50 lattice spacings. (Adapted from Reference 95.)

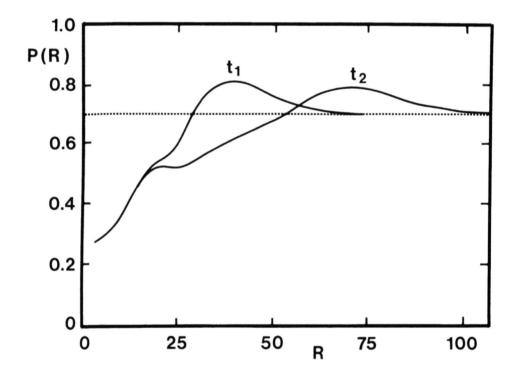

FIGURE 33. Circularly averaged radial distribution function of dye impurities, P(R), as a function of linear dimension, R, at low temperatures. The data are obtained from Monte Carlo simulations on the growth model of Section VI.B.2 for impurity-controlled fractal solidification in lipid monolayers. The results refer to an impurity concentration of 70%. The ratio of solidification time scale to that of impurity diffusion is τ_S/τ_D, = 2. For two consecutive times, $t_1 < t_2$, the solid aggregate contains 1500 and 5000 acyl chains, respectively. (Adapted from Reference 93.)

interface gets. That the morphologies are in fact described by fractal geometry[207] is seen in Figure 34 which gives an analysis of the particle content, N(R), of the solid domains vs. their linear extension, R, in terms of the power law:

$$N(R) \sim R^D. \tag{39}$$

D is the so-called fractal dimension. If $D < d$, where d = 2 is the spatial dimension, the

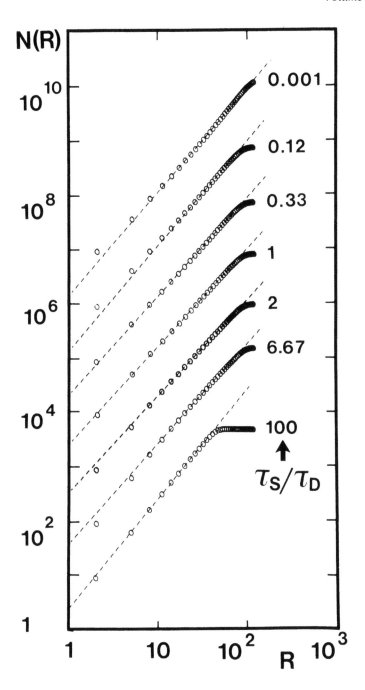

FIGURE 34. Double-logarithmic plot of the number of acyl chains, N(R), vs. linear dimension, R, of low-temperature lipid monolayer solids formed during an impurity-controlled solidification process according to the growth model of Section VI.B.2. The results are obtained form Monte Carlo simulations at an impurity concentration of 70% for different time scale ratios, τ_S/τ_D, of acyl chain solidification and dye impurity lateral diffusion. For the sake of clarity, each data set has been shifted one decade upward relative to the one below. The dotted lines denote fits to $N(R) \sim R^D$, Equation 39. (Adapted from Reference 95.)

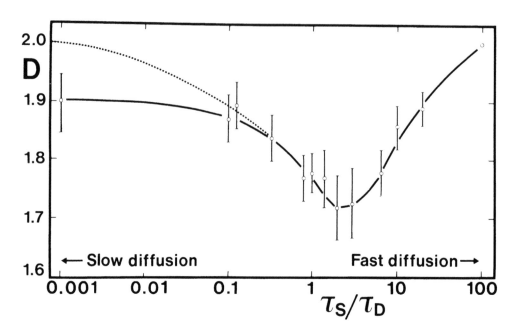

FIGURE 35.   Semilogarithmic plot of the low-temperature fractal dimension, D in Equation 39, vs. time scale ratio, τ_S/τ_D, for solid lipid monolayer domains grown according to the impurity-controlled solidification model of Section VI.B.2, cf. also Figures 32 and 34. The concentration of dye impurities is 70%. The solid line is a guide to the eye. The dashed line indicates for slow diffusion crossover to the cluster-cluster aggregation regime. (Adapted from Reference 95.)

structure is not described by a single-length scale, but rather possesses a scaling symmetry according to Equation 39. The effective fractal dimension as defined by the fits in Figure 34 is shown in Figure 35 as a function of time scale ratio. It is seen that D is dependent on the time scale ratio. The lowest value of D obtained is similar to that characterizing standard diffusion-limited aggregation.[207]

The solid domain monolayer patterns shown in Figure 32 correspond to a very low growth temperature. Obviously, these patterns are nonequilibrium structures which will rearrange and compactify as time lapses or as the temperature is raised. In Figure 36 are shown the effects of the growth temperature. The growth patterns are displayed as they appear in the early time regime of the process. At later times, each of the structures seen in Figure 36 will rearrange and compactify and the growth will proceed in a stable compact manner.

The Monte Carlo computer simulation study[93] of the far-from-equilibrium solidification process in impure lipid monolayers has hence shown that the fractal growth is controlled by impurity diffusion, in agreement with the interpretation of the experimental observations by Miller et al.[202,203] In fact, elevated levels of fluorescent dye were found experimentally in the growth zone using densitometric methods.[203] Moreover, the simulated patterns are very similar to those seen in the experiments, cf. Figure 31A and B, and so are the effective fractal exponents derived from the model and from analysis of the experimental data.[203,206] The computer simulation results furthermore illustrate the crossover from nonequilibrium fractal growth to equilibrium compact growth both as a function of time and temperature. The variation of the effective fractal exponent D (cf. Figure 35) with the diffusion rate of the impurity suggests that it will be interesting to study experimentally the solidification process for a monolayer with fluorescent proteins which have quite a different diffusion constant.

Finally, it should be noted that Suresh et al.[206] have interpreted their findings of fractal

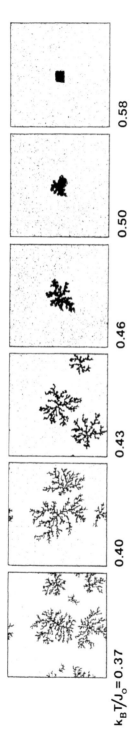

FIGURE 36.   Typical solid domains formed in impure lipid monolayers at early times for different reduced temperatures, $k_B T/J_o$. The data are obtained from Monte Carlo simulations on the impurity-controlled solidification model of Section VI.B.2 at an impurity concentration of 70%. Both fluid and solid lipid chains are denoted by black dots. The connected structure are the solid domains. The ratio of time scales of acyl chain solidification and impurity lateral diffusions is $\tau_S/\tau_D = 1$. The lattice contains 256×256 sites. (Adapted from Reference 94).

solid patterns in monolayers of myristic acid in terms of a diffusion-driven instability taking into account the reduced line tension near the critical point rather than impurity diffusion. This interpretation is supported by the finding that the patterns are not sensitive to the impurity concentration. Suresh et al.[206] furthermore performed a computer simulation study of a noise-reduced diffusion-limited aggregation model to substantiate and support their interpretation.

VII. EFFECTS OF INTRINSIC MOLECULES ON LIPID MEMBRANE COOPERATIVE PHENOMENA

The theoretical approaches to modeling the interactions between lipid membranes and intrinsic molecules have recently been reviewed by Abney and Owicki.[12] Most of these approaches have been shaped by the experimental spectroscopists' preoccupation[120,208,209] with a study of the changes in acyl chain conformational and orientational order (statically and dynamically) of the lipids near the intrinsic molecules. For integral proteins in particular, this has led to theoretical concepts regarding the protein as a rigid body which poses a boundary condition with which the acyl chain ordering has to comply.[210] To a lesser extent, the focus has been on modeling the phase equilibria in mixed membrane systems, presumably because the experimental information on phase diagrams is rather sparse and inaccurate.

The same theoretical bias toward a description of the influence on single intrinsic molecules on the bilayer acyl chain order has been translated into most of the computer simulation approaches to lipid-intrinsic molecule interactions in membranes. This is particularly true of the Monte Carlo simulation of order parameter profiles by Scott[75,77] and the molecular dynamics calculations by Edholm et al.[81,82] (The reader is referred to the article by Scott elsewhere in this volume.) A substantial part of the computer simulation work has dealt with simulation of protein lateral diffusion[72-74,78] and the lateral distribution of proteins in membranes.[67-71] None of these studies are concerned with the cooperative phenomena and the phase equilibria of lipid membranes with intrinsic molecules. The only computer simulations to date, which have attempted to analyze cooperative phenomena in many-component membranes, are of the Monte Carlo type. The models which have been studied are exclusively two-dimensional multistate Pink models on lattices where intrinsic molecules such as cholesterol[58,64] and protein and polypeptides[65,66] are assumed to occupy one or more sites of the lattice. Since these models, as earlier pointed out in the present review, are equally good models of lipid monolayers, the computer simulation results to be reported below will also have some validity for monolayers with intrinsic molecules to a degree which depends on the molecular species in question.

A. LIPID BILAYERS CONTAINING CHOLESTEROL

It is only recently that a reasonably clear experimental picture has emerged of the phase diagram for the phosphatidylcholine-cholesterol system. (For a list of references to the relevant experimental literature, see Reference 211.) This phase diagram is reproduced in Figure 37A. The diagram is still not complete since the phases related to the ripple phase[212] have not been included. The theoretical interpretation and understanding of the experimental phase diagram have to a large extent been helped along by use of the multistate Pink model with crystalline variables[113,211,213] and a phenomenological model[211] which accounts for both chain degeneracies and cholesterol solubility in the two lipid phases. Within the framework of the multistate Pink model with crystalline variables, cholesterol has been modeled by Ipsen et al.,[211] cf. Figure 37B, as a molecule which on the one hand interacts favorably with the acyl chain conformations of the solid-ordered (so) phase, but on the other hand dissolves most easily in the liquid-disordered (ℓd) phase and hence acts as a crystal breaker in the so phase. These conflicting interactions lead to the peculiar properties of the phase

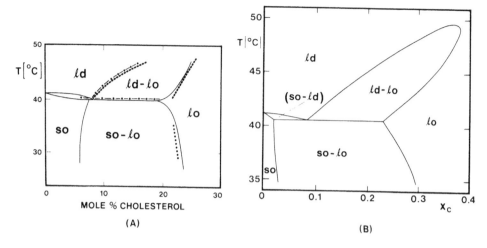

FIGURE 37.   Phase diagram of DPPC bilayers containing cholesterol. The various phases are denoted by so (solid-ordered), ℓd (liquid-disordered), and ℓo (liquid-ordered). (A) Experimental phase diagram as obtained by NMR spectroscopy and differential scanning calorimetry (——), EPR spectroscopy (------), freeze-fracture (⋯⋯), and micromechanics (-·-·-·-). (Adapted from Reference 211.) (B) Theoretical phase diagram obtained from the mean-field solution to the ten-state Pink model with crystalline variables. (Adapted from Reference 213.)

diagram in Figure 37 for DPPC-cholesterol bilayers. At low cholesterol concentrations, x_C ≤ 8 to 10 mol%, the two opposite effects of cholesterol on the lipid bilayer are in balance leading to only a slight freezing-point depression. For higher concentrations, cholesterol has effectively decoupled the acyl chain ordering from the crystallization which leads to formation of a new phase, the liquid-ordered (ℓo) phase. Massive phase separation then sets in both above and below the pure bilayer main transition temperature, T_m. The diagram for DMPC cholesterol is expected to be very similar to that of Figure 37. The model by Ipsen et al.[211] has also been able to explain calorimetric[213] and NMR spectroscopic data.[113] So far no computer simulations have been performed on this model.

1. Model and Phase Diagram

The first computer simulation of a lipid-cholesterol mixture is that of Mouritsen et al.,[58] who used a two-state Pink model with exclusively acyl chain conformational degrees of freedom. Only interactions between lipid chains in the lower state and cholesterol were considered. It was found from the simulations that such a simple model provides an incorrect description of the phase transition. In an attempt to model more accurately some aspects of the cooperative phenomena in membranes containing cholesterol, without having to adopt the full ten-state model with crystalline variables, Cruzeiro-Hansson et al.[64] recently studied a somewhat simpler model which is designed to give the correct phase behavior in the low concentration regime where the peculiar properties of the ℓo phase have not yet manifested themselves, i.e., for concentrations x_C ≤ 10 mol%.

The model studied by Cruzeiro-Hansson et al.[64] adds to the standard ten-state Pink model a term,

$$\mathcal{H}_6 = \Pi A_C \sum_{i=1}^{N} \mathcal{L}_{Ci} - \frac{J_o}{2} \sum_{i,j}^{N} \sum_{\alpha=1}^{10} V_\alpha S_\alpha I_C (\mathcal{L}_{\alpha i} \mathcal{L}_{Cj} + \mathcal{L}_{\alpha j} \mathcal{L}_{Ci}) - \frac{J_o}{2} \sum_{i,j}^{N} I_C^2 \mathcal{L}_{Ci} \mathcal{L}_{Cj} \quad (40)$$

which accounts for lipid-cholesterol as well as cholesterol-cholesterol interactions in the spirit of shape-dependent, nematic interactions, cf. Equation 21. In Equation 40, I_C is the (constant) shape factor assigned to the cholesterol molecule. It is related to the van der

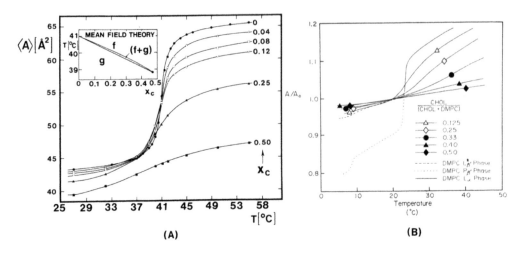

FIGURE 38.   Cross-sectional area, $\langle A(T) \rangle$, per molecule of the mixture for a lipid bilayer containing cholesterol in different concentrations, x_C. (A) Theoretical data obtained from Monte Carlo simulations on the ten-state Pink model for DPPC bilayers with lipid-cholesterol interactions, cf. Equation 40, for a lattice with 10,000 sites. The insert shows the corresponding phase diagram calculated in the mean-field approximation, g and f denote gel and fluid lipid phases, respectively. (Adapted from Reference 64.) (B) Experimental data for the relative membrane area of single DMPC-cholesterol vesicles studied by micromechanical techniques. (From Needham, D., McIntosh, T. J., and Evans, E., *Biochemistry*, 27, 4668, 1988. With permission.)

Waals' interaction between the hydrophobic part of the cholesterol molecule and the corresponding part of a lipid chain or another cholesterol molecule. $\mathcal{L}_{Ci} (= 0, 1)$ is the occupation variable of the cholesterol molecules. The cholesterol cross-sectional area[214] is $A_C = 32 \text{ Å}^2$ and the cholesterol concentration is given by

$$x_C = \langle \mathcal{L}_{Ci} \rangle / (2 - \langle \mathcal{L}_{Ci} \rangle). \tag{41}$$

In fact, the interactions of Equation 40 are not specific for cholesterol, but may equally well represent the interaction with other small and stiff membrane-bound amphiphilic molecules which are hydrophobically smooth. Relative to the pure lipid bilayer model, $\mathcal{H} = \mathcal{H}_1 + \mathcal{H}_2 + \mathcal{H}_3$, cf. Equations 20, 21, and 25, the present model, $\mathcal{H} = \mathcal{H}_1 + \mathcal{H}_2 + \mathcal{H}_3 + \mathcal{H}_6$, involves only a single new parameter, I_C. I_C was fixed by Cruzeiro-Hansson et al.[64] by the requirement that the phase diagram of the model resembles that of DPPC-cholesterol mixtures, cf. Figure 37, for x_C up to about 10 mol%, i.e., with a very narrow coexistence region and a modest freezing-point depression. A simple mean-field calculation suggests $I_C = 0.45$ to be a suitable choice and leads to the phase diagram shown as an insert in Figure 38A. The coexistence region between gel and fluid bilayer phases terminates according to this model in a critical endpoint at $x_C \simeq 0.48$. Despite the fact that the model of Cruzeiro-Hansson et al.[64] should not be considered a proper model of the phase equilibria in the DPPC-cholesterol system above $x_C \simeq 0.1$, results will be presented below for concentrations beyond this limit. The reason for this is twofold. Firstly, the model describes general aspects of lipid membranes with intrinsic molecules, and secondly the model may in fact also at high concentrations account for the dominant effect of cholesterol on the phase behavior since these are tightly coupled to the three-phase line which the simple phase diagram of Figure 38 follows rather closely.

2. Membrane Area, Chain Statistics, and Lateral Compressibility

The Monte Carlo data for the average cross-sectional area per molecule of the mixture, $\langle A(T) \rangle$, are shown in Figure 38 together with the experimental results for DMPC obtained

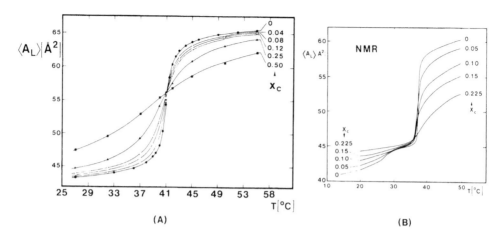

(A)   (B)

FIGURE 39.   Cross-sectional area per lipid molecule, $\langle A_L(T)\rangle$ in Equation 42 for a DPPC lipid bilayer containing cholesterol in different concentrations, x_C. (A) Theoretical results obtained from Monte Carlo simulations on the ten-state Pink model with lipid-cholesterol interactions, cf. Equation 40, for a lattice with 10,000 sites. (Adapted from Reference 64.) (B) Experimental data derived from ^{2}H-MNR measurements of the first moment M_1 for d_{62}-DPPC bilayers by using Equations 19 and 32 to 34. (Adapted from Reference 113.) The experimental data are those of Vist. (From Vist, M. R., Partial Phase Behavior of Perdeuterated Dipalmitoylphosphatidylcholine/Cholesterol Model Membranes, M.Sci., thesis, University of Guelph, Ontario, 1984. With permission.) Note that the main transition temperature of d_{62}-DPPC bilayers is $T_m = 37°C$.

by Needham et al.[215] from micromechanic measurements on giant single vesicles. Despite the difference in lipid type and despite the fact that the model is not designed to be valid at high concentrations, there is an amazing similarity between the two data sets. It should be noted that the micromechanic measurements do not yield absolute area values but only fractional changes and that the experimental data set for each concentration has therefore been scaled to a common point below the transition region. Figure 38 shows that cholesterol leads to a broadening of the transition and that there is a rather complicated relationship between $\langle A(T)\rangle$ and x_C below the transition. A more clear picture of the effect of cholesterol on the membrane area is obtained by suppressing the mere dilution effect on $\langle A(T)\rangle$ by calculating the cross-sectional area per lipid molecule:

$$\langle A_L(T)\rangle = (\langle A(T)\rangle - x_C A_C)/(1 - x_C).$$

(42)

The Monte Carlo data for $\langle A_L(T)\rangle$ are given in Figure 39A. This figure now clearly shows the expected systematic expansion effect of cholesterol below the transition and the condensation effect above the transition. It is not possible experimentally to measure $\langle A_L(T)\rangle$ directly. However, an approximate experimental value of $\langle A_L(T)\rangle$ may be obtained from ^{2}H-NMR spectroscopy[113] via the first moment, M_1, of the quadrupolar spectrum, cf. Section V.A.3, Equations 33 and 34. Experimental data derived in this way are shown in Figure 39B for d_{62}-DPPC multilayer systems. Suppressing the experimental effects due to the ripple phase, we again find a good agreement between the experimental data and the computer simulation results.

The changes observed in the average cross-sectional area per lipid molecule, $\langle A_L(T)\rangle$ in Figure 39, as the cholesterol concentration is varied, reflect of course the influence of cholesterol on the acyl chain orientational order. This is also clearly demonstrated by the effect on the chain state occupation variables, as seen in Figure 40 for $x_C = 0.12$. By comparison with the similar results for the pure system, Figure 5, it is noted that the intermediate chain states are promoted in the transition region by cholesterol. Furthermore, the all-*trans* state is suppressed below the transition and the fluid chain state is suppressed

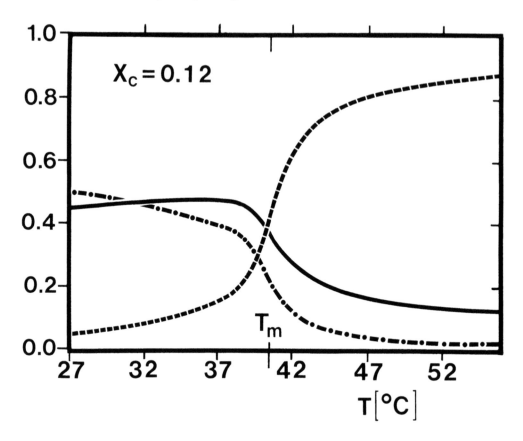

FIGURE 40.   Temperature dependence of chain state occupation variables as obtained from Monte Carlo simulations on the ten-state Pink model of a DPPC bilayer with cholesterol in concentration of $x_C = 0.12$: (—·—·—·—),
all-*trans* state $\langle \mathscr{L}_{1i} \rangle$; (------), fluid state $\langle \mathscr{L}_{10i}$, and (——), intermediate states $\Sigma_{\alpha=2}^{9} \langle \mathscr{L}_{\alpha i} \rangle$. The data are obtained
from a lattice with 10,000 sites (Adapted from Reference 64.)

above the transition. These findings are in accord with the usual interpretation of spectroscopic data.[216]

Turning then to the effects of cholesterol on the lateral isothermal compressibility, $\chi(T)$,
the Monte Carlo data in Figure 41 demonstrate that the pronounced peak at the transition
temperature changes in a very characteristic way: the peak height is reduced as x_C is increased
and at the same time the intensity of $\chi(T)$ is increased away from the transition. Hence, the
lateral density fluctuations are suppressed at the transition point, but are enhanced away
from the transition. This is a rather remarkable effect which is supported by similar results
for the specific heat. Since there are no signs of a phase separation within the resolution
limits of the computer simulation,[64] the peak position of $\chi(T)$ can be associated with the
transition temperature. The compressibility has been measured experimentally by
micromechanics[215] for DMPC vesicles containing cholesterol. It was found that $\chi(T)$ decreases with x_C at high concentrations, in agreement with the Monte Carlo results in Figure
41. The experimental data are not able to discern the enhancement in the wings of $\chi(T)$ at
low concentrations. The suppression of the intensity of $\chi(T)$ at the transition point is inti-
mately related to the model assumption of cholesterol being mobile in the membrane. For
a stationary dilution of cholesterol, the phenomenological model study by Jähnig[217] shows
that the peak intensity rather is increased by cholesterol (driven towards criticality) in
contradiction with experiment.[215]

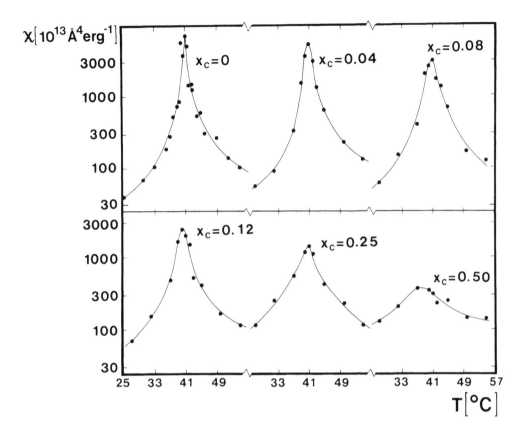

FIGURE 41. Semilogarithmic plot of the isothermal lateral compressibility, $\chi(T)$ in Equation 5, for a DPPC bilayer with different concentrations, x_C, of cholesterol. The data are obtained from Monte Carlo simulations on the ten-state Pink model including lipid-cholesterol interactions, cf. Equation 40, for a lattice with 10,000 sites. (Adapted from Reference 64.)

3. Lateral Density Fluctuations and Lipid Domain Formation

Cruzeiro-Hansson et al.[64] have extended their study[62] of the heterogeneous dynamic membrane structure formed near the main transition in pure lipid bilayers (cf. Section V.B) to bilayers containing cholesterol. Snapshots obtained from Monte Carlo calculations on the ten-state Pink model showing the influence of cholesterol are presented in Figure 42 for low cholesterol concentrations. Only the lipid domain boundaries and the lateral distribution of cholesterol molecules are indicated on this figure. It is seen that the presence of cholesterol leads to larger and more ramified domains and even induces a clustering among the domains themselves.

A quantitative analysis of the domain distributions is given in Figure 43 in terms of the average domain size $\bar{\ell}(T,x_C)$ (in units of molecules) as calculated from the lipid domain distribution function, $n_\ell^i(T,x_C)$, i = gel or fluid. The overall behavior of $\bar{\ell}$ as a function of T and x_C is very similar to that of the lateral compressibility in Figure 41. In particular, cholesterol at low concentrations decreases the peak intensity at the transition, but increases $\bar{\ell}$ away from the transition. The enhancement in the wings persists up to about $x_C \simeq 0.25$, whereas at $x_C = 0.50$, cholesterol suppresses $\bar{\ell}$ at all temperatures. This finding is consistent with the presence of a critical point in this model in between these two concentration values.

It is not possible to directly monitor the lipid domain formation phenomena in bilayers. However, in lipid monolayers, it has been observed by epifluorescence microscopy[218] that cholesterol leads to a ramification of the solid domain interfaces.

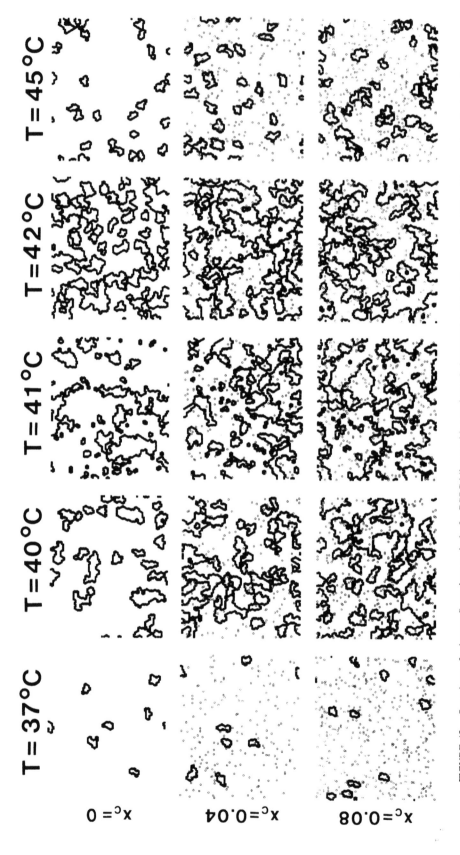

FIGURE 42. Snapshots of microconfigurations typical of a DPPC bilayer with a variety of cholesterol concentrations. x_C, for different temperatures in the region of the main transition. The data are obtained from Monte Carlo simulations on the ten-state Pink model including lipid-cholesterol interactions, cf. Equation 40, for a lattice with 10,000 sites. Only the interfacial regions (the solid network) and the cholesterol distribution (○) are shown. (Adapted from Reference 64.)

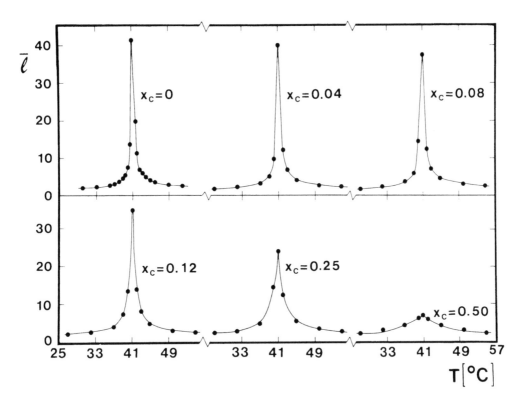

FIGURE 43. Average lipid domain size, $\bar{\ell}(T,x_C)$ in Equation 36, as a function of temperature and cholesterol concentration, x_C, in a DPPC bilayer, $\bar{\ell}$ denotes the number of lipid molecules in the average-sized domain of the minority phase. The results are obtained from Monte Carlo simulations on the ten-state Pink model with lipid-cholesterol interactions according to Equation 40 for a lattice with 10,000 sites. (Adapted from Reference 64.)

4. Cholesterol at Lipid-Domain Interfaces

A closer inspection of the snapshots of microconfigurations in Figure 42 indicates that the cholesterol molecules are not randomly distributed in the plane of the membrane, but exhibit a tendency to accumulate at the lipid-domain interfaces. Cruzeiro-Hansson et al.[64] performed a detailed analysis along the lines described for the pure lipid bilayer case in Section V.B.2. In this analysis, the fractional interfacial area, a_i is divided into a lipid and a cholesterol part, $a_i = a_{iL} + a_{iC}$. It was found[64] that at the transition for low x_C, there is hardly any change in a_{iL} when cholesterol is introduced, whereas a_{iL} increases with x_C at temperatures away from transition. In contrast, a_{iC} increases steadily with x_C at all temperatures. This effect is most clearly seen by examining the excess fractional interfacial area:

$$a_{iL}^{excess}(x_C) = a_{iL}(x_C) - a_{iL}(x_C = 0) \qquad (43)$$

which is a measure of the change due to cholesterol in the lipid part of the interfacial area relative to the pure system. The Monte Carlo data for $a_{iL}^{excess}(T,x_C)$ are shown in Figure 44. This figure clearly demonstrates that at low cholesterol concentrations and away from the transition temperature not only is the total interfacial area increased, but also the lipid part of this area is increased. This means that the interface is not simply increased with an amount corresponding to the accumulated cholesterol. This is a highly nontrivial result which is caused by the cooperative behavior of the lipid-cholesterol mixture. This result has some important consequences for the permeability of the cholesterol-containing membranes. The subtle temperature dependence of a_{iL}^{excess} in Figure 44 may be rationalized in physical terms

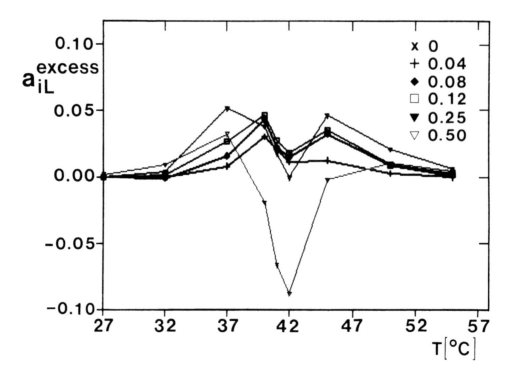

FIGURE 44.   Excess fractional interfacial area, a_{iL}^{excess} in Equation 43 of the lipid part of the interfacial area as a function of temperature for a DPPC bilayer containing different concentrations of cholesterol, x_C. The results are derived from Monte Carlo simulations on the ten-state Pink model including lipid-cholesterol interactions, cf. Equation 40, for a lattice with 10,000 sites. (Adapted from Reference 64.)

by remarking that cholesterol acts so as to lower the interfacial tension between the lipid domains and the bulk. In general the interface acts as a sink for impurities. The reason why the effects of cholesterol in low concentrations are so weak at the very transition is due to the fact that the interfacial tension at this point is already small due to the proximity to a pseudo-critical point, cf. Section V.A.4.

The claimed accumulation of cholesterol at the lipid-domain interfaces is made quantitative by the data presented in Figure 45 which show that the level of cholesterol in the interfacial region is more than twice that of cholesterol in the bulk for low global cholesterol concentrations, x_C. This accumulating effect is found to be sharply localized in the first interfacial layer[64] and the decay to the bulk distribution is very rapid.

The finding from the Monte Carlo simulations of a cholesterol-induced increase in the lipid part of the interfacial area away from the transition has the consequence that the passive ion permeability, as predicted from the simple model described in Section V.B.3, varies with x_C and T as seen in Figure 46. There are at present no experimental data available in the low concentration region to assess the validity of this prediction. For high-cholesterol concentrations, the experimental measurements[135] show, however, in agreement with Figure 46, that the permeability is lowered in the presence of 50 mol% cholesterol. As pointed out by Cruzeiro-Hansson and Mouritsen,[62] the influence of the cholesterol on the interfacial regions in membranes may also inhibit permeation of other molecular species. The experimental finding of a lowered water permeation in membranes containing large amounts of cholesterol[154,219] is in accordance with this suggestion. Moreover, the quantitative result in Figure 46 of a strong suppression of the permeability at high cholesterol concentrations is in line with the general idea of cholesterol being a molecular agent which assures high mechanical coherence and low leakiness of membranes.[215,220]

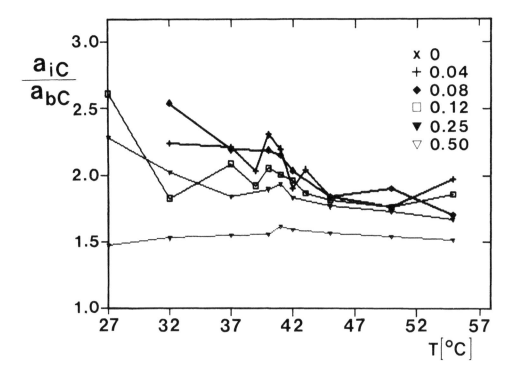

FIGURE 45.   Ratio, a_{iC}/a_{bC}, between the cholesterol concentration in the interfaces and in the bulk for different cholesterol concentrations, x_C in a DPPC bilayer. The data are obtained from Monte Carlo simulations on the 10-state Pink model with lipid-cholesterol interactions, cf. Equation 40, for a lattice with 10,00 sites. (Adapted from Reference 64.)

Experimental measurements of the kinetics of the phase transition in lipid bilayers containing cholesterol have been interpreted in terms of cluster-formation phenomena.[221,222] For example, it has been found that for $x_C = 0.075$, the kinetic processes associated with domain formation are suppressed at the transition, but enhanced away from the transition in agreement with Figure 43. At higher cholesterol concentrations, the kinetics associated with the cooperative domain-formation processes are fully suppressed.[222] Furthermore, extrapolation of the interpretation of specific-heat anomalies in terms of domain distributions[122] to the specific heat measure for cholesterol-containing membranes[223,224] bears further testimony to the model results in Figure 43.

Finally, it should be pointed out that the finding of the ability of cholesterol to modulate the interfacial regions of membranes is of marked interest in relation to studies of interfacially active enzyme processes.[141,225,226] The specific example mentioned in Section V.B.2 of pancreatic phospholipase[150] is particularly interesting in this context. In the presence of cholate, which has a structure similar to that of cholesterol, it was found[226] that small amounts of cholate increase the rate of activation of the phospholipase away from the phase transition. Since it has been suggested[150] that the rate of activation is closely linked to the lipid-membrane fluctuations and the formation of a particular interfacial environment which supports the active conformation of the enzyme, the effect of cholate is in good agreement with the results of the computer simulation on the simple model of cooperative phenomena membranes with small intrinsic molecules.

B. LIPID BILAYERS CONTAINING PROTEINS AND POLYPEPTIDES

Going from lipid membranes containing small intrinsic molecules to membranes with large proteins implies a substantial complication in the theoretical model formulation as well

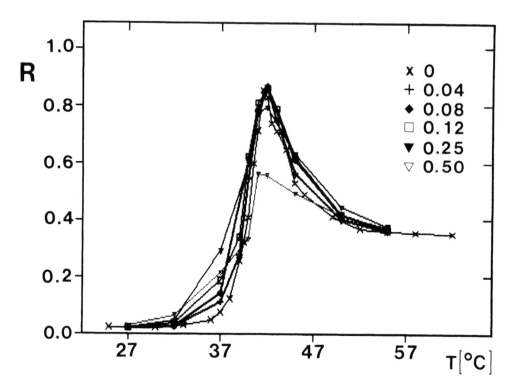

FIGURE 46.   Reduced permeability, $R(T)$ in Equation 38 of Na^+ ions in DPPC liposomes as a function of temperature and cholesterol concentration, x_C. $R(T)$ is given in arbitrary units. The data are obtained from Monte Carlo simulations on the ten-state Pink model with lipid-cholesterol interactions, cf. Equation 40, on a lattice with 10,000 sites. (Adapted from Reference 64.)

as in the computer simulation of the properties of these models. Modeling complicated objects such as transmembrane proteins usually involves a number of drastic assumptions and unknown parameters. The simulation of the cooperative phenomena and phase equilibria in such models is hampered by the requirement of large system sizes to model mixtures of molecular species of very different sizes. Furthermore the general difficulty in applying thermodynamic criteria to computer simulation data in order to determine phase equilibria is a severe one, considering the fact that most lipid-protein systems have phase diagrams with regions of massive phase separation. All these difficulties have implied that very little computer simulation work has been done on cooperative phenomena in membranes containing proteins and polypeptides. In fact, to date only two original articles[65,66] have appeared on this topic. Since this work is reviewed by Pink in Chapter 1.A.4, (as well as in an earlier review by Pink[17]), the present Section is only intended, for the sake of completeness, to describe the main results of these simulations.

Both simulation studies build on the two-state Pink model (in the version with temperature-dependent properties of the lower state[17]) for the pure DPPC or DMPC bilayers. In the work by Lookmann et al.[66] the proteins are considered as hexagons on a superlattice imposed on the underlying triangular lattice. Each hexagon covers several lipid sites corresponding to molar weights around 15,000 Da. The interaction between the lipid and protein molecules is given by a single constant measuring the strength of the interaction between the protein and a lipid chain in the fluid conformational state. The value of this constant is fixed in accordance with NMR order parameter measurements which generally show[208] that the protein does not change $\langle S \rangle$ above the transition. Thermodynamic and structural properties are then calculated to be compared with DSC and freeze-fracture experiments. We shall

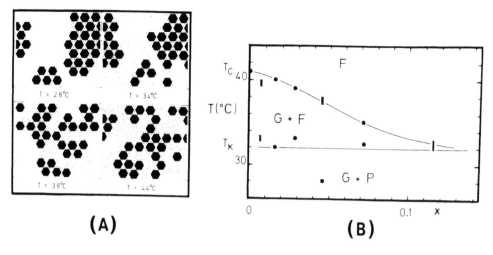

(A)   **(B)**

FIGURE 47.   Phase behavior of a DPPC bilayer model membrane with proteins of molecular weight of ~15,000 Da. (A) Lateral organization at different temperatures. Black hexagons denote the proteins and dots represent lipid chains in the fluid conformational state. White regions indicate the gel lipid matrix. (B) Phase diagram. F and G denote fluid and gel lipid phases and P denotes a protein-rich phase. (From Lookman, T., Pink, D. A., Grundke, E. W., Zuckermann, M. J., and de Verteuil, F., *Biochemistry*, 21, 5593, 1982. With permission.)

here only focus on the phase equilibria, cf. Figure 47. From direct inspection of snapshots like those of Figure 47A, and from observations of short-time fluctuations, Lookmann et al.[66] inferred a phase diagram of the type in Figure 47B. Obviously, the phase boundaries of this diagram cannot be very precise since no objective thermodynamic criteria have been applied. This problem lies at the root of determining the thermodynamic phase of a system from a Monte Carlo simulation in the canonical ensemble. In order to get accurate phase boundaries, grand canonical sampling has to be invoked introducing a chemical potential to control the protein concentration. This is not a difficulty which arises from computer simulation alone. In fact, the same problem comes up in almost every attempt to use experimental measurements, be it calorimetric or spectroscopic, to derive the phase diagram for a multicomponent mixture.[227] Still, the results presented in Figure 47B are very informative and in close agreement with the interpretation of experiments on many membranes reconstituted with different integral proteins, e.g., Ca^{2+}-Mg^{2+}-ATPase.[66] The computer simulation work also provides some interesting information on the melting behavior of acyl chains trapped within patches of proteins.[66]

The second piece of work by MacDonald and Pink[65] is on an even more complicated system, i.e., glycophorin in DMPC bilayers. This system has a rather complicated phase behavior due to the large extramembrane moiety of glycophorin. Within the model, the protein is assigned two different states corresponding to this moiety either standing out from the membrane or lying on the membrane polar surface. These two states are represented by two different hexagon sizes in the spirit of the previous model.[66] It was found that the effect of these two different protein states on the adjacent lipid correspond to a difference in the internal lateral pressure exerted on the lipids. This in turn leads to a phase diagram strikingly similar to the experimental one.[228]

VIII. CONCLUDING REMARKS AND OUTLOOK

The insight so far gained in the function of biological membranes from computer simulation calculation of cooperative phenomena is still modest. On the other hand, the knowledge about the physical properties, i.e., structure and dynamics, of model membranes has increased substantially by computer simulation of microscopic interaction models of lipid bilayers and monolayers. This knowledge is a prerequisite for further work toward a theoretical understanding of the fundamental relationships between function and structure and how the physical properties of lipid membranes modulate their physiological function.

The theoretical models studied are by nature very simplified from a biological and biochemical point of view, but rather complicated from the point of view of fundamental physics and physical chemistry. The modern computer simulation techniques described in this review meet these two conflicting viewpoints by making it feasible and meaningful from a physical point of view to study quantitatively certain models which are sufficiently realistic and hence complex to merit the results in the eyes of the experimental membranologists.

The particular focus in the present review has been on the phase transitions and cooperative phenomena in lipid membranes and how these phenomena are influenced by other membrane components such as cholesterol and proteins. A major hypothesis of the review is that the cooperative processes and the resulting membrane lateral heterogeneity may form a basis for understanding and interpreting a variety of experimental observations of membrane function and structure without having to invoke subtle and complicated mechanisms. In this way, the computer simulation approach to membranology becomes, by its simplistic nature, an important assay to clarify to which extent observed membrane phenomena are "simple" consequences of the mere fact that the membrane consists of a large ensemble of mutually interacting molecules.

The many advantages of the computer simulation approach to membrane cooperative phenomena copiously outbalance the drawbacks. Still, these drawbacks hamper the progress which is betoken by the fast development of computer hardware. Among these drawbacks is the approximate nature of the simulation models and the variety of unknown model parameters these models usually imply. As far as membrane cooperative phenomena are concerned, most of the simulations are therefore not on models which are material specific, but rather on models which emphasize the general behavior of a class of related compounds. Obviously, this is a severe limitation. On the other hand it is, at the present stage of theoretical modeling, of major importance to focus on general behavior in order to determine the type of parameters and physical features which are the relevant ones for characterizing a specific phenomenon.

Undoubtedly, the computer simulation approach to the study of cooperative phenomena in lipid membranes is going to gain more importance in the future along with the rapid development of faster computers and the advances in theoretical design of more refined models. This importance will be shaped by an anticipated very strong interplay between computer modeling and those experimental activities which exploit powerful and modern physical measurements. It is expected that the progress will follow two routes which are interrelated. One route involves refinement of lattice models of membranes with more material specific potentials and a refined description of membrane-bound molecules, such as polypeptides, anesthetics, sterols, and proteins. Another route involves simulation on larger systems of molecules in a membrane assembly building on as realistic spatially dependent potentials as possible. This last route also implies taking better account of water molecules, ions, and electrostatic forces.

ACKNOWLEDGMENTS

A large part of the research work on which this review is based has been carried out in collaboration with a number of colleagues. In particular, I wish to thank the following scientists for stimulating and exciting collaboration: Myer Bloom, Leonor Cruzeiro-Hansson, Hans C. Fogedby, John Hjort Ipsen, Erik Schwartz Sørensen, and Martin J. Zuckermann. My own research work is supported by the Danish Natural Science Research Council under grant J.nr. 5.21.99.52.

APPENDIX 1

ABBREVIATIONS USED

AC   Alternating current
DHPE   Dihexadecylphosphatidylethanolamine
DMPC   Dimyristoylphosphatidylcholine
DMPA   Dimyristoylphosphatidic acid
DPPC   Dipalmitoylphosphatidylcholine
DPPE   Dipalmitoylphosphatidylethanolamine
DSC   Differential scanning calorimetry
EPR   Electron paramagnetic resonance
NMR   Nuclear magnetic resonance

REFERENCES

1. **Tanford, C.,** *The Hydrophobic Effect. Formation of Micelles and Biological Membranes,* John Wiley & Sons, New York, 1973.
2. **Israelachvili, J. N., Marčelja, S., and Horn, R. G.,** Physical principles of membrane organization, *Q. Rev. Biophys.,* 13, 121, 1981.
3. **Evans, E. A. and Skalak, R. S.,** *Mechanics and Thermodynamics of Biomembranes,* CRC Press, Boca Raton, FL, 1980.
4. **Evans, E. and Needham, D.,** Physical properties of surfactant bilayer membranes: thermal transitions, elasticity, rigidity, cohesion, and collodial interactions, *J. Phys. Chem.,* 91, 4219, 1987.
5. **Sackmann, E.,** Physical basis of trigger processes and membrane structures, in *Biological Membranes,* Chapman, D., Ed., Vol. 5, Academic Press, New York, 1984, 105.
6. **Quinn, P. J. and Chapman, D.,** The dynamics of membrane structure, *CRC Crit. Rev. Biochem.,* 8, 1, 1980.
7. **Mouritsen, O. G.,** Physics of biological membranes, in *Physics in Living Matter,* Baeriswyl, D., Droz, M., Malapinas, A., and Martinoli, P., Eds., Springer-Verlag, New York, 1987, 76.
8. **Phillips, M. C. and Chapman, D.,** Monolayer characteristics of saturated 1,2-diacyl phosphatidylcholines (lecithins) and phosphatidylethanolamines at the air-water interface, *Biochim. Biophys. Acta,* 163, 301, 1968.
9. **Albrecht, O., Gruler, H., and Sackmann, E.,** Polymorphism of phospholipid monolayers, *J. Phys. (Paris),* 39, 301, 1978.
10. **MacDonald, R. C. and Simon, S. A.,** Lipid monolayer states and their relationships to bilayers, *Proc. Natl. Acad. Sci. U.S.A.,* 84, 4089, 1987.
11. **Cullis, P. R., Hope, M. J., de Kruijff, B., Verkeij, A. J., and Tilcock, C. P. S.,** Structural properties and functional roles of phospholipids in biological membranes, in *Phospholipids and Cellular Regulation,* Vol. 1, Kuo, J. F., Ed., CRC Press, Boca Raton, FL, 1985, 1.
12. **Abney, J. R. and Owicki, J. C.,** Theories of protein-lipid and protein-protein interactions in membranes, in *Progress in Protein-Lipid Interactions,* Vol. 1, Watts, A. and De Pont, J. J. H. H. M., Eds., Elsevier, New York, 1985, 1.
13. **Nagle, J. F.,** Theory of the main lipid bilayer phase transition, *Annu. Rev. Phys. Chem.,* 31, 157, 1980.
14. **Mouritsen, O. G.,** *Computer Studies of Phase Transitions and Critical Phenomena,* Springer-Verlag, New York, 1984.
15. **Heermann, D. W.,** *Computer Simulation Methods,* Springer-Verlag, New York, 1986.
16. **Pink, D. A.,** Theoretical models of phase changes in one- and two-component lipid bilayers, in *Biological Membranes,* Chapman, D., Ed., Academic Press, London, 1981, 131.
17. **Pink, D. A.,** Theoretical studies of phospholipid bilayers and monolayers. Perturbing probes, monolayer phase transitions, and computer simulations of lipid-protein bilayers, *Can. J. Biochem. Cell Biol.,* 62, 760, 1984.
18. **Berendsen, H. J. C.,** Biological molecules and membranes, in *Proc. Int. School ''Enrico Fermi'', Course XCVII on Molecular-Dynamics Simulations of Statistical-Mechanical Systems,* Ciccotti, G. and Hoover, W. G., Eds., North-Holland, Amsterdam, 1986, 496.

19. **Hoover, W. G.,** *Molecular Dynamics,* Springer-Verlag, New York, 1986.
20. **Binder, K., Ed.,** *Monte Carlo Method in Statistical Physics,* Vol. 2, Ed., Springer-Verlag, New York, 1986.
21. **Binder, K., Ed.,** *Applications of the Monte Carlo Method in Statistical Physics,* Springer-Verlag, New York, 1984.
22. **Edholm, O., Nilsson, L., Berg, O., Ehrenberg, M., Claesens, F., Gräslund, A., Jönsson, B., and Teleman, O.,** Biomolecular dynamics, *Q. Rev. Biophys.,* 17, 125, 1984.
23. **McCammon, J. A. and Harvey, S. C.,** *Dynamics of Proteins and Nucleic Acids,* Cambridge University Press, New York, 1987.
24. **Jönsson, B., Edholm, O., and Teleman, O.,** Molecular dynamics simulations of a sodium octanoate micelle in aqueous solution, *J. Chem. Phys.,* 85, 2259, 1986.
25. **Whittington, S. G. and Chapman, D.,** Effect of density on configurational properties of long-chain molecules using a Monte Carlo method, *Trans. Faraday Soc.,* 62, 3319, 1966.
26. **Belle, J., Bothorel, P., and Lemaire, B.,** Melting entropy and structure of aliphatic chains in mono and bilayers, *FEBS Lett.,* 39, 115, 1974.
27. **Lemaire, B. and Bothorel, P.,** Conformational analysis of aliphatic chains at interfaces. Influence of the radius of curvature, *Macromolecules,* 13, 311, 1980.
28. **Clark, A. T. and Lal, M.,** Effect of surface coverage on the configurational properties of adsorbed chains, *J. Chem. Soc. Faraday Trans.,* 74, 1857, 1978.
29. **Frischleder, H. and Peinel, G.,** Monte Carlo investigation of phospholipid fatty acid chain fluidity, *Chem. Phys. Lipids,* 27, 71, 1980.
30. **Day, J. and Willis, C. R.,** Determination of the single chain density of states for membrane systems, *J. Teor. Biol.,* 88, 693, 1981.
31. **Lemaire, B. and Bothorel, P.,** Statistical mechanics of aliphatic chain layers, influence of chain-length mixing, *J. Polym. Sci. Polym. Phys. Ed.,* 20, 867, 1982.
32. **O'Shea, P. S. and Matela, R.,** Computer simulations of the dynamic state of phospholipid membranes, *Biochem. Soc. Trans.,* 14, 1119, 1986.
33. **Tevlin, P., Jones, F. P., Lafleur, S., and Trainor, L. E. H.,** Derivation of the conformational density of states of a normal hydrocarbon, *J. Chem. Phys.,* 85, 4052, 1986.
34. **Marčelja, S.,** Chain ordering in liquid crystals. II. Structure of bilayer membranes, *Biochim. Biophys. Acta,* 367, 165, 1974.
35. **Gruen, D. W. R.,** A statistical mechanical model of the lipid bilayer above its phase transition, *Biochim. Biophys. Acta,* 595, 161, 1980.
36. **Cotterill, R. M. J.,** Computer simulation of model lipid membrane dynamics, *Biochim. Biophys. Acta,* 433, 264, 1976.
37. **Jacobs, R. E., Hudson, B., and Andersen, H. C.,** A theory of the chain melting phase transition of aqueous phospholipid dispersions, *Proc. Natl. Acad. Sci. U.S.A.,* 72, 3993, 1975.
38. **Taxværd, S.,** The equation of state of dense fluid monolayers, *J. Chem. Phys.,* 67, 2056, 1977.
39. **Werge, C. and Binder, H.,** Molecular dynamics and Monte Carlo calculations on a two-dimensional system of asymmetrical molecules, *Stud. Biophys.,* 93, 219, 1983.
40. **Fraser, D. P., Chantrell, R. W., Melville, D., and Tildesley, D. J.,** Two-dimensional Monte Carlo studies of lipid molecules in a bilayer membrane, *Liquid Crystals,* 3, 423, 1988.
41. **Chen, Z.-Y., Talbot, J., Gelbart, W. M., and Ben-Shaul, A.,** Phase transitions in systems of grafted rods, *Phys. Rev. Lett.,* 61, 1376, 1988.
42. **Scott, H. L.,** Monte Carlo studies of the hydrocarbon region of lipid bilayers, *Biochim. Biophys. Acta,* 469, 264, 1977.
43. **Busico, V. and Vacatello, M.,** Lipid bilayers in the "fluid" state: computer simulation and comparison with model compounds, *Mol. Cryst. Liq. Cryst.,* 97, 195, 1983.
44. **Vacatello, M. and Busico, V.,** The structure and conformation of n-hydrocarbon chains in bilayer systems in the "fluid" phase, *Mol. Cryst. Liq. Cryst.,* 107, 341, 1984.
45. **Kox, A. J., Michels, J. P. J., and Wiegel, F. W.,** Simulation of a lipid monolayer using molecular dynamics, *Nature (London),* 287, 317, 1980.
46. **Northrup, S. H. and Curvin, M. S.,** Molecular dynamics simulation of disorder transitions in lipid monolayers, *J. Phys. Chem.,* 89, 4707, 1985.
47. **Bareman, J. P., Cardini, G., and Klein, M. L.,** Characterization of structural and dynamical behavior in monolayers of long-chain molecules using molecular dynamics calculations, *Phys. Rev. Lett.,* 60, 2152, 1988.
48. **van der Ploeg, P. and Berendsen, H. J. C.,** Molecular Dynamics simulation of a bilayer membrane, *J. Chem. Phys.,* 76, 3271, 1982.
49. **van der Ploeg, P. and Berendsen, H. J. C.,** Molecular dynamics of a bilayer membrane, *Mol. Phys.,* 49, 233, 1983.

50. **Khalatur, P. G., Balabaev, N. K., and Pavlov, A. S.,** Molecular dynamics study of a lipid bilayer and a polymer liquid, *Mol. Phys.,* 59, 753, 1986.
51. **Khalatur, P. G., Pavlov, A. S., and Balabaev, N. K.,** Molecular motions in liquid-crystalline lipid bilayer. Molecular dynamics simulation, *Makromol. Chem.,* 188, 3029, 1987.
52. **Egberts, E. and Berendsen, H. J. C.,** Molecular dynamics simulation of a smectic liquid crystal with atomic detail, *J. Chem. Phys.,* 89, 3718, 1988.
53. **Georgallas, A. and Pink, D. A.,** Phase transition in monolayers of saturated lipids. Exact results and Monte Carlo simulations, *J. Colloid Interface Sci.,* 89, 107, 1982.
54. **Mouritsen, O. G. and Zuckermann, M. J.,** Acyl chain ordering and crystallization in lipid monolayers, *Chem. Phys. Lett.,* 135, 294, 1987.
55. **Mouritsen, O. G., Ipsen, J. H., and Zuckermann, M. J.,** Lateral density fluctuations in the chain-melting phase transition of lipid monolayers, *J. Colloid Interface Sci.,* 129, 32, 1989.
56. **Ipsen, J. H., Mouritsen, O. G., and Zuckermann, M. J.,** Decoupling of crystalline and conformational degrees of freedom in lipid monolayers, *J. Chem. Phys.,* 91, 1855, 1989.
57. **Mouritsen, O. G.,** Studies on the lack of cooperativity in the melting of lipid bilayers, *Biochim. Biophys. Acta,* 731, 217, 1983.
58. **Mouritsen, O. G., Boothroyd, A., Harris, R., Jan, N., Lookman, T., MacDonald, L., Pink, D. A., and Zuckermann, M. J.,** Computer simulation of the main gel-fluid transition of lipid bilayers, *J. Chem. Phys.,* 79, 2027, 1983.
59. **Mouritsen, O. G. and Zuckermann, M. J.,** Softening of lipid bilayers, *Eur. Biophys. J.,* 12, 75, 1985.
60. **Mouritsen, O. G. and Zuckermann, M. J.,** Model of interfacial melting, *Phys. Rev. Lett.,* 58, 389, 1987.
61. **Zuckermann, M. J. and Mouritsen, O. G.,** The effects of acyl chain ordering and crystallization on the main phase transition of wet lipid bilayers. A theoretical study, *Eur. Biophys. J.,* 15, 77, 1987.
62. **Cruzeiro-Hansson, L. and Mouritsen, O. G.,** Passive ion permeability of lipid membranes modelled via lipid-domain interfacial area, *Biochim. Biophys. Acta,* 944, 63, 1988.
63. **Georgallas, A., Hunter, D. L., Lookman, T., Zuckermann, M. J., and Pink, D. A.,** Interactions between two sheets of a bilayer membrane and its internal lateral pressure, *Eur. Biophys. J.,* 11, 79, 1984.
64. **Cruzeiro-Hansson, L., Ipsen, J. H., and Mouritsen, O. G.,** Intrinsic molecules in lipid membranes change the lipid-domain interfacial area: cholesterol at domain interfaces, *Biochim. Biophys. Acta,* 979, 166, 1989.
65. **MacDonald, A. L. and Pink, D. A.,** Thermodynamics of glycophorin in phospholipid bilayer membranes, *Biochemistry,* 26, 1909, 1987.
66. **Lookman, T., Pink, D. A., Grundke, E. W., Zuckermann, M. J., and de Verteuil, F.,** Phase separation in lipid bilayers containing integral proteins. Computer simulation studies, *Biochemistry,* 21, 5593, 1982.
67. **Freire, E. and Snyder, B.,** Estimation of the lateral distribution of molecules in two-component lipid bilayers, *Biochemistry,* 19, 88, 1980.
68. **Freire, E. and Snyder, B.,** Monte Carlo studies of the lateral organization of molecules in two-component lipid bilayers, *Biochim. Biophys. Acta,* 600, 643, 1980.
69. **Freire, E. and Snyder, B.,** Quantitative characterization of the lateral distribution of membrane proteins within the lipid bilayer, *Biophys. J.,* 37, 617, 1982.
70. **Jan, N., Lookman, T., and Pink, D. A.,** On Computer simulation methods used to study models of two-component lipid bilayers, *Biochemistry,* 23, 3227, 1984.
71. **Laidlaw, D. J. and Pink, D. A.,** Protein lateral distribution in lipid bilayer membranes. Applications to ESR studies, *Eur. Biophys. J.,* 12, 143, 1985.
72. **Pink, D. A., Lookman, T., MacDonald, A. L., Zuckermann, M. J., and Jan, N.,** Lateral diffusion of gramicidin S, M-13 coat protein and glycophorin in bilayers of saturated phospholipids. Mean field and Monte Carlo studies, *Biochim. Biophys. Acta,* 687, 42, 1982.
73. **Pink, D. A.,** Constraints on protein lateral diffusion, *Trends Biochem. Sci.,* 10, 230, 1985.
74. **Pink, D. A., Laidlaw, D. J., and Crisholm, D. M.,** Protein lateral movement in lipid bilayers. Monte Carlo simulation studies of its dependence upon attractive protein-protein interactions, *Biochim. Biophys. Acta,* 863, 9, 1986.
75. **Scott, H. L. and Cherng, S.-L.,** Monte Carlo studies of phospholipid lamellae. Effects of proteins, cholesterol, bilayer curvature, and lateral mobility on order parameters, *Biochim. Biophys. Acta,* 510, 209, 1978.
76. **Binder, H.,** Monte Carlo simulation of one- and two-component systems: physical properties of model membranes, *Stud. Biophys.,* 93, 217, 1983.
77. **Scott, H. L.,** Monte Carlo calculations of order parameter profiles in models of lipid-protein interactions in bilayers, *Biochemistry,* 25, 6122, 1986.
78. **Saxton, M. J.,** Lateral diffusion in an archipelago. The effect of mobile obstacles, *Biophys. J.,* 52, 989, 1987.

79. **Fraser, D. P.**, Theoretical Studies of Lipid-Protein Interactions in Biological Membranes, Ph.D. thesis, Lancashire Polytechnic, England, 1987.

80. **Mountain, R. D., Mazo, R. M., and Volwerk, J. J.**, Molecular dynamics simulation study of a two-dimensional fluid mixture system: a model for biological membranes, *Chem. Phys. Lipids*, 40, 35, 1986.

81. **Edholm, O. and Johansson, J.**, Lipid bilayer polypeptide interactions studied by molecular dynamics simulation, *Eur. Biophys. J.*, 14, 203, 1987.

82. **Edholm, O. and Jähnig, F.**, The structure of a membrane-spanning polypeptide studied by molecular dynamics, *Biophys. Chem.*, 30, 279, 1988.

83. **Scott, H. L.**, Monte Carlo studies of a general model for lipid bilayer condensed phases, *J. Chem. Phys.*, 80, 2197, 1984.

84. **Scott, H. L.**, The ripple phase in lipid bilayers: Theory and computer simulation, *Comments Mol Cell. Biophys.*, 2, 197, 1984.

85. **Georgallas, A. and Zuckermann, M. J.**, Lipid vertical motion and related steric effects in bilayer membranes, *Eur. Biophys. J.*, 14, 53, 1986.

86. **Scott, H. L.**, Anisotropic Ising model with four-spin interactions: application to lipid bilayers, *Phys. Rev. B*, 37, 263, 1988.

87. **MacDonald, A. L. and Pink, D. A.**, Equilibrium thermodynamics of models of hydrogen bonding in lipid bilayer membranes: the amide model, *Phys. Rev. B*, 37, 3552, 1988.

88. **Frischleder, H. and Peinel, G.**, Quantum-chemical and statistical calculations on phospholipids, *Chem. Phys. Lipids*, 30, 121, 1982.

89. **Binder, H. and Peinel, G.**, Behavior of water at membrane surfaces — a molecular dynamics study, *THEOCHEM*, 24, 155, 1985.

90. **Scott, H. L.**, Monte Carlo studies of lipid/water interfaces, *Biochim. Biophys. Acta*, 814, 327, 1985.

91. **Hussin, A. and Scott, H. L.**, Density and bonding profiles of interbilayer water as functions of bilayer separation: a Monte Carlo study, *Biochim. Biophys. Acta*, 897, 432, 1987.

92. **Mouritsen, O. G., Fogedby, H. C., Sørensen, E. S., and Zuckermann, M. J.**, Pattern formation in lipid membranes, in *Time-Dependent Effects in Disordered Materials*, Pynn, R. and Riste, T., Eds., Plenum Press, New York, 1987, 457.

93. **Fogedby, H. C., Sørensen, E. S., and Mouritsen, O. G.**, Fractal growth in impurity-controlled solidification in lipid monolayers, *J. Chem. Phys.*, 87, 6706, 1987.

94. **Sørensen, E. S., Fogedby, H. C., and Mouritsen, O. G.**, Crossover from non-equilibrium fractal growth to equilibrium compact growth, *Phys. Rev. Lett.*, 61, 2770, 1988.

95. **Sørensen, E. S., Fogedby, H. C., and Mouritsen, O. G.**, Computer simulation of temperature-dependent growth of fractal and compact domains in diluted Ising models, *Phys. Rev. A*, 39, 2194, 1989.

96. **Jönsson, B., Wennerström, H., and Halle, B.**, Ion distributions in lamellar liquid crystals. A comparison between results from Monte Carlo simulations and solutions to the Poisson-Boltzmann equation, *J. Phys. Chem.*, 84, 2179, 1980.

97. **Wennerström, H., Jönsson, B., and Linse, P.**, The cell model for polyelectrolyte systems. Exact statistical mechanical relations, Monte Carlo simulations and the Poisson-Boltzmann approximation, *J. Chem. Phys.*, 76, 4665, 1982.

98. **Guldbrand, L., Jönsson, B., Wennerström, H., and Linse, P.**, Electrical double layer forces. A Monte Carlo study, *J. Chem. Phys.*, 80, 2221, 1984.

99. **Metropolis, N., Rosenbluth, A. W., Rosenbluth, M. N., Teller, A. H., and Teller, E.**, Equation of state calculations by fast computing machines, *J. Chem. Phys.*, 21, 1087, 1953.

100. **Limoge, Y. and Bocquet, J. L.**, Monte Carlo simulation in diffusion studies: time scale problems, *Acta Metall.*, 36, 1717, 1988.

101. **Ryckaert, J.-P. and Bellemans, A.**, Molecular dynamics of liquid alkanes, *Faraday Discuss. Chem. Soc.*, 66, 95, 1978.

102. **Ryckaert, J.-P., Cicotti, G., and Berendsen, H. J. C.**, Numerical integration of the Cartesian equations of motion of a system with constraints: molecular dynamics of *n*-alkanes, *J. Comp. Phys.*, 25, 327, 1977.

103. **van Gunsteren, W. F. and Berendsen, H. J. C.**, Algorithms for macromolecular dynamics and constraint dynamics, *Mol. Phys.*, 34, 1311, 1977.

104. **Doniach, S.**, Thermodynamic fluctuations in phospholipid bilayers, *J. Chem. Phys.*, 68, 4912, 1978.

105. **Caillé, A., Rapini, A., Zuckermann, M. J., Cros, A., and Doniach, S.**, A simple model for phase transitions in monolayers and bilayers of lipid molecules, *Can. J. Phys.*, 56, 348, 1978.

106. **Pink, D. A., Green, T. J., and Chapman, D.**, Raman scattering in bilayers of saturated phosphatidylcholines. Experiment and theory, *Biochemistry*, 19, 349, 1980.

107. **Caillé, A., Pink, D., de Verteuil, F., and Zuckermann, M. J.**, Theoretical models for quasi-two-dimensional mesomorphic monolayers and membrane bilayers, *Can. J. Phys.*, 58, 581, 1980.

108. **Flory, P. J.**, Spatial configuration of macromolecular chains, *Science*, 188, 1268, 1975.

109. **Träuble, H. and Haynes, D. H.**, The volume change in lipid bilayer lamellae at the crystalline-liquid crystalline phase transition, *Chem. Phys. Lipids*, 7, 324, 1971.

110. **Tardieu, A., Luzatti, V., and Reman, F. C.,** Structure and polymorphism of the hydrocarbon chains of lipids: a study of lecithin-water phases, *J. Mol. Biol.*, 75, 711, 1973.
111. **Wulf, A.,** Short-range correlations and the effective orientational energy in liquid crystals, *J. Chem. Phys.*, 67, 2254, 1977.
112. **Salem, L.,** Forces between polyatomic molecules. II. Short-range repulsive forces, *J. Chem. Phys.*, 37, 2100, 1962.
113. **Ipsen, J. H., Mouritsen, O. G., and Bloom, M.,** Relationships between lipid membrane area, hydrophobic thickness, and acyl-chain orientational order: the effects of cholesterol, *Biophys. J.*, 57, 405, 1990.
114. **Grest, G. S., Anderson, M. P., and Srolovitz, D. J.,** Domain-growth kinetics for the Q-state Potts model in two and three dimensions, *Phys. Rev. B*, 38, 4752, 1988.
115. **Davis, J. H.,** Deuterium magnetic resonance study of the gel and liquid crystalline phases of dipalmitoyl phosphatidylcholine, *Biophys. J.*, 27, 339, 1979.
116. **MacKay, A. L.,** A proton NMR moment study of the gel and liquid-crystalline phases of dipalmitoyl phosphatidylcholine, *Biophys. J.*, 35, 301, 1981.
117. **Evans, E. and Kwok, R.,** Mechanical calorimetry of large dimyristoylphosphatidylcholine vesicles in the phase transition region, *Biochemistry*, 21, 4874, 1982.
118. **Albon, N. and Sturtevant, J. M.,** Nature of the gel to liquid crystal transition of synthetic phosphatidylcholines, *Proc. Natl. Acad. Sci. U.S.A.*, 75, 2258, 1978.
119. **Vist, M. R. and Davis, J. H.,** Phase equilibria of cholesterol/dipalmitcylphosphatidylcholine mixtures: ^{2}H nuclear magnetic references and differential scanning calorimetry, *Biochemistry*, 29, 451, 1990.
120. **Seelig, J. and Seelig, A.,** Lipid conformation in model membranes and biological membranes, *Q. Rev. Biophys.*, 13, 19, 1980.
121. **Mountcastle, D. B., Biltonen, R. L., and Halsey, M. J.,** Effect of anesthetics and pressure on the thermotropic behavior of multilamellar dipalmitoylphosphatidylcholine liposomes, *Proc. Natl. Acad. Sci. U.S.A.*, 75, 4906, 1978.
122. **Freire, E. and Biltonen, R. L.,** Estimation of molecular averages and equilibrium fluctuations in lipid bilayer systems from excess heat capacity function, *Biochim. Biophys. Acta*, 514, 54, 1978.
123. **Mitaku, S., Jippo, T., and Kataoka, R.,** Thermodynamic properties of the lipid bilayer transition. Pseudocritical phenomena, *Biophys. J.*, 42, 137, 1983.
124. **Hatta, I., Suzuki, K., and Imaizumi, S.,** Pseudo-critical heat capacity of single lipid bilayers, *J. Phys. Soc. Jpn.*, 52, 2790, 1983.
125. **Imaizumi, S. and Garland, C. W.,** AC calorimetric studies of main transition in dipalmitoylphosphatidylcholine (DPPC), *J. Phys. Soc. Jpn.*, 56, 3887, 1987.
126. **Hatta, I., Imaizumi, S., and Akutsu, Y.,** Evidence for weak first-order nature of lipid bilayer phase transition from analysis of pseudo-critical specific heat, *J. Phys. Soc. Jpn.*, 53, 882, 1984.
127. **Biltonen, R. L.,** private communication, 1988.
128. **Lis, L. J., McAlister, M., Fuller, N., Rand, R. P., and Parsegian, V. A.,** Measurement of the lateral compressibility of several bilayers, *Biophys. J.*, 37, 667, 1982.
129. **Kwok, R. and Evans, E.,** Thermoelasticity of large lecithin bilayer vesicles, *Biophys. J.*, 35, 637, 1981.
130. **Mitaku, S., Ikegami, A., and Sakanishi, A.,** Ultrasonic studies of lipid bilayer. Phase transition in synthetic phosphatidylcholine liposomes, *Biophys. Chem.*, 8, 295, 1978.
131. **Mitaku, S. and Date, T.,** Anomalies of nanosecond ultrasonic relaxation in the lipid bilayer transition, *Biochim. Biophys. Acta*, 688, 411, 1982.
132. **Genz, A. and Holzwarth, J. F.,** Dynamic fluorescence measurements on the main phase transition of dipalmitoylphosphatidylcholine vesicles, *Eur. Biophys. J.*, 13, 323, 1986.
133. **Hawton, M. H. and Doane, J. W.,** Pretransitional phenomena in phospholipid/water multilayers, *Biophys. J.*, 52, 401, 1987.
134. **Ruggiero, A. and Hudson, B.,** Critical density fluctuations in lipid bilayers detected by fluorescence lifetime heterogeneity, *Biophys. J.*, 55, 1111, 1989.
135. **Papahadjopoulos, D., Jacobsen, K., Nir, S., and Isac, T.,** Phase transitions in phospholipid vesicles, Fluorescence polarization and permeability measurements concerning the effects of temperature and cholesterol, *Biochim. Biophys. Acta*, 311, 330, 1973.
136. **Sillerud, L. O. and Barnett, R. E.,** Lack of transbilayer coupling in phase transition of phosphatidylcholine vesicles, *Biochemistry*, 21, 1756, 1982.
137. **McCammon, J. A. and Deutch, J. M.,** "Semiempirical" models for biomembrane phase transitions and phase separations, *J. Am. Chem. Soc.*, 97, 6675, 1975.
138. **Tsong, T. Y., Greenberg, M., and Kanehisa, M. I.,** Anesthetic action on membrane lipids, *Biochemistry*, 16, 3115, 1977.
139. **March, D., Watts, A., and Knowles, P. F.,** Cooperativity of the phase transition in single- and multilayer lipid bilayers, *Biochim. Biophys. Acta*, 465, 500, 1977.
140. **Kanehisa, M. I. and Tsong, T. Y.,** Cluster model of lipid phase transitions with application to passive permeation of molecules and structure relaxations in lipid bilayers, *J. Am. Chem. Soc.*, 100, 424, 1978.

141. **Lee, A. G.**, Lipid phase transitions and phase diagrams. I. Lipid phase transitions, *Biochim. Biophys. Acta,* 472, 237, 1977.

142. **Forsyth, P. A., Marčelja, S., Mitchell, D. J., and Ninham, B. W.**, Phase transition in charged lipid membranes, *Biochim. Biophys. Acta,* 469, 335, 1977.

143. **March, D., Watts, A., and Knowles, P. F.**, Evidence for phase boundary lipid. Permeability of Tempocholine into dimyristoylphosphatidylcholine vesicles at the phase transition, *Biochemistry,* 15, 3570, 1976.

144. **Black, S. G. and Dixon, G. S.**, AC calorimetry of dimyristoylphosphatidylcholine multilayers: hysteresis and annealing near the gel to liquid-crystal transition, *Biochemistry,* 20, 6740, 1981.

145. **Mabrey, S. and Sturtevant, J. M.**, High-sensitivity differential scanning calorimetry in the study of biomembranes and related model systems, *Methods Membrane Biol.,* 9, 237, 1978.

146. **Hui, S. W. and Parsons, D. F.**, Direct observation of domains in wet lipid bilayers, *Science,* 190, 383, 1975.

147. **Linden, C. D., Wright, K. L., and McConnell, H. M.**, Lateral phase separations in membrane lipids and the mechanism of sugar transport in *Escherichia coli, Proc. Natl. Acad. Sci. U.S.A.,* 70, 2271, 1973.

148. **Op den Kamp, J. A. F., Kauertz, M. T., and van Deenen, L. L. M.**, Action of pancreatic phospholipase A_2 on phosphatidylcholine bilayers in different physical states, *Biochim. Biophys. Acta,* 406, 169, 1975.

149. **Gabriel, N. E., Agman, N. V., and Roberts, M. F.**, Enzymatic hydrolysis of short-chain lecithin/long-chain phospholipid unilamellar vesicles: sensitivity of phospholipases to matrix phase state, *Biochemistry,* 26, 7409, 1987.

150. **Menashe, M., Romero, G., Biltonen, R. L., and Lichtenberg, D.**, Hydrolysis of dipalmitoylphosphatidylcholine small unilamellar vesicles by porcine pancreatic phospholipase A_2, *J. Biol. Chem.,* 261, 5328, 1986.

151. **Nagle, J. F. and Scott, H. L.**, Lateral compressibility of lipid mono- and bilayers. Theory of membrane permeability, *Biochim. Biophys. Acta,* 513, 236, 1978.

152. **Marčelja, S. and Wolfe, J.**, Properties of bilayer membranes in the phase transition or phase separation region, *Biochim. Biophys. Acta,* 557, 24, 1979.

153. **Georgallas, A., MacArthur, J. D., Ma, X.-P., Nguyen, C. V., Palmer, G. R., Singer, M. A., and Tse, M. Y.**, The diffusion of small ions through phospholipid bilayers, *J. Chem. Phys.,* 86, 7218, 1987.

154. **Carruthers, A. and Melchior, D. L.**, Studies of the relationship between bilayer water permeability and bilayer physical state, *Biochemistry,* 22, 5759, 1983.

155. **Tsong, T. Y.**, Kinetics of the crystalline-liquid phase transition of dimyristoyl L_α-lecithin bilayers, *Proc. Natl. Acad. Sci. U.S.A.,* 71, 2684, 1974.

156. **Gruenewald, B.**, On the phase transition kinetics of phospholipid bilayers. Relaxation experiments with detection of fluorescence anisotropy, *Biochim. Biophys. Acta,* 687, 71, 1982.

157. **Elamrani, K. and Blume, A.**, Phase transition kinetics of phosphatidic acid bilayers. A pressure-jump relaxation study, *Biochemistry,* 22, 3305, 1983.

158. **Tsong, T. Y. and Kanehisa, M. I.**, Relaxation phenomena in aqueous dispersions of synthetic lecithins, *Biochemistry,* 16, 2674, 1977.

159. **Elamrani, K. and Blume, A.**, Phase transition kinetics of phosphatidic acid bilayers. A stopped-flow study of the electrostatically induced transition, *Biochim. Biophys. Acta,* 769, 578, 1984.

160. **Caffrey, M. and Bilderback, D. H.**, Kinetics of the main phase transition of hydrated lecithin monitored by real-time X-ray diffraction, *Biophys. J.,* 45, 627, 1984.

161. **Wu, W.-G., Chong, P. L.-G., and Huang, C.-H.**, Pressure effect on the rate of crystalline phase formation of L-α-dipalmitoylphosphatidylcholines in multilamellar dispersions, *Biophys. J.,* 47, 237, 1985.

162. **Caffrey, M.**, Kinetics and mechanism of the lamellar gel/lamellar liquid-crystal and lamellar/inverted hexagonal phase transition in phosphatidylethanolamine: a real-time X-ray diffraction study using synchrotron radiation, *Biochemistry,* 24, 4826, 1985.

163. **Lis, L. J. and Quinn, P. J.**, A time-resolved synchrotron X-ray study of a crystalline phase bilayer transition and packing in a saturated monogalactosyldiacylglycerol-water system, *Biochim. Biophys. Acta,* 862, 81, 1986.

164. **Johnson, M. L., van Osdol, W. W., and Biltonen, R. L.**, The measurement of the kinetics of lipid phase transitions: a volume-perturbation kinetic calorimeter, *Methods Enzymol.,* 130, 534, 1986.

165. **Kodama, M., Hashigami, H., and Seki, S.**, Static and dynamic calorimetric studies on the three kinds of phase transitions in the systems of L- and DL-dipalmitoylphosphatidylcholine/water, *Biochim. Biophys. Acta,* 814, 300, 1985.

166. **Tsuchida, K., Hatta, I., Imaizumi, S., Ohki, K., and Nazowa, Y.**, Kinetics near the pretransition of a multilamellar phospholipid studied by ESR, *Biochim. Biophys. Acta,* 812, 249, 1985.

167. **Tenchov, B. G., Lis, L. J., and Quinn, P. J.**, Mechanism and kinetics of the subtransition in hydrated L-dipalmitoylphosphatidylcholine, *Biochim. Biophys. Acta,* 897, 143, 1987.

168. **Broughton, J. Q. and Gilmer, G. H.**, Thermodynamic criteria for grain-boundary melting: a molecular dynamics study, *Phys. Rev. Lett.,* 56, 2692, 1986.

169. **Deymier, P. and Kalonji, G.**, Effects of grain boundary melting on sliding in bicrystals: a molecular dynamics study, *Scr. Metall.*, 20, 13, 1986.

170. **Melchior, D. L., Bruggemann, E. P., and Steim, J. M.**, The physical state of quick-frozen membranes and lipids, *Biochim. Biophys. Acta*, 690, 81, 1982.

171. **Costello, M. J. and Gulik-Krzywicki, T.**, Correlated X-ray diffraction and freeze-fracture studies of membrane model systems, *Biochim. Biophys. Acta*, 455, 412, 1976.

172. **Sackmann, E., Rüppel, D., and Gebhardt, C.**, Defect structure and texture of isolated bilayers of phospholipids and phospholipid mixtures, in *Springer Series in Chemical Physics*, Vol. 11, Helfrich, W. and Heppke, G., Eds., 309, 1980.

173. **Pink, D. A., MacDonald, A. L., and Quinn, B.**, Anisotropic interactions in hydrated cerebrosides. A theoretical model of stable and metastable states and hydrogen-bond formation, *Chem. Phys. Lipids*, 47, 83, 1988.

174. **Hatta, I., Kato, S., Ohki, K., Orihara, H., and Tsuchida, K.**, Defects in the ripple structure of phospholipids, *Mol. Cryst. Liq. Cryst.*, 146, 367, 1987.

175. **Scott, H. L.**, Lecithin bilayers: a theoretical model which describes the main and lower transitions, *Biochim. Biophys. Acta*, 643, 161, 1981.

176. **Wardlaw, J. R., Sawyer, W. H., and Ghiggino, K. P.**, Vertical fluctuations of phospholipid acyl chains in bilayers, *FEBS Lett.*, 223, 20, 1987.

177. **Pearce, P. A. and Scott, H. L.**, Statistical mechanics of the ripple phase in lipid bilayers, *J. Chem. Phys.*, 77, 951, 1982.

178. **Bak, P.**, Commensurate phases, incommensurate phases, and the devil's staircase, *Rep. Prog. Phys.*, 45, 587, 1982.

179. **Gaines, G. L.**, *Insoluble Monolayers on the Liquid-Gas Interface*, Interscience, New York, 1966.

180. **Verger, R. and Pattus, F.**, Lipid-protein interactions in monolayers, *Chem. Phys. Lipids*, 30, 189, 1982.

181. **Heckl, W. M., Lösche, M., Scheer, H., and Möhwald, H.**, Protein/lipid interactions in phospholipid monolayers containing the bacterial protein B800-850, *Biochim. Biophys. Acta*, 810, 73, 1985.

182. **Cadenhead, D. A., Kellner, B. M. J., and Phillips, M. C.**, The miscibility of dipalmitoyl phosphatidylcholine and cholesterol in monolayers, *J. Colloid Interface Sci.*, 57, 224, 1976.

183. **Albrecht, O., Gruler, H., and Sackmann, E.**, Pressure-composition phase diagrams of cholesterol/lecithin, cholesterol/phosphatidic acid, and lecithin/phosphatidic acid mixed monolayers: a Langmuir film balance study, *Colloid Interface Sci.*, 79, 319, 1981.

184. **Beurer, G. and Galla, H.-J.**, Anaesthetic-phospholipid interaction. The effect of chlorpromazine on phospholipid monolayers, *Eur. Biophys. J.*, 14, 403, 1987.

185. **Pallas, N. R. and Pethica, B. A.**, Liquid-expanded to liquid-condensed transitions in lipid monolayers at the air/water interface, *LANGMUIR*, 1, 509, 1985.

186. **Nagle, J. F.**, Theory of lipid monolayer and bilayer chain-melting phase transitions, *Faraday Discuss. Chem. Soc.*, 81, 151, 1986.

187. **von Tcharner, V. and McConnell, H. M.** An alternative view of phospholipid phase behavior at the air-water interface. Microscope and film balance studies, *Biophys. J.*, 36, 409, 1981.

188. **Lösche, H. and Möhwald, H.**, Fluorescence microscopy on monomolecular films at an air/water interface, *Colloids Interfaces*, 10, 217, 1984.

189. **Lösche, M. and Möhwald, H.**, Impurity controlled phase transitions of phospholipid monolayers, *Eur. Biophys. J.*, 11, 35, 1984.

190. **Weis, R. M. and McConnell, H. M.**, Two-dimensional chiral crystals of phospholipid, *Nature (London)*, 310, 47, 1984.

191. **Moy, V. T., Keller, D. J., Gaub, H. E., and McConnell, H. M.**, Long-range molecular orientational order in monolayer solid domains of phospholipid, *J. Phys. Chem.*, 90, 3198, 1986.

192. **Moy, V. T., Keller, D. J., and McConnell, H. M.**, Molecular order in finite two-dimensional crystals of lipid at the air/water interface, *J. Phys. Chem.*, 92, 5233, 1988.

193. **Kjaer, K., Als-Nielsen, J., Helm, C. A., Laxhuber, L. A., and Möhwald, H.**, Ordering in lipid monolayers studied by synchrotron X-ray diffraction and fluorescence microscopy, *Phys. Rev. Lett.*, 58, 2224, 1987.

194. **Helm, C. A., Möhwald, H., Kjaer, K., and Als-Nielsen, J.**, Phospholipid monolayers between fluid and solid states, *Biophys. J.*, 52, 381, 1987.

195. **Dutta, P., Peng, J. B., Lin, B., Ketterson, J. B., Prakash, M., Georgopoulos, P., and Erhlich, S.**, X-ray diffraction studies of organic monolayers on the surface of water, *Phys. Rev. Lett.*, 58, 2228, 1987.

196. **Helm, C. A., Möhwald, H., Kjaer, K., and Als-Nielsen, J.**, Phospholipid monolayer density distribution perpendicular to the water surface. A synchrotron X-ray reflectivity study, *Europhys. Lett.*, 4, 697, 1987.

197. **Als-Nielsen, J. and Möhwald, H.**, Synchrotron X-ray scattering studies of Langmuir films, in *Handbook of Synchrotron Radiation*, Vol. 4, Ebashi, S., Rubenstein, E., and Koch, M., Eds., North-Holland, in press.

198. **Zuckermann, M. J., Pink, D. A., Costas, M., and Sanctuary, B. C.,** A theoretical model for phase transitions in lipid monolayers, *J. Chem. Phys.,* 76, 4206, 1982.

199. **Fischer, A., Lösche, M., Möhwald, H., and Sackmann, E.,** On the nature of the lipid monolayer phase transition, *J. Phys. Lett. (Paris),* 45, L-785, 1984.

200. **Georgallas, A. and Pink, D. A.,** A new theory of the liquid condensed-liquid expanded phase transition in lipid monolayers, *Can. J. Phys.,* 60, 1678, 1982.

201. **Nelson, D. R. and Halperin, B. I.,** Dislocation-mediated melting in two dimensions, *Phys. Rev. B,* 19, 2457, 1979.

202. **Miller, A., Knoll, W., and Möhwald, H.,** Fractal growth of crystalline phospholipid domains in monomolecular layers, *Phys. Rev. Lett.,* 56, 2633, 1986.

203. **Miller, A. and Möhwald, H.,** Diffusion limited growth of crystalline domains in phospholipid monolayers, *J. Chem. Phys.,* 86, 4258, 1987.

204. **Sander, L. M.,** Fractal growth processes, *Nature (London),* 322, 789, 1986.

205. **Witten, T. A. and Cates, M. E.,** Tenuous structures from disorderly growth processes, *Science,* 232, 1607, 1986.

206. **Suresh, K. A., Nittmann, J., and Rondelez, F.,** Pattern formation during phase transition in Langmuir monolayers near critical temperature, *Europhys. Lett.,* 6, 437, 1988.

207. **Meakin, P.,** The growth of fractal aggregates and their fractal measures, in *Phase Transitions and Critical Phenomena,* Domb, C. and Lebowitz, J. L., Eds., Academic Press, New York, 1988, 335.

208. **Bloom, M. and Smith, I. C. P.,** Manifestations of lipid-protein interactions in deuterium NMR, in *Progress in Protein-Lipid Interactions,* Vol. 1, Watts, A. and De Pont, J. J. H. H. M., Eds., Elsevier, New York, 61, 1985.

209. **Devaux, P. F.,** ESR and NMR studies of lipid-protein interactions in membranes, in *Biological Magnetic Resonance,* Vol. 5, Berliner, L. J. and Reuben, J., Eds., Plenum Press, New York, 1983, 183.

210. **Mouritsen, O. G. and Bloom, M.,** Mattress model of lipid-protein interactions in membranes, *Biophys J.,* 46, 141, 1984.

211. **Ipsen, J. H., Karlström, G., Mouritsen, O. G., Wennerström, H., and Zuckermann, M. J.,** Phase equilibria in the phosphatidylcholine-cholesterol system, *Biochim. Biophys. Acta,* 905, 162, 1987.

212. **Mortensen, K., Pfeiffer, W., Sackmann, E., and Knoll, W.,** Structural properties of a phosphatidylcholine-cholesterol system as studied by small angle neutron scattering: ripple structure and phase diagram, *Biochim. Biophys. Acta,* 945, 221, 1988.

213. **Ipsen, J. H., Mouritsen, O. G., and Zuckermann, M. J.,** Theory of thermal anomalies in the specific heat of lipid bilayers containing cholesterol, *Biophys. J.,* 56, 661, 1989.

214. **Engelman, D. M. and Rothman, J. E.,** The planar organization of lecithin-cholesterol bilayers, *J. Biol. Chem.,* 247, 3694, 1972.

215. **Needham, D., McIntosh, T. J., and Evans, E.,** Thermomechanical and transition properties of dimyristoylphosphatidylcholine/cholesterol bilayers, *Biochemistry,* 27, 4668, 1988.

216. **Presti, F. T.,** The role of cholesterol in regulating membrane fluidity, in *Membrane Fluidity in Biology,* Vol. 4, Aloia, R. C. and Boggs, J. M., Eds., Academic Press, New York, 1985, 97.

217. **Jähnig, F.,** Critical effects from lipid-protein interaction in membranes. II. Interpretation of experimental results, *Biophys. J.,* 36, 347, 1981.

218. **Weis, R. M. and McConnell, H. M.,** Cholesterol stabilizes the crystal-liquid interface in phospholipid monolayers, *J. Phys. Chem.,* 89, 4453, 1985.

219. **Blok, M. C., van Deenen, L. L. M., and de Gier, J.,** The effect of cholesterol incorporation on the temperature dependence of water permeation through liposomal membranes prepared from phosphatidylcholines, *Biochim. Biophys. Acta,* 464, 509, 1977.

220. **Bloom, M. and Mouritsen, O. G.,** The evolution of membranes, *Can. J. Chem.,* 66, 706, 1988.

221. **Blume, A. and Hillmann, M.,** Dimyristoylphosphatidic acid/cholesterol bilayers. Thermodynamic properties and kinetics of the phase transition as studied by the pressure jump relaxation technique, *Eur. Biophys. J.,* 13, 343, 1986.

222. **Genz, A., Holzwarth, J. F., and Tsong, T. Y.,** The influence of cholesterol on the main phase transition of unilamellar dipalmitoylphosphatidylcholine vesicles. A differential scanning calorimetry and iodine laser T-jump study, *Biophys. J.,* 50, 1043, 1986.

223. **Mabrey, S., Mateo, P. L., and Sturtevant, J. M.,** High-sensitivity scanning calorimetric study of mixtures of cholesterol with dimyristoyl- and dipalmitoylphosphatidylcholines, *Biochemistry,* 17, 2464, 1978.

224. **Estep, T. N., Mountcastle, D. B., Biltonen, R. L., and Thompson, T. E.,** Studies on the anomalous thermotropic behavior of aqueous dispersions of dipalmitoylphosphatidylcholine-cholesterol mixtures, *Biochemistry,* 17, 1984, 1978.

225. **Sandermann, H.,** Regulation of membrane enzymes by lipids, *Biochim. Biophys. Acta,* 515, 209, 1978.

226. **Gheriani-Gruszka, N., Almog, S., Biltonen, R. L., and Lichtenberg, D.,** Hydrolysis of phosphatidylcholine in phosphatidylcholine-cholate mixtures by porcine pancreatic phospholipase A$_2$, *J. Biol. Chem.,* 263, 11808, 1988.

227. **Ipsen, J. H. and Mouritsen, O. G.,** Modelling the phase equilibria in two-component membranes of phospholipids with different acyl chain lengths, *Biochim. Biophys. Acta,* 944, 121, 1988.
228. **Rüppel, D., Kapitza, H.-G., Galla, H. J., Sixtl, F., and Sackmann, E.,** On the microstructure and phase diagram of dimyristoylphosphatidylcholine-glycophorin bilayers. The role of defects and the hydrophilic lipid-protein interactions, *Biochim. Biophys. Acta,* 692, 1, 1982.

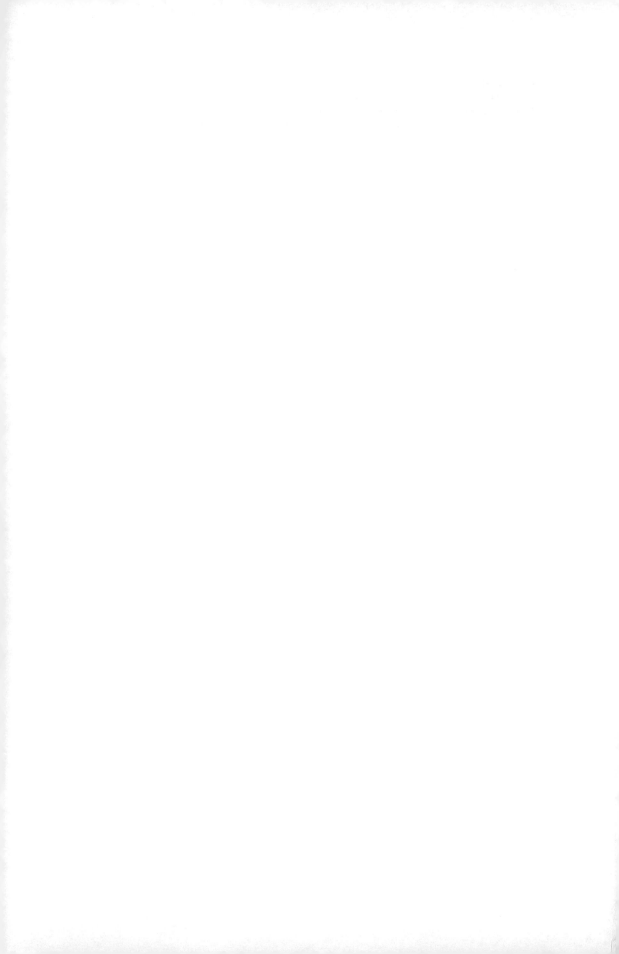

Chapter 1.A.2

COMPUTER-AIDED INVESTIGATIONS OF THE HYDROPHOBIC CORE OF THE LIPID MONOLAYER

Isak Bivas, Bernard Lemaire, and Pierre Bothorel

TABLE OF CONTENTS

I. INTRODUCTION

When we use the term "living matter", we usually think about some organic substances (proteins, nucleic acids, etc.) interacting in a definite way. One main structure, ensuring these interactions is the biological membrane. This is the reason for the continuously growing interest in this subject among biologists, chemists, physicists, and physical chemists.

Biological membranes are complicated formations having various functions, as their study usually passes through the stage of examination of simplified models, carrying their main properties. Further, these models should become complicated in order to approach closely the real object. For this way of development to be followed, we need some knowledge about the organization of the molecules in the membrane.

It is accepted nowadays that biological membranes consist of proteins, the space between them being filled by lipid molecules.[1-5] Figuratively, one may say that the membrane is a "lipid sea", in which the integral proteins "float". To avoid contact of the hydrophobic chains with the water, the lipid areas of the membrane are organized in bilayers. The model described is known in the literature as fluid mosaic.[5] We note that in illustrating this model it is a very popular picture among membranologists that the lipid bilayer is quite ordered and looks like a two-dimensional crystal. In fact, in the functioning membrane it is usually in a less ordered state, nearer to a two-dimensional liquid. Based on this concept, it is possible for simplified models of the biological membrane to be proposed.

Suppose the integral proteins are removed from the membrane. Only the lipid bilayer will remain. It will preserve many of the properties of the membrane, its mechanical characteristics, the passive permeability, etc. The lipid bilayer is a comparatively easy to prepare object, either as a black lipid membrane or as a large or giant liposome. It is much easier for theoretical or experimental study.

The lipid bilayer consists of two interacting monolayers. However, the interaction of one molecule with the nearest neighbors of the same monolayer is much stronger than the interactions with any molecules belonging to the other monolayer. Consequently, the approximation that the two monolayers of the bilayer are not interacting seems reasonable. In this way, we get a still simpler model of the biomembrane, the lipid monolayer. It can be situated either at the air-water interface or at the oil-water one. Experiments show that some of the properties of the bilayer are better preserved in monolayers of the first type, and others are better preserved in monolayers of the second type. If some proteins and other biologically active substances are added to the monolayer, the model of the biomembrane becomes quite realistic.

The lipids are a type of amphiphilic molecules of the kind presented on Figure 1. Their molecule consists of a hydrophilic head and two hydrophobic chains. They can differ in the kind of the head, in the lengths of the chains, and in the presence or absence of double bonds in them. The properties of the monolayer, built up of lipid molecules, are determined by the interactions between the hydrophilic and the hydrophobic parts of the molecules with the liquid substratum and by these interactions: heads-heads, heads-chains, and chains-chains. It is clear that even such a simplified model of the biomembrane as the monolayer contains a tremendous quantity of inter- and intramolecular interactions.

The hydrophilic heads of the lipids represent a glycerine skeleton with attached to it hydrophobic chains and hydrophilic parts. Because of the flexibility of the skeleton, the chains behave practically as if they were independent. Consequently, the hydrophobic core of the lipid monolayer can be assumed to consist of independent single hydrophobic chains.

Let us now consider an imaginary monolayer consisting of single hydrophobic chains. The examination of a model system of this kind should determine the contribution of the chain-chain interaction to the macroscopic properties of the real monolayer. For the theoretical study of the idealized monolayer of this kind, different theoretical approaches have

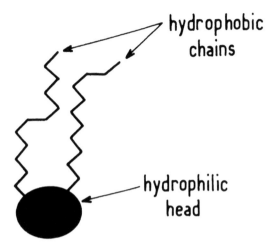

FIGURE 1.   Schematic representation of the lipid molecule.

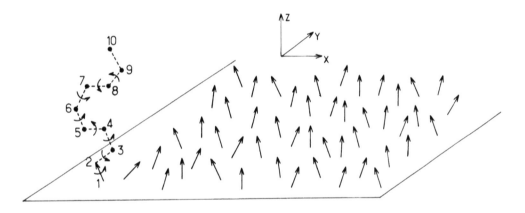

FIGURE 2.   Translational and rotational degrees of freedom of molecular chains at the interface.

been used: mean field approximation, decomposition in series around critical points, and simplified and oversimplified molecular models. These methods give the qualitative behavior of the object, but in most cases, it is not a good quantitative description. Moreover, adjustable parameters are often introduced in theories dealing with the inter- and intramolecular interactions that are not compatible with the fact that these interactions determine entirely the macroscopic behavior of the system.

Even the hydrophobic chains of the simplest type, $(CH_2)_{n-1}CH_3$, have many degrees of freedom. That is why Monte Carlo simulations and molecular dynamics simulations are natural candidates for the study of systems composed of them, in particular the above-mentioned idealized monolayer.

At this point it is probably useful, for the remainder of this study, to make a complete description of the set of degrees of freedom of the ensemble of molecules composing a model of aliphatic interface (Figure 2). On the figure, all the CH_2 and CH_3 groups of each chain are arbitrarily numbered, the first of which being the group lying on the plane interface. For each chain, any bond of the C^i–C^{i+1} type, for $i \geqslant 2$, can freely rotate around the preceeding one, C^{i-1}–C^i, keeping geometrical constraints of the molecule as valence angles and bond lengths constant. In addition the first C–C bond (see vectors of Figure 2) of each chain and consequently the whole molecule can take any direction in the three-dimensional

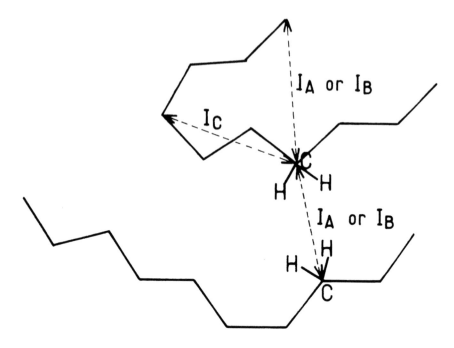

FIGURE 3.   Interactions between atoms or groups.

space, according to the steric restrictions due to the neighboring molecules. Finally, each molecule can translate along the plane interface according to its "free surface" and fluctuate along the Z-direction, perpendicular to the plane.

The successive models developed at the Centre de Recherche Paul Pascal (CNRS), Talence, France have taken into account more and more of the degrees of freedom described above. The aim of the present work is to make a review of these results, obtained essentially by means of Monte Carlo simulations of the behavior of a monolayer, consisting of identical saturated hydrophobic chains. In the last and more complete one, all the degrees of freedom described above have been considered, except the fluctuations around the Z-axis. These newest studies will be also described, connected with an improvement of the Monte Carlo method, permitting the calculation of the free energy of the system when the Metropolis algorithm is used. The last results are obtained in collaboration between the Centre de Recherche Paul Pascal and the Institute of Solid State Physics, Bulgarian Academy of Sciences, Sofia, Bulgaria. Finally, possible ways for perfecting the model and perspectives for its development will be discussed.

II. INTER- AND INTRAMOLECULAR INTERACTIONS

Later we will consider only saturated hydrophobic chains of the kind $(CH_2)_{n-1}CH_3$. The value of the number of carbon atoms n will always be specified when this is necessary. We distinguish the following kind of interactions (Figure 3):

1. Interactions between hydrogens and carbon atoms not belonging to the same or neighboring CH_2 and/or CH_3 groups of one chain — The interactions are of the type of Lennard-Jones:[6]

$$u = u_0[(\frac{r_1}{r})^{12} - 2(\frac{r_1}{r})^6]$$

(1)

TABLE 1
Values of the Constant in the Lennard-Jones Potential of Interaction Between Carbon and/ or Hydrogen Atoms of Aliphatic Chains (see Equation 1)

	u_0 in cal/mol	r_1 in Å
H – H	4.5	2.936
C – C	19.6	4.228
H – C	9.4	2.74

TABLE 2
Values of the Constant in the Lennard-Jones Potential of Interaction Between Spheres Presenting the CH_2 and/or CH_3 Groups of Aliphatic Chains (see Equation 2)

	u_0' in kJ/mol	r_1' in nm
CH_2 - CH_2	0.4301	0.374
CH_2 - CH_3	0.5255	0.324
CH_3 - CH_3	0.6423	0.274

where r is the distance between the centers of the respective atoms. For the constants u_0 and r_1, the values proposed by Lifson and Warshel[7] have been used (Table 1).

2. In the last part of this work, one simplified version of the interactions of Section II.A will be used. The CH_2 and CH_3 groups are treated as parts of spheres with centers coinciding with the centers of the respective carbon atoms. The spheres that are not neighbors of the same chains interact via the Lennard-Jones potential u' of the type:

$$u' = 4u_0'[(\frac{r_1'}{r'})^{12} - (\frac{r_1'}{r'})^6]$$ (2)

where r' is the distance between the interacting spheres; the values of the constants u_0' and r_1' are identical with these used by van der Ploeg et al.[8-10] and are given in Table 2.

3. Interactions between neighboring CH_2 groups. Let us examine four successive CH_2 groups (the last of them can be possibly CH_3 group) belonging to one and the same hydrocarbon chain. For facility's sake, we number their carbon atoms as C^1, C^2, C^3, and C^4. In the model used by us, all the angles between successive C–C bonds are tetrahedral. Let φ be the angle between the planes determined by the atoms C^1, C^2, C^3, and $C^2 C^3 C^4$, respectively; φ is equal to zero when all the four atoms lie on one plane and C^1 and C^4 are from different sides toward the line determined by C^2 and C^3. Then, following Ryckaert and Bellemans,[11] we attribute to the bond C^2–C^3 the energy of $u^r(\varphi)$:

$$u^r(\varphi) = \sum_{i=0}^{5} C_i(\cos \varphi)^i$$ (3)

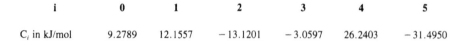

TABLE 3
Values of the Coefficients in the Expression for the Energy of C–C Bond
Due to Its Rotation (see Equation 3)

i	0	1	2	3	4	5
C_i in kJ/mol	9.2789	12.1557	−13.1201	−3.0597	26.2403	−31.4950

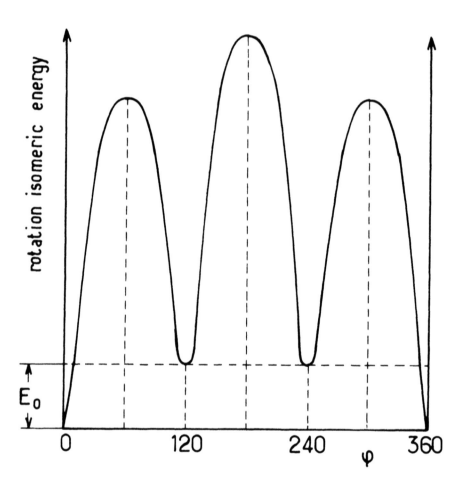

FIGURE 4.   Dependence of the internal rotational energy of a C–C bond on the rotation angle, φ.

The values of the six coefficients C_i are given in Table 3. For these values of C_i, the dependence of u^r on φ is given on Figure 4.

For chains of the kind $(CH_2)_{n-1}CH_3$ there are $n - 3$ such energies. The energy $u^r(\varphi)$ has local minima for $\varphi = 0$ and $\varphi = \pm\ 2\pi/3$. The difference between the energies u^r $(\pm 2\pi/3) - u^r(0)$ is 2.9288 kJ/mol. Through the apparatus of the statistical mechanics, all the macroscopic properties of the above-mentioned imaginary monolayer could be obtained. In what follows, approximations and simplifications of the mathematical expressions and equations will be proposed, in order to obtain quantitatively these macroscopic properties.

III. ROTATIONAL ISOMERIC MODEL

One broadly used approximation for the intramolecular interactions of saturated hydrophobic chains is the rotational isomeric model[12] taken from the polymer science. The main point of this model is the assumption that the angle φ defined before in Equation 3 takes a discrete set of values. These are the values for which the function $u^r(\varphi)$ reaches its minima, namely, $\varphi = 0$ and $\varphi = \pm 2\pi/3$. The state of the bond with $\varphi = 0$ is called *trans*, and those with $\varphi = + 2\pi/3$ or $\varphi = - 2\pi/3$, respectively, are called *gauche* plus (g^+) and *gauche* minus (g^-). In addition to the energies of the C–C bonds, taking into account the interactions between the atoms of the first neighbors CH_2 groups, interactions exist between the atoms of the CH_2 and CH_3 groups that are not neighbors. Let us number the carbon atoms of the $(CH_2)_{n-1}CH_3$ chains in a way that the most outlying from the CH_3 group is the first and the carbon atom of the CH_3 group is the nth. We accept that the C–C bond between the first and the second carbon atom is always *trans*. Then the interactions between the atoms of not neighboring groups can be taken approximatively into account via the condition that the state of one C–C bond cannot be $g\pm$ if the state of the preceeding C–C bond is $g\mp$. We denote

$$E_0 = u^r(\pm\frac{2\pi}{3}) - u^r(0) \tag{4}$$

$$\sigma = \exp(-\frac{E_0}{kT})$$

where k is the Boltzmann constant and T is the absolute temperature. We accept the probability for *trans* conformation of the C–C bond to be equal conditionally to 1. With w_{ij} we denote the probability for the appearance of the conformation j on some of the C–C bonds if the state of the preceeding C–C bond is i $(i,j = trans, g^+, g^-)$. Let us juxtapose to *trans*, g^+, and g^-, respectively, the numbers 1, 2, 3. Then the values of w_{ij} can be arranged in a matrix of the kind:

$$W = \begin{vmatrix} 1 & \sigma & \sigma \\ 1 & \sigma & 0 \\ 1 & 0 & \sigma \end{vmatrix} \tag{5}$$

The values of the matrix W give in summary the essence of the rotational isomeric model applied for the studied hydrophobic chains.

IV. ISOLATED CHAINS

Let us suppose that our monolayer consists of noninteracting chains.[13] Then, using the rotational isomeric model, the partition function q per saturated carbon chains with n carbon atoms can be calculated. It is

$$q = [1,0,0]W^{n-3} \begin{bmatrix} 1 \\ 1 \\ 1 \end{bmatrix} \tag{6}$$

where W is the matrix (Equation 5).

The matrix W has the following eigenvalues:

$$\lambda_1 = \frac{1}{2}[1 + \sigma + \sqrt{(1+\sigma)^2 + 4\sigma}] \tag{7}$$

$$\lambda_2 = \frac{1}{2}[1 + \sigma - \sqrt{(1+\sigma)^2 + 4\sigma}]$$

$$\lambda_3 = \sigma$$

Then,

$$q = A\lambda_1^{n-3} + B\lambda_2^{n-3} = \lambda_1^{n-3}C_{n-3} \tag{8}$$

with

$$A = -\frac{\lambda_2 - 1 - 2\sigma}{\lambda_1 - \lambda_2} \tag{9}$$

$$B = \frac{\lambda_1 - 1 - 2\sigma}{\lambda_1 - \lambda_2}$$

$$C_{n-3} = A + B\left(\frac{\lambda_2}{\lambda_1}\right)^{n-3}$$

Using the well-known relations between the partition function and the entropy per chain S^{ch}, we get:

$$S^{ch} = k[\ln q + T(\frac{\partial}{\partial t} \ln q)_p] \tag{10}$$

$$S^{ch} = (n-3)[k \ln \lambda_1 + \frac{\sigma E_0}{2T\lambda_1}(1 + \frac{3+\sigma}{\sqrt{(1+\sigma)^2 + 4\sigma}})] + \tag{11}$$
$$+ k \ln C_{n-3} + kT\frac{\partial \ln C_{n-3}}{\partial T}$$

At given temperature, a phase transition occurs in the hydrophobic core of the real lipid bilayer from ordered state (when almost all the chains are in all-*trans* conformation) to disordered state (when the number of g $\pm$ increases with a jump). The entropy of the transition can be measured experimentally. By independent experiment, the quantity E_0 can be measured, too. (It is of order of 600 cal/mol.) It is curious that if calculations are carried out according to Equation 11 with $E_0 = 1400$ cal/mol, very good agreement will be obtained with the measured values of the entropy for the above-mentioned transition (Figure 5). The cooperativity due to the interactions between the chains manifests in effective increase of E_0.

V. INTERACTING CHAINS

The numerical results of the model calculations will be more realistic as more completely the inter- and intramolecular interactions are included. (In our work, the role of the molecules is played by the hydrocarbon chains.) In this section, we describe the refinement of the models used in order to approximate this aim.

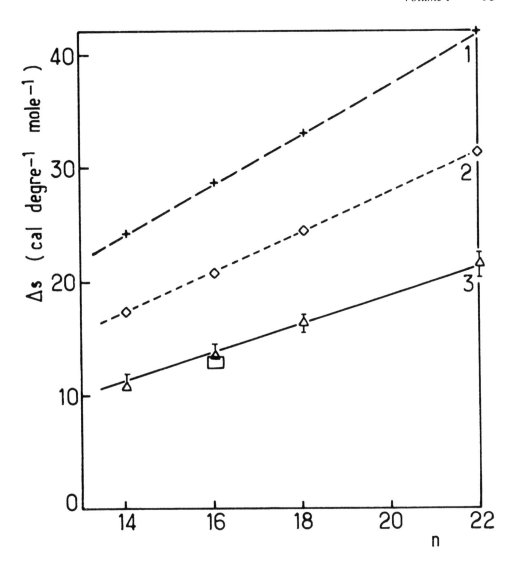

FIGURE 5. Variation of melting entropy of the chains in terms of their number n of carbon atoms. Experimental values: Δ, Reference 14; $\square$, our results. Theoretical curves: $E_0 = 0$ (1), 600 cal/mol (2), and 1400 cal/mol (3).

A. Rotational Isomeric Model with Chain Interactions (WIRI model)

This model[15-17] takes partially into account the interactions between the molecules. The first carbon atoms of two identical chains lie in a plane with a distance d between them (Figure 6). They can get different (but identical for both chains) conformations permitted by the rotational isomeric model. The atoms of the two chains interact, when d is low enough. The three initial atoms of each of the two chains are immobilized and assure that the beginnings of the chains are perpendicular to the plane where the first carbon atoms lie. The chains are closed in a cylinder with a generant perpendicular to the plane of the first carbon atoms and depending on d dimensions of the cross section, as shown in Figure 7.

The energy of the conformation is assumed to be infinite, if the center of any carbon or hydrogen atom is situated out of the cylinder. In this way, the interaction of the two chains with the surrounding molecules is imitated. When the conformations assure for the chains to be in the cylinder, their interaction energies (the interactions of all the pairs of carbon and/or hydrogen atoms not belonging to the same chain) are calculated according to

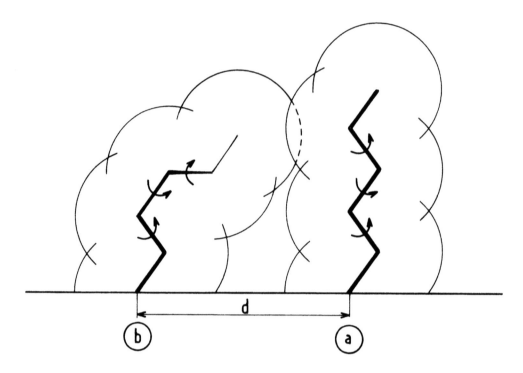

FIGURE 6.   Distance *d* between the two chains *a* and *b* in the WIRI model.

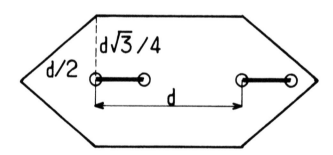

FIGURE 7.   Dimensions of the box where the two chains of the WIRI model are closed. The projection of this box on the plane of the monolayer is shown.

Equation 1. The partition function q_{pair} for the couple of chains is

$$q_{pair} = \sum_{\substack{\text{all conformations} \\ \text{in the cylinder}}} \exp\left(-\frac{E_k^{tot}}{kT}\right) \tag{12}$$

E_k^{tot} includes the interchain interactions plus the energies of all C–C bonds for the kth permitted conformation.

    This model is applied for chains with six carbons atoms. The mean internal energy $\overline{E^{int}}$ and the entropy per chain S^{ch} are calculated as functions of d. The entropy is calculated according to formula (11) and the energy according to the formula:

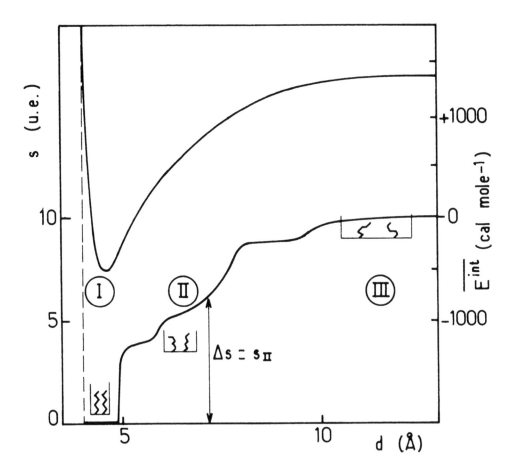

FIGURE 8. Theoretical variation of the internal energy and entropy in terms of the distance *d* between the chains for a chain with six carbon atoms. Calculation with the WIRI model.

$$\overline{E^{int}} = q_{pair}^{-1} \sum_{\substack{\text{all conformations} \\ \text{in the cylinder}}} E_k^{tot} \exp\left(-\frac{E_k^{tot}}{kT}\right) \tag{13}$$

The results for $S^{ch}(d)$ and $\overline{E^{int}}(d)$ are given in Figure 8.

We should like to note that the jumps of the calculated entropy are a result of the constraints imposed on the model: the distance between the chains is fixed for given dimensions of the cross section of the cylinder and the conformations accepted are among only those permitted by the rotational isomeric model. Due to these two factors, distances *d* exist having the property that for their infinitesimal changes, the number of conformations permitted (and the connected with this number entropy) changes with a jump.

In spite of its imperfection, the (WIRI) model gives a qualitative explanation of some experimental results. Let us define the thickness of the monolayer as the mean value of the distance between the plane of the first carbon atoms and the carbon atom lying farthest out for a given conformation. The calculated thickness depends weakly on the distance *d* between the chains. The experimental data confirm such a behavior. The birefrengence of the core,[18] both the experimental one and the one predicted by the WIRI model, depends strongly on *d*.

The calculation of different quantities in the frame of the WIRI model can be carried out according to the described procedure if all the permitted conformations are taken into account. Even with the help of a computer, this can be done if the number of carbon atoms in the chain is not too high. The conformational analysis of longer chains needs some statistical approach. The method proposed by Metropolis et al.[19] (Metropolis algorithm) is used in this case. The set of the accepted conformations is considered as a space of sets of a Markovian chain. The transition from one state to another is carried out through the modification of the local conformations of some C–C bonds of the chain. These deformations are realized at random. Two simulations are carried out. In the first one, used to evaluate average quantities, the Metropolis algorithm for the acceptance or rejection of a new conformation is applied taking into account all the inter- and intrachain interactions. In the second one used to obtain the number of permitted conformations, acceptance and rejection of the new conformation do not involve any interaction. With the help of this formalism, the entropies of the chains are calculated as functions of the interchain distance d for different chains having n carbon atoms with n between 14 and 22.

In the development of the modeling of interacting chains so far described, two essential disadvantages exist. The first of them is that the translational entropy due to the lateral displacement of the chains as a whole is disregarded. The second one is the too crude treatment of the interaction of the chain with its neighbors. In the following, improvements are made with the aim to overcome at least partially these shortcomings.

B. MODEL OF A MONOLAYER, BUILT UP OF INTERACTING CHAINS WITH COOPERATIVE CONFORMATIONAL STATES OF NEAR NEIGHBORS

In this model,[20-24] as in the WIRI one, the C–C bonds of the hydrophobic chains building up the monolayer can be in *trans*, g^+, or g^- states with energies as described in Section III. The difference from the rotational isomeric model is that the sequence $g^\pm g^\mp$ of two consecutive bonds is not forbidden any more, but an additional energy of 1900 cal/mol is attributed to it.[25]

The hydrogen and carbon atoms belonging to different chains interact with Lennard-Jones potential of the kind in Equation 1. The first carbon atoms of all the chains lie in a plane, called conditionally "interface". When the chains are in an all-*trans* state, their axes are perpendicular to the "interface" and pierce it in points that form a regular triangular lattice (Figure 9).

Later, we call the axis of the all-*trans* state of one chain simply the axis of the chain. The first calculations were done with the assumption that the planes determined by the first three carbon atoms of the chain (later we call these planes simply planes of the chains) are mutually parallel for all the chains and they are situated with respect to the triangular lattice as shown on Figure 9. The angle, θ, denoted on the Figure, is equal to $\pi/6$. The so-described planes of the chains with $\theta = \pi/6$ are called reference planes.

Later, the same calculations were carried out with the additional degree of freedom allowing the planes of the chains to rotate around the chain axes in the interval $[-\pi/6, +\pi/6]$ toward the reference planes. The latter results will be presented here.

Each chain of the monolayer has a definite conformation and is surrounded by six first neighbors having the same conformation. There is no correlation between the rotation angles of the planes for the chain and its neighbors. The main hypothesis used in the model is that the partition function q for one chain can be presented in the form:

$$q = q_{transl} \times q_{conf} \times q_{vib} \tag{14}$$

where q_{vib} is the component of the partition function due to the molecular vibrations, q_{transl} is the component due to their lateral translation, and q_{conf} is the component due to the conformational changes and the rotation of the chain. The three parts of q are assumed to

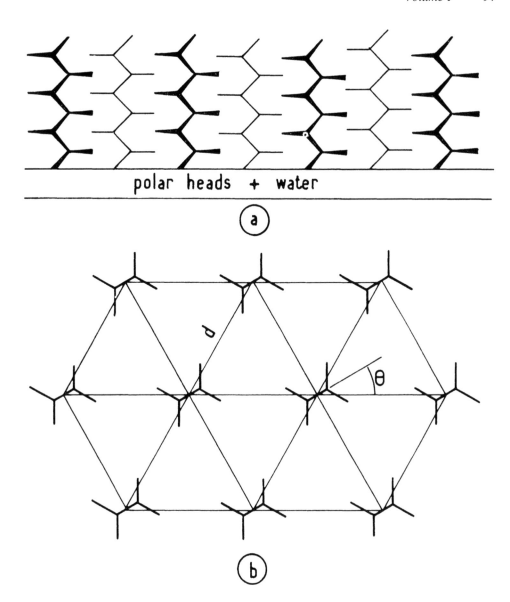

FIGURE 9.   Disposition of the hydrocarbon chains in the model of chains with cooperative conformational states of near neighbors. θ is the angle that the projection of the plane of the chain makes with the elements of the triangular lattice. For the definition of the plane of the chain, see the text. On the figure, the projections of the C–C and C–H bonds are drawn when the chains are in all-*trans* state, and the angle θ is equal to $\frac{\pi}{6}$. The projection of the plane of the chain coincides with the projection of its C–C bonds, when the chain is in an all-*trans* state.

be independent. The part q_{vib} depends only on the temperature and does not contribute to the properties of the monolayer when the temperature is fixed.

The calculation of the conformational part q_{conf} of the partition function continues to be a difficult problem even after the drastic restriction that all the chains have the same conformations. The procedure used for the calculation includes the following approximations. Because of the large number of conformations of the chain, again we study not all of the conformations, but apply an importance sampling algorithm to carry out the statistical sampling.

Let us examine one of the chains with its six first neighbors for a given distance d

between their axes. First of all, the rotational angles of the planes of the seven chains with respect to their reference planes are chosen at random within the interval mentioned. This determines the positions of the first three carbon atoms of each of the chains. The C–C bond between the first and the second carbon atom is in *trans* conformation. The conformation of the bond between the mth and $(m + 1)$-th carbon atoms ($2 \leqslant m \leqslant n - 2$, where n is the number of carbon atoms in the chain) should determine the positions of the $(m + 2)$-th carbon atom. For the choice of this conformation of the bond under consideration of the central molecule, the three energies $u_{m,i}^{tot}$ ($i = 1, 2, 3$) are calculated with $i = 1$ for *trans*, $i = 2$ for g^+, and $i = 3$ for g^- conformation. In $u_{m,i}^{tot}$ are included both the energy of the bond (zero for *trans* or 600 cal/mol for $g^\pm$ plus 1900 cal/mol for $g^\pm$ isomers following $g^\mp$ isomers of the preceeding C–C bond) and the interaction energies of the atoms of the $(m + 2)$-th CH_2 (or CH_3 group with all the atoms of the $(m + 1)$ groups of the six neighbors. These last energies are calculated by means of Equation 1. After that, the three probabilities p_i^m are calculated:

$$P_i^m = \frac{\exp[-\frac{u_{m,i}^{tot}}{kT}]}{\sum\limits_{i=1}^{3}\exp[-\frac{u_{m,i}^{tot}}{kT}]} \quad, i = 1,2,3 \tag{15}$$

Then the state of the bond under consideration is chosen at random in accordance with these probabilities. The same conformation is ascribed to the respective bonds of the neighbors. We denote with Ξ the set of angles of rotation of θ of the planes of the seven chains and with μ the set of the generated conformations of the C–C bonds. We introduce the quantities:

$$P(\Xi,\mu) = \prod_{m=2}^{n-2} P_i^m \tag{16}$$

$$u^{tot}(\Xi,\mu) = \sum_{m=2}^{n-2} u_{m,i}^{tot} \tag{17}$$

in Equations 16 and 17 for each m are taken p_i^m and $u_{m,i}^{tot}$ of the chosen conformations.

Let M be the number of the chosen sets Ξ and let for each of these sets M' conformations of the chain to be generated. Then for the estimation of the conformational partition function q_{conf} per chain, the following expression is used:

$$q_{conf} = \frac{1}{MM'}\sum_{k=1}^{M}\sum_{j=1}^{M'}\exp[-\frac{u^{tot}(\Xi_k,\mu_j)}{kT}]P^{-1}(\Xi_k,\mu_j) \tag{18}$$

The mean values of $\overline{G}$ of any molecular quantity $G(\Xi,\mu)$ are defined in a similar way:

$$\overline{G} = \frac{\sum\limits_{k=1}^{M}\sum\limits_{j=1}^{M'}G(\Xi_k,\mu_j)\exp[-\frac{u^{tot}(\Xi_k,\mu_j)}{kT}]P^{-1}(\Xi_k,\mu_j)}{\sum\limits_{k=1}^{M}\sum\limits_{j=1}^{M'}\exp[-\frac{u^{tot}(\Xi_k,\mu_j)}{kT}]P^{-1}(\Xi_k,\mu_j)} \tag{19}$$

We should like to note that the ideas of the mean field approximation are used implicitly for the construction of the last expressions. Really the requirement that the conformations of one chains and its neighbors are identical should have as a consequence that for all the macroscopic ensemble representing the monolayer, only one conformation is permitted, this with minimal internal energy, if rigorous statistical mechanical calculations are carried out.

The exact calculations of the translational partition function q_{transl} is possible if the free area for each conformation has been obtained. This is connected with great difficulties because of the dependence of the interchain interactions both on the chain conformations and on the distance between chains. That is why for the estimation of q_{transl} we make an approximation. Let δ be the mean thickness of the layer calculated by means of q_{conf}, where for given Ξ and μ, the thickness of the layer is defined as the distance between the interface and the most outlying carbon atom. Let d be the interchain distance, i.e., the step of the lattice on Figure 9. It is clear, that δ depends on d, $\delta = \delta(d)$. Let V be the volume of one hydrophobic chain. The assumption is made that V does not depend on d. We introduce the quantity $\mathcal{D}(d)$ having the meaning of the diameter of a mean circular cylinder with height δ and volume V:

$$\frac{\pi[D(d)]^2\delta(d)}{4} = V \tag{20}$$

The volume V is determined by independent experiments. Then the mean free area A_{free} of the chain can be estimated as:

$$A_{free} = \pi[d - D(d)]^2 \tag{21}$$

We denote with f_{transl} the translational free energy:

$$f_{transl} = -kT \ln q_{transl} \tag{22}$$

Using a simple model,[26] we can express f_{transl} via A_{free}:

$$f_{transl} = -kT \ln A_{free} + const(T) \tag{23}$$

On Figure 10 are given the values of $f_{conf} = -kT \ln q_{conf}$ calculated according the described procedure for different values of the interchain distance and for various number n of carbon atoms per chain.

On Figure 11 is given the dependence of the total free energy per chain $f = -kT \ln$ as well as the mean internal energy, $\overline{u_I^{int}}$ including all the inter- and intrachain interactions calculated for a chain with 16 carbon atoms. The dependence of the different quantities on the radius of curvature of the interface may be included in the model described above. To do this, we view the first carbon atoms of the chains as situated not on a plane, but on a spherical surface (Figure 12).

A sphere with a given radius R touches a plane hexagon in its center. The intersection points of the lines, passing through the center of the sphere and the apices of the hexagon, with the spherical surface determine the positions of the six neighbors of the chain situated in the center of the hexagon. These lines are also the axes of the neighbors. The axis of the central chain is the line passing through the center of the sphere and the center of the hexagon.

The calculation of all the quantities are carried out in exactly the same way as for the plane interface. The results obtained are different because the axes of the molecules are not parallel, but splayed.[23] When the quantity $\mathcal{D}(d)$ is calculated, an expression for the volume of a circular cone is used:

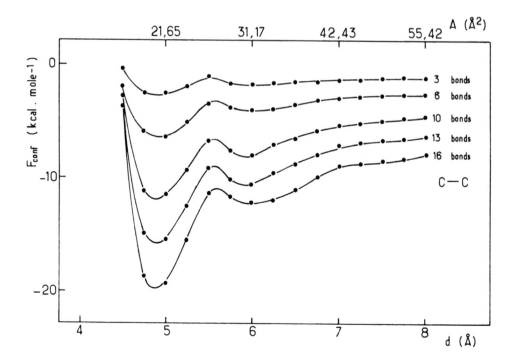

FIGURE 10.   Conformational free energy per chain for various chain lengths vs. the distance between chains, for a plane layer, calculated with the model of chains with cooperative conformational states of near neighbors.

$$V = \frac{\pi [D(d)]^2}{12} \delta(d)(3 + 3X + 3X^2) \tag{24}$$

where X is expressed via the radius R of curvature of the interface as:

$$X = \frac{\delta(D)}{R} \tag{25}$$

Figure 13 presents the dependence of the conformational free energy f_{conf} per chain for chain with 17 carbon atoms on the distance d between the chains for different radii of curvature R of the interface. With s we denote the mean area per chain in the monolayer, s can be expressed by means of d:

$$s = \frac{3\sqrt{3}}{8} d^2 \tag{26}$$

The knowledge of the dependence of the free energy per chain $\mathscr{F}_1$ on the interchain distance (and consequently on the mean area per chain s) permits the calculation of the important mechanical characteristics of the monolayer, its stretching elastic modulus k_s.

$$k_s = -s \frac{\partial^2 \mathscr{F}_1}{\partial s^2} \tag{27}$$

The values k_s for the minimal values of s with the property $\delta \mathscr{F}_1/\partial s = 0$ is of the order 1000 to 1500 dyn/cm. For comparison, we can note that for a lipid bilayer of egg yolk lecithin, this value is considerably less, about 140 dyn/cm.[27] This model can be generalized for monolayers consisting of two kinds of chains with different lengths.[24]

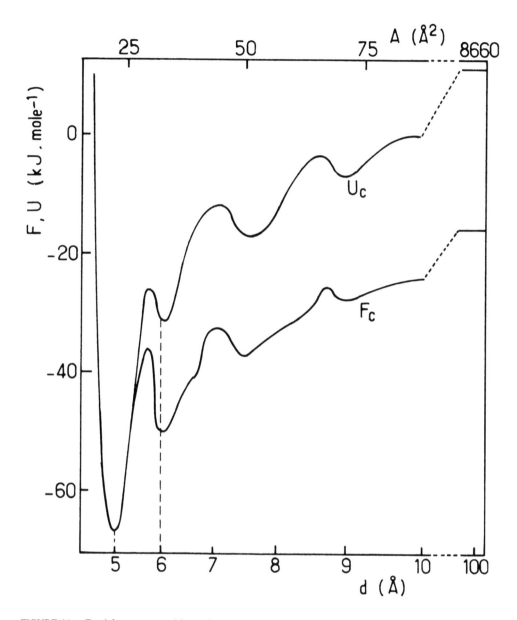

FIGURE 11.   Total free energy and internal energy per chain vs. the distance between the chains for a flat layer built up of chains with 16 carbon atoms, calculated with the model of chains with cooperative conformational states of near neighbors.

The model accounts for the effects of chain length mixing on the thermodynamical and structural properties of plane and curved layers. For all the quantities under study, it is sufficient to evaluate the main contribution of each chain surrounded by a mean distribution of neighboring molecules. Mixtures of C_{17} and C_4 chains, with varying proportions, have been studied. It can be observed that the loss of free energy due to mixing of chain lengths is greatly reduced by curvature. In addition the results suggest the existence of a natural radius of curvature and that penetration of the curved interface by organic solvent or by another curved layer is possible up to the limit of a hard sphere radius defined by the short chains.

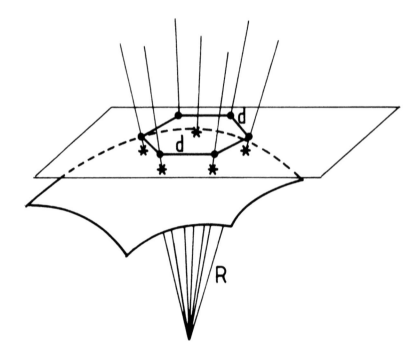

FIGURE 12.   Position of the chain axes for a spherically deformed interface.

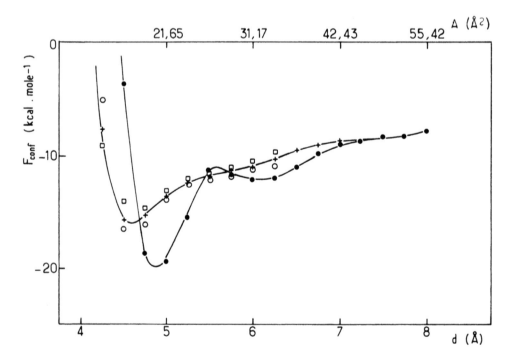

FIGURE 13.   Conformational free energy per chain vs. the distance between the chains for various radii of curvature of the interface. The chain contains 17 carbon atoms: (●) R = ∞; (○) R = 95 Å; (+) R = 75 Å; (□) R = 55 Å.

VI. PRESENT STATE OF ART OF THE COMPUTER MODELING OF THE HYDROPHOBIC CORE OF THE LIPID MONOLAYER

The study[28] presented in this section is aimed at decreasing as much as possible the hypotheses used in the models developed up to now. A Monte Carlo simulation is carried out for a "macroscopic" sample containing 100 molecules. Because of the size of the sample, we avoid most of the approximations necessary for the preceeding approaches.

A. DESCRIPTION OF THE MODEL

The flat monolayer under consideration consists of saturated hydrocarbon chains of the kind $(CH_2)_{n-1}CH_3$. The chains and their groups interact between them, but not with the water substrate. (The possibility of taking into consideration the interaction between the molecules and the substrate will be discussed.) The fact the monolayer is flat is accounted for by having the centers of the first CH_2 group (the outermost from the CH_3 group) of all the molecules lying in a plane. (We can call this plane conditionally "water-hydrocarbon chains interface".)

One of the most difficult problems in the derivation of the state equation of a system is the consideration of the steric repulsion between the molecules. For a two-dimensional system of hard noninteracting circular disks, for example, this equation can be obtained only numerically, via molecular dynamics computer simulation. However, when the mean free area per disk is low enough, an ultrasimplified model of this system can be used: the disks are arranged so that their centers coincide with the centers of the cells of one honeycomb-like hexagonal grid, whose dimension is chosen so that in each cell there is exactly one disk (i.e., the cell dimension depends on the mean area per disk). After that, instead of the real system, another one is considered, in which each disk can move in the space which remains when all the others are "centered" in their cells (approximation of the excluded volume interactions). Asymptotically, the equations of state of the two systems are identical when the free surface per disk tends to zero.

Such an approximation will be used by us, too. Instead of the true system, we consider another one, in which we put the neighbors of each chain in the centers of the cells of a hexagonal lattice, and this chain can move laterally in the space left by its neighbors. The validity of this approximation follows from the fact that because of the great number of degrees of freedom, when the conformation and the position of the neighbors are fixed, the chain under consideration will have the tendency to fill in the free volume, so that its free surface will be very low (the free surface, which allows for translational movements in the plane of the interface). So we have a situation very similar with a hard disk system, in which the mean area per disk is very near to the minimal one. Here we do not use a constraint accounting for the conservation of the volume of the chain.

To carry out the simulation, additional simplifications are assumed in the inter- and intramolecular interactions. The hydrocarbon chain is considered to be constituted of CH_2 groups and one CH_3 group; they are represented as parts of the spheres (Figure 14).

Each CH_2 group is characterized with a radius $R = 1.96$ Å and a volume $V_{CH_2} = 27$ Å^3. The CH_3 group has the same radius R, but a different volume $V_{CH_3} = 54$ Å^3. The interactions between the CH_2–CH_2, CH_2–CH_3, and CH_3–CH_3 groups are presented by Equation 2 with the parameters given in Table 2.

The interaction between two neighboring group is given by Equation 3 with the values of the coefficients given in Table 3. The interactions between all the CH_2 and CH_3 groups of one chain that are not nearest neighbors are also taken into account in the total energy of interaction.

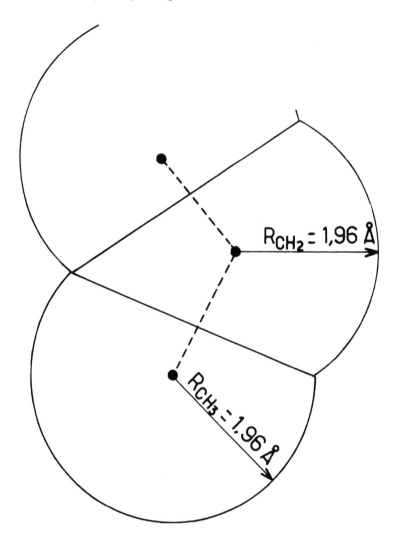

FIGURE 14. Presentation of the CH_2 and CH_3 groups as parts of spheres.

B. DESCRIPTION OF THE SYSTEM FOR WHICH MONTE CARLO SIMULATIONS ARE CARRIED OUT

Let us consider a system consisting of N of the mentioned above chains, situated on a surface S; a frame XY is introduced in the same plane. In this frame, a honeycomb-like hexagonal lattice is drawn as shown in Figure 15.

Each cell of this lattice has surface S/N; there are N such cells. One chain having some conformation is situated in each cell. The centers of the spheres of the first CH_2 groups (the outermost from the CH_3 groups) of each molecule lie in the plane XY. Let Z be an axis, perpendicular to the plane XY and let for this plane $z = 0$.

Then we impose the constraint that the zth coordinate of the centers of all the other CH_2 and CH_3 groups is not negative. Let us consider now a cylinder whose cross section, perpendicular to its generant, is a regular hexagon. Let the generant of the cylinder be perpendicular to the plane XY. For the conformation of the ith molecule, let us choose the cylinder with the minimal possible cross section, such that all the molecule is contained inside. (This means that no part of the spheres representing the CH_2 or CH_3 groups is out of the cylinder.) We call the cylinder with this property "minimal cylinder". Let us situate

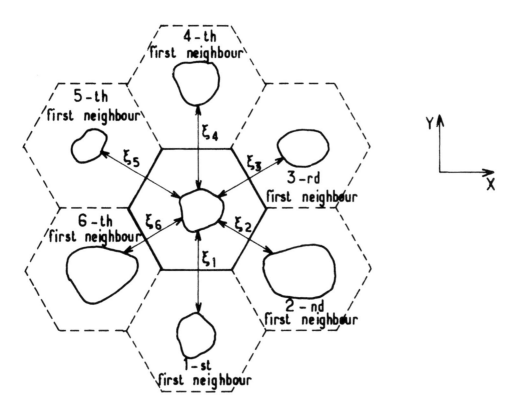

FIGURE 15. Honeycomb-like lattice. In each cell of the lattice, there is one chain that can move inside the cell. Each chain is surrounded by its six first neighbors. The free surface per chain with a given conformation is calculated assuming that the neighbors are centered in their cells. With ξ_i, $i = 1, 2, \ldots, 6$, we denote the maximal displacement of the central chain to its ith neighbor, when there is still no overlapping between the chains.

each chain in its cell so that the axis of its corresponding minimal cylinder passes through the center of the cell. For a given set $m_1, m_2, \ldots, m_N$ of conformations of the N chains, we say that it is permitted if, after the disposition of all the N conformations in the described above manner, there is no overlapping between the spheres representing the CH_2 or CH_3 groups of any two different chains. For a permitted set of conformations, we call this disposition of chains "centered".

Because we work with a finite number N of chains, we choose N to be equal to the square of some natural number, arrange the cells so that they constitute a lozenge with an acute angle $\pi/3$, and impose periodic boundary conditions. In order to determine the free surface available for the ith chain in its m_ith conformation, when the other chains have conformations $m_1, m_2, \ldots, m_N$, we apply the following procedure. We start from the centered disposition of the chains. After that we allow the ith chain to move, keeping its six neighbors in their former places. We consider only permitted states, for which there is no overlapping between the chain under consideration and its neighbors. In doing this, we change the position of the cross-point of the axis of the minimal cylinder with the plane XY. Let us call this point the "center" of the conformation. The free surface for the conformation is then the surface available for its center. We denote it with $S^i_{m_1, m_2 \ldots, m_N}$. For the calculation of this quantity, we use one more approximation. Let the center of the chain move to the center of its lth neighbor ($l = 1, 2, \ldots, 6$, see Figure 15). Let ξ_l be the maximal permitted shift when there is still no overlapping of the molecule with anyone of its six neighbors. Then we assume that:

$$S^i_{m_1,m_2,\ldots,m_N} \sim (\xi_1 \cdot \xi_2 \cdot \xi_3 \cdot \xi_4 \cdot \xi_5 \cdot \xi_6)^{1/3} \tag{28}$$

The coefficient of proportionality plays no role in the following calculations. The approximation (Equation 28) is in conformity with the assumption that the set of conformations $m_1, m_2, \ldots, m_N$ is permitted, if there is no overlapping when the chains are centered. The energy $U^{tot}(m_1, m_2, \ldots, m_N)$ of a permitted set of conformations is calculated when the system is centered. The energy is presented as:

$$U^{tot}(m_1, m_2, \ldots, m_N) = U^{inter}(m_1, m_2, \ldots, m_N) + \tag{29}$$

$$U^{intra}(m_1, m_2, \ldots, m_N)$$

where $U^{inter}(m_1, m_2, \ldots, m_N)$ is the sum of the energies of interaction between all the pairs of CH_2 and/or CH_3 groups of first neighbor chains plus the sum of interactions of nonneighboring pairs of CH_2 and CH_3 groups belonging to one and the same molecule; $U^{intra}(m_1, m_2, \ldots, m_N)$ is the sum of the rotational energies of all the C–C bonds of one chain with respect to the all-*trans* state. Evidently,

$$U^{intra}(m_1, m_2, \ldots, m_N) = u^{intra}(m_1) + u^{intra}(m_2) + \cdots + u^{intra}(m_N) \tag{30}$$

where $u^{intra}(m_i)$ is the conformational energy due to rotations of the m_ith conformation calculated according to Equation 3. Without loss of generality, we can assume that the number M of possible conformations that one chain can take is very large but finite. Note that for our chains $(CH_2)_{n-1}CH_3$ each conformation can be characterized with two steric angles, specifying the orientation of the line connecting the centers of the first and the third CH_2 groups, and $n-3$ rotation angles determining the mutual orientation between two CH_2 groups. The assumption that M is finite is equivalent with the assumption that each of these angles can take a finite number of values. We can now write the statistical sum Q of the system. For simplicity, we denote:

$$S_{m_1,m_2,\ldots,m_N} = \prod_{i=1}^{N} S^i_{m_1,m_2,\ldots,m_N} \tag{31}$$

The partition function Q of the system can then be written in the form:

$$Q = \sum_{\substack{m_1,m_2,\ldots,m_N = 1 \\ (m_1,m_2,\ldots,m_N - \text{permitted})}}^{M} S_{m_1,m_2,\ldots,m_N}\, e^{-\frac{U^{tot}(m_1,m_2,\ldots,m_N)}{KT}} \tag{32}$$

From Equations 29, 30, and 32,

$$Q = \sum_{\substack{m_1,m_2,\ldots,m_N = 1 \\ (m_1,m_2,\ldots,m_N - \text{permitted})}}^{M} \left\{ \prod_{i=1}^{N} \left(e^{-\frac{u^{intra}(m_i)}{KT}} \right) \right\} S_{m_1,m_2,\ldots,m_N}\, e^{-\frac{U^{inter}(m_1,m_2,\ldots,m_N)}{KT}} \tag{33}$$

Let us now change the set of conformations $(1, 2, \ldots, M)$, where the figures mean the number of the corresponding conformation, with another one:

$$(\quad \underbrace{1,1,\ldots,1}_{F.e^{-\frac{u^{intra}(1)}{KT}} \text{ - times}} \quad , 2,2,\ldots,2,\ldots, \quad \underbrace{M,M,\ldots,M}_{F.e^{-\frac{u^{intra}(M)}{KT}} \text{ - times}} \quad)$$

where F is a large enough number, and denote this set with $(1', 2', \ldots, M')$, where

$$M' = F \sum_{i=1}^{M} e^{-\frac{u^{intra}(i)}{KT}}$$

Obviously,

$$Q = F^{-N} \sum_{\substack{m'_1, m'_2, \ldots, m'_N = 1 \\ (m'_1, m'_2, \ldots, m'_N \text{ - permitted})}}^{M'} S_{m'_1, m'_2, \ldots, m'_N} e^{-\frac{U^{inter}(m'_1, m'_2, \ldots, m'_N)}{KT}} \qquad (34)$$

and because F^{-N} is a constant, the system with statistical sum Q',

$$Q' = \sum_{\substack{m'_1, m'_2, \ldots, m'_N = 1 \\ (m'_1, m'_2, \ldots, m'_N \text{ - permitted})}}^{M'} S_{m'_1, m'_2, \ldots, m'_N} e^{-\frac{U^{inter}(m'_1, m'_2, \ldots, m'_N)}{KT}} \qquad (35)$$

will have the same physical properties as the system with a statistical sum Q. We introduce a size l_j of the minimal cylinder of the j'th conformation possible for one chain, this is the length l from Figure 16 of the cross section of the cylinder with the plane XY: l varies in some interval (l_{min}, l_{max}).

We divide this interval via $p - 1$ points to p subintervals $(l_{min}, l_1), (l_1, l_2), \ldots, (l_{p-2}$ $l_{max})$ and number these intervals with $1, 2, \ldots, p$. Then each conformation m' can be characterized with the number of the interval h, $1 \leq h \leq p$ in which its size will fall. Let in the kth interval there be M'_k conformations. Then $M'_1 + \ldots + M'_p = M'$. Equation 35 can be rewritten in the form:

$$(36)$$

$$Q' = \sum_{\substack{h_1, h_2, \ldots, h_N = 1}}^{p} \sum_{\substack{m'_1 \in h_1, m'_2 \in h_2, \ldots, m'_N \in h_N \\ (m'_1, m'_2, \ldots, m'_N \text{ - permitted})}} S_{m'_1, m'_2, \ldots, m'_N} e^{-\frac{U^{inter}(m'_1, m'_2, \ldots, m'_N)}{KT}}$$

Let us now make a uniformly distributed random choice of L conformations from a set $(1', 2', \ldots, M')$ belonging to each of the p intervals. It will constitute a set of conformations:

$$\left(\underbrace{1'', 2'', \ldots, L''}_{\text{first interval}}, \underbrace{(L+1)'', (L+2)'', \ldots, (2L)''}_{\text{second interval}}, \ldots, \underbrace{(L(p-1)+1)'', (L(p-1)+2)'', \ldots, (Lp)''}_{\text{p-th interval}} \right)$$

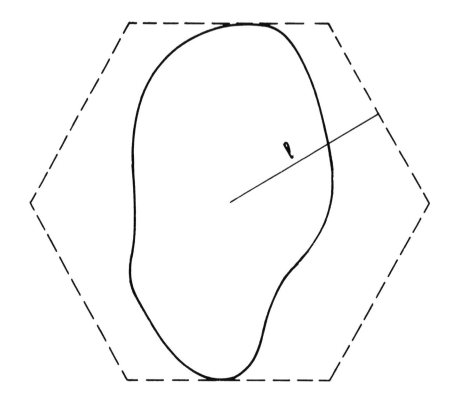

FIGURE 16.   Projection of one of the conformations of the chain on the plane of the monolayer. With dashed line is given the projection of the minimal cylinder with hexagonal cross section, containing this conformation, and a generant perpendicular to the plane; *l* is the "size" of the conformation.

If L is a large enough number, Q' can then be estimated as:

$$Q' \sim \sum_{h_1, h_2, \ldots, h_N = 1}^{p} \frac{M'_{h_1}}{L} \cdot \frac{M'_{h_2}}{L} \cdots \frac{M'_{h_N}}{L} \sum_{\substack{m''_1 \in h_1, m''_2 \in h_2, \ldots, m''_N \in h_N \\ (m''_1, m''_2, \ldots, m''_N - \text{permitted})}} \tag{37}$$

$$S_{m''_1, m''_2, \ldots, m''_N} e^{-\frac{U^{inter}(m''_1, m''_2, \ldots, m''_N)}{kT}}$$

In Equation 37, h_i is the number of the subinterval to which the m''_ith conformation of the ith molecule belongs. We denote

$$U_0(m''_1, m''_2, \ldots, m''_N) = -kT \ln(S_{m''_1, m''_2, \ldots, m''_N}) \tag{38}$$
$$+ \sum_{i=1}^{N} -kT \ln(M'_{h_i})$$

$$U(m''_1, m''_2, \ldots, m''_N) = U^{inter}(m''_1, m''_2, \ldots, m''_N) + \tag{39}$$
$$U_0(m''_1, m''_2, \ldots, m''_N)$$

Let $M'' = L.p$. Then a system with the statistical sum Q'' of the kind:

$$Q'' = \sum_{\substack{m_1'', m_2'', \ldots, m_N'' = 1 \\ (m_1'', m_2'', \ldots, m_N'' - \text{permitted})}}^{M''} e^{-\frac{U(m_1'', m_2'', \ldots, m_N'')}{KT}} \tag{40}$$

permits us to determine the properties of the primary system with the statistical sum Q. Note that for one permitted set of conformations $(m_N'', m_N'', \ldots, m''N)$, the quantity $U(m_1'', m_2'', \ldots, m_{N_1}'')$ can be calculated, if the factors Mh_i are known. Let

$$s = S/N \tag{41}$$

be the mean area per chain in the system. S and s without indices refer to the real area of the system and the real mean area per chain, while this letter with indices refers to auxiliary variables. s is equal to the surface of one cell of the lattice in Figure 15. Let $P(s,N)$ be the number of permitted sets of conformations $(m_1'', m_2'', \ldots, m_N'')$ for our system of N molecules, when the mean area per molecule is s. Then Equation 40 can be transformed as follows:

$$Q'' = \frac{P(s, N)}{\sum\limits_{m_1'', m_2'', \ldots, m_N''=1}^{M''} e^{+\frac{U(m_1'', m_2'', \ldots, m_N'')}{KT}} w(m_1'', m_2'', \ldots, m_N'', s)} \tag{42}$$

where $w(m_1'', m_2'', \ldots, m_N'', s)$ is the probability for the set of conformations $(m_1'', m_2'', \ldots, m_N'')$ when the mean area per molecule is s. The denominator in Equation 42 is in fact the mean value of the quantity $e^{+\frac{U}{KT}}$. This mean value can be presented in the form:

$$\int_{-\infty}^{+\infty} w(U, s, N) e^{+\frac{U}{KT}} \, dU \tag{43}$$

In Equation 43, $w(U,s,N)$ is the probability density for the quantity U in a system with mean are per molecule s. This function is of the kind presented in Figure 17.

It is well known that if $\overline{U}$ is the mean value of U, then $\overline{U(s,N)} = N\overline{u(s)}$, where $\overline{u(s)}$ does not depend on N. The basic idea used later on is that $w(U,s,N)$ can be expressed for large enough N as follows:[29]

$$w(U, s, N) = \frac{e^{-\frac{Nf(U/N, s)}{KT}}}{\int_{-\infty}^{+\infty} e^{-\frac{Nf(U/N, s)}{KT}} \, dU} \tag{44}$$

This idea is grounded on the statistical mechanical consideration of the macrocanonical distribution. Let us denote $u = U/N$.

Because the function $f(u,s)$ has a minimum at $u = \overline{u(s)}$, it can be expanded in a series of the kind:

$$f(u, s) = f(\overline{u(s)}, s) + \frac{1}{2} \left. \frac{\partial^2 f(u, s)}{\partial u^2} \right|_{u=\overline{u(s)}} [u - \overline{u(s)}]^2 + \cdots \tag{45}$$

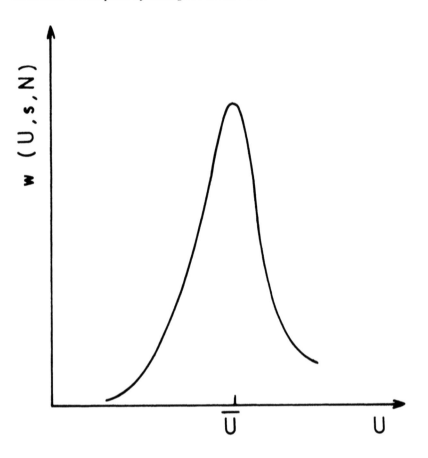

FIGURE 17. General dependence of the quantity $w(U,s,N)$ on U.

Then Equation 43 can be presented as follows:

$$\frac{N\int_{-\infty}^{+\infty}\left[e^{-\frac{Nf(u,s)}{KT}}e^{\frac{Nu}{KT}}\right]du}{N\int_{-\infty}^{+\infty}e^{-\frac{Nf(u,s)}{KT}}du} \tag{46}$$

Let $u_1(s)$ be the value of u for which

$$\frac{\partial}{\partial u}\left[f(u,s)-u\right]\big|_{u=u_1(s)} = 0 \tag{47}$$

However, Q'' is a function of s and N. Only this part of the function whose logarithm is proportional to N is important for the calculation of the free energy of the system with large enough N. In Equation 42, the logarithm of the numerator $P(s,N)$ is obviously proportional to N, if the finite size effect of the system is neglected (i.e., if N is large enough). Consequently, we can keep only these terms in the denominator Equation 43 as well. The final result is then:

$$Q''(s,N) \approx \frac{P(s,N)}{e^{\frac{N\overline{u(s)}}{kT}}e^{\frac{N\{f[\overline{u(s)},s]-f[u_1(s),s]-\overline{u(s)}+u_1(s)\}}{kT}}} \tag{48}$$

Consequently, if the functions $P(s,N)$ and $f(u,s)$ are known, the statistical sum $Q''(s,N)$ can be calculated. Knowing it, we can obtain the equation of state of the system. In what follows, we will describe the way of choosing the set of conformations $\{1'', 2'', \ldots, M''\}$ and the calculation of these two functions.

C. CHOOSING THE SET OF CONFORMATIONS

First of all, we divide the interval l_{min}, l_{max} of possible sizes of the conformations, in p subintervals. For the definition of the size of conformations, see the text before Equation 36. l_{min} is the minimal cylinder for the all-*trans* state, and l_{max} is of the order of half the length of the all-*trans* conformation. After that, we choose randomly the two angles specifying the orientation of the line connecting the first and third CH_2 groups. For the chains of the kind $(CH_2)_{n-1}CH_{n-3}$ angles ϕ_i, $i = 1, \ldots, n - 3$ are chosen in the interval $(0, 2\pi)$ using the probability function $g(\phi)$:

$$\sim e^{-\frac{u^r(\phi)}{kT}} \tag{49}$$

with $u^r(\phi)$ from Equation 3. With these $n - 1$ angles, we try to construct a conformation. If there is an overlapping between the nonneighboring CH_2 and/or CH_3 groups, or if there are groups for which the coordinate z of their center is negative, we abandon the conformation. If the conformation is accepted, we determine its size and the subinterval in which it falls. This procedure is repeated many times until a large enough number of conformations is accumulated in each interval. The so obtained set of conformations corresponds to the set $(1', 2', \ldots, M')$ discussed after Equation 33. Really the ratio of the probabilities of two conformation L_1' and L_2' is equal to

$$e^{-\frac{u^{intra}(L_1') - u^{intra}(L_2')}{kT}}$$

as follows from the rule of generation of the set. The number of conformations in the kth interval, divided by the total number of conformations, will give a value proportional to the factor appearing in Equation 37. Following the described procedure, from each interval we choose randomly equal number L of conformations. So the set of conformations $(1'', 2'', \ldots, M'')$ is constructed.

D. CALCULATION OF THE NUMBER OF STATES OF THE SYSTEM

Let $s_1, s_2, \ldots, s_p$ be hexagons having sizes $l_1, l_2, \ldots, l_p$, respectively. The definition of the size of a hexagon is given before Equation 36 and is shown on Figure 16. Let $P(s,N,s_j)$ be the number of the permitted sets of conformations, in which sets each conformation belongs to the interval with a number $\leq j$. If $s_j \leq s$, then

$$P(s, N, s_j) = (jL)^N \tag{50}$$

Having in mind that $l_p = l_{max}$, it is clear that

$$P(s, N, s_p) = P(s, N) \tag{51}$$

In what follows, we will suppose that s is chosen so that a number n_0 exists with the property $s = s_{n_0}$. Let us now do a Monte Carlo simulation of the system of the following kind. The initial state is a permitted state with a set of centered conformations belonging, for example, to the intervals with numbers less than n_0. Let $k \leq p$. We choose randomly one conformation whose size is less than or equal to l_k. If the new conformation centered at the place of some randomly chosen molecule does not overlap with six neighbors, it is accepted. In the new set of conformations, the conformation with the highest size is found and the number of the interval to which it belongs is determined. This number is used to label the new set of conformations. If it is not accepted, the procedure must be repeated. So we will obtain an array of A sets of possible conformations of the system of N chains, to which corresponds an array of A labels. Note that the array of states is filled in only when the new conformation is accepted. The labels are between 1 and j. Let a_i be the number of the labels equal to i, . . . , and a_{j-i} the number of labels equal to $j - i$. Then,

$$A = a_1 + a_2 + \cdots + a_j \tag{52}$$

If A is large enough so that a_j and a_{j-i} are large enough too, then,

$$\frac{P(s, N, s_j)}{P(s, N, s_{j-i})} = \frac{a_1 + a_2 + \cdots + a_j}{a_1 + a_2 + \cdots + a_{j-i}} \tag{53}$$

Because $P(s,N,s_{n_0})$ is known from Equation 50 and knowing the ratios (Equation 53) (after a sufficient number of simulations for different j), we have the possibility to calculate $P(s,N)$. In order to simplify the calculations, we assume that j is a continuous variable; consider a function $g(j) = P(s,N,s_j)$ and calculate the derivative $dg(j)/dj$:

$$\frac{g(j + \Delta j)}{g(j)} = \frac{a_1 + \cdots + a_j + a_{j+1} + \cdots + a_{j+\Delta j}}{a_1 + a_2 + \cdots + a_j} \tag{54}$$

However,

$$\frac{g(j + \Delta j)}{g(j)} = 1 + \frac{1}{g(j)} \frac{d[g(j)]}{dj} \Delta j = 1 + \frac{d \ln[g(j)]}{dj} \Delta j \tag{55}$$

Consequently,

$$\frac{d \ln[g(j)]}{dj} = \frac{a_{j+1} + a_{j+2} + \cdots + a_{j+\Delta j}}{a_1 + \cdots + a_j} \frac{1}{\Delta j} \tag{56}$$

The derivatives (Equation 56) were determined for a finite number of j and after that were interpolated for all the $j, n \leq j \leq p$, considered as a continuous variable. A simple integration gives then the values of $\ln[g(j)]$ and of $g(j)$ itself, using $g(n_0) = (n_0 L)^N$.

$$P(s, N) = (n_0 L)^N \frac{g(p)}{g(n_0)} = g(p) \tag{57}$$

In fact, for the calculation of the free energy $\mathcal{F}$ of the system, we need exactly $\ln[g(p)]$ because $\mathcal{F} = -kT \ln Q''$.

E. CALCULATION OF THE PROBABILITY FUNCTION OF THE SYSTEM

Starting from one permitted set of conformations, we realize the following Monte Carlo simulation. First of all, we calculate the energy U of the system; after that we choose randomly one chain and one conformation, put the new conformation in the place of the chain, and verify if the obtained set of conformations of the whole system is permitted. If the conformation is not permitted, the procedure is repeated without adding any new set of conformations in the array of the generated sets of conformations of the systems. If the conformation is permitted, then the value of U for the new set of conformations is calculated, and the Metropolis algorithm is applied. In the array, either the old or the new set of conformations is put with probability given by Metropolis algorithm. From the array generated, the mean value $\overline{U}$ of U is calculated.

Let us now choose some number $a > \overline{U(s,N)/N} = \overline{u(s)}$. Let the energy U of the initial state of the system (see the beginning of this paragraph) be such that $U \geqslant N.a$. Let the simulation be realized only on the set of conformations, for which $U \geqslant N.a$. To assure this, it is sufficient to abandon each new conformation (and the corresponding state) for which this inequality is not valid. In such a system, the probability $w(U,s,N)$ from Equation 44 will be transformed to $w(U,s,N,a)$ of the following kind:

$$w(U,s,N,a) = \frac{e^{-\frac{Nf(u,s)}{kT}}}{N\int_a^\infty e^{-\frac{Nf(u,s)}{kT}} \, du} \tag{58}$$

With the probability (Equation 58), the mean value $\overline{u(s,a)}$ can be calculated, and because exponential is a very rapidly decreasing function, when $a > \overline{u(s)}$, the $f(u,s)$ can be presented in the form:

$$f(u,s) \approx f(a,s) + \left.\frac{\partial f(u,s)}{\partial u}\right|_{u=a} (u-a) \tag{59}$$

Then,

$$\overline{u(s,a)} = \frac{1}{N}\int_a^\infty U w(U,s,N,a) dU \tag{60}$$

$$= \frac{\int_a^\infty u e^{-\frac{N\frac{\partial f}{\partial u}\big|_{u=a}(u-a)}{kT}} \, du}{\int_a^\infty e^{-\frac{N\frac{\partial f}{\partial u}\big|_{u=a}(u-a)}{kT}} \, du}$$

$$= a + \frac{kT}{N\frac{\partial f}{\partial u}\big|_{u=a}}$$

Consequently, the quantity $\overline{Nu(s,a)} - Na$, which can be determined numerically, gives immediately information for $\left.\frac{\partial f(u,s)}{\partial u}\right|_{u=a}$; but knowing the derivative including the point $\overline{u(s)}$ where the first derivative is 0 and the second is also calculated, we can obtain the function $f(u,s)$. Without loss of generality, $f[\overline{u(s)},s] = 0$. Consequently,

$$f(u,s) = \frac{1}{2}\left.\frac{\partial^2 f}{\partial u^2}\right|_{u=\overline{u(s)}} [u - \overline{u(s)}]^2 \tag{61}$$

+ higher orders whose number depends on

number of the points where $\dfrac{\partial f}{\partial u}$ **is calculated**

Then $u_1(s)$ can be determined for which $\left.\dfrac{\partial f(u,s)}{\partial u}\right|_{u=u_1(s)} = 1$; so the denominator of Equation 48 is also calculated. The free energy per molecule, as a function of s and N, is

$$\mathcal{F}_1(s) = \frac{1}{N}(-kT)\ln[\mathcal{Q}''(s, N)] \qquad (62)$$

F. RESULTS AND DISCUSSION

The Monte Carlo simulations were carried out for a system of $N = 100$ chains, each of them having $n = 10$ carbon atoms. This choice on n was done in order to obtain results that could be compared with those of van der Ploeg et al.[10] These authors have carried out molecular dynamics simulations for mono- and bilayers built up of similar molecules. The temperature of the system was chosen to be 29°C. Our simulations were done for mean area per chain in the interval [25 to 35 Å^2]. We obtain the following numerical results.

1. Order Parameters

They are calculated first for one single CH_2 group (of the nine CH_2 groups) as $\left(\dfrac{3}{2}\cos^2\psi_j^{m''} - \dfrac{1}{2}\right)$ where m'' denotes the conformation, and $\psi_j^{m''}$ denotes the angle between the normal, determined by the centers of the two hydrogens atoms and the carbon atom of the ith CH_2 group with the axis Z. For all the conformations it is $\dfrac{1}{8}\sum\limits_{j=2}^{9}\left(\dfrac{3}{2}\cos^2\psi_j^{m''} - \dfrac{1}{2}\right)$.

After the simulation, the statistical weight of each conformation is determined and the mean order parameters for the system are calculated. The dependence of the order parameter of each of the CH_2 groups for different values of the mean area per chain is given on Figure 18. On this figure, the well-known plateau for the groups between four and seven can be seen. Figure 19 presents the mean order parameter for all the chains as a function of the mean area per chain. The comparison with the molecular dynamics simulations shows that all of our values are higher, particularly for bonds near the interface. This suggests that probably in our model chains are more tightly attached to the flat interface.

2. Distribution of the Density Along the Thickness of the Core

Knowing the statistical weight of each conformation, we simply calculate the mean number of CH_2 groups, having the Z-coordinate of their center between z_0 and $z_0 + \Delta z$ for different values of z_0. The results are presented on Figure 20. This quantity is almost constant along the thickness of the core. Taking the mean thickness of the core as the Z-coordinate such that the density is 0.5, it can be seen that the variation Δe of this quantity is very slight vs. the mean area per chain.

3. Correlation Function ξ^k for the First Neighbors, Second Neighbors, etc. (k = 1, 2, ...)

We define it as:

$$\xi^k = \frac{\overline{S^i_{m_1'',m_2',...,m_N''}\, S^{i+k}_{m_1'',m_2',...,m_N''}} - \overline{S^i_{m_1'',m_2',...,m_N''}} \times \overline{S^{i+k}_{m_1'',m_2',...,m_N''}}}{\left[\overline{(S^i_{m_1'',m_2',...,m_N''})^2} \times \overline{(S^{i+k}_{m_1'',m_2',...,m_N''})^2}\right]^{\frac{1}{2}} - \overline{S^i_{m_1'',m_2',...,m_N''}} \times \overline{S^{i+k}_{m_1'',m_2',...,m_N''}}} \qquad (63)$$

The dependence of the correlation as a function of the remoteness of the neighbors for different mean areas per chain is plotted on Figure 21. The correlation between the first neighbors still exists, while for the second neighbors, it is practically zero. These last results show that the WIRI model considers the chains quite independent, while the model with

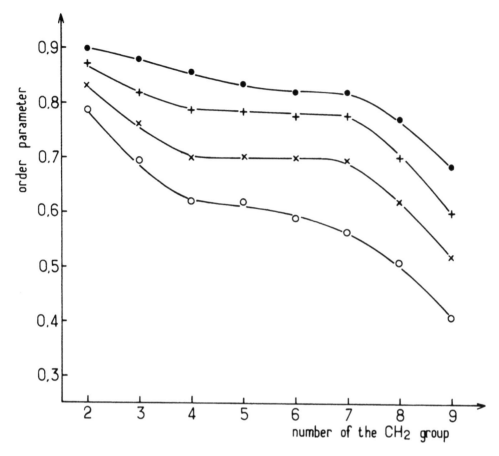

FIGURE 18. Numerical results for the dependence of the order parameters of CH_2 groups obtained by Monte Carlo simulation for different mean areas s per chain: (●), $s = 26$ Å²; (+), $s = 28$ Å²; (×), $s = 31$ Å²; (○), $s = 35$ Å².

cooperative conformational states of neighbors overestimates this correlation. These results on the correlation function can be obtained, in our model, with a precision better than in the molecular dynamics simulations.[9]

4. Mean Internal Energy of the System

It is defined as:

$$\overline{u_1^{int}(s)} = [\overline{U^{inter}(s, N)} + \overline{U^{intra}(s, N)}] \tag{64}$$

Its dependence on the mean area per chain s is given in Figure 22.

5. Free Energy per Chain

This is the most important quantity that can be calculated with our method. It is defined via Equation 62. Its dependence on the mean area per chain is shown on Figure 23. We have also plotted in Figure 24 the lateral pressure $\Pi_1 = -\dfrac{\partial \mathscr{F}_1(s)}{\partial s}$ vs. the mean area per chain.

Here we could include the interaction of the hydrophobic core with the water substratum. If our idealized monolayer of hydrophobic chains is situated on a water substratum, the "interface" water chains can be considered approximately as oil-water interface with free

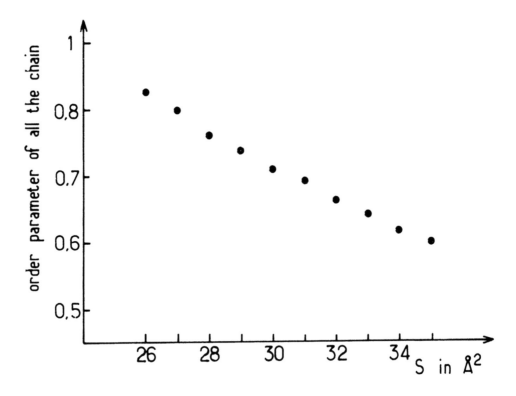

FIGURE 19.   Dependence of the mean order parameter of all the chain on the mean area per chain.

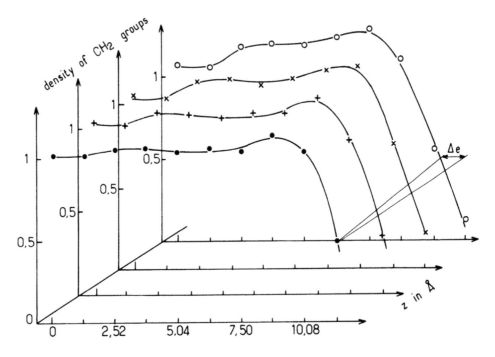

FIGURE 20.   Distribution of the density along the thickness of the core for different mean areas per chain, with Δe indicating a reliable variation of the mean thickness: ($\bullet$), $s = 26$ Å^2; ($+$), $s = 28$ Å^2; ($\times$), $s = 31$ Å^2; ($\circ$), $s = 35$ Å^2.

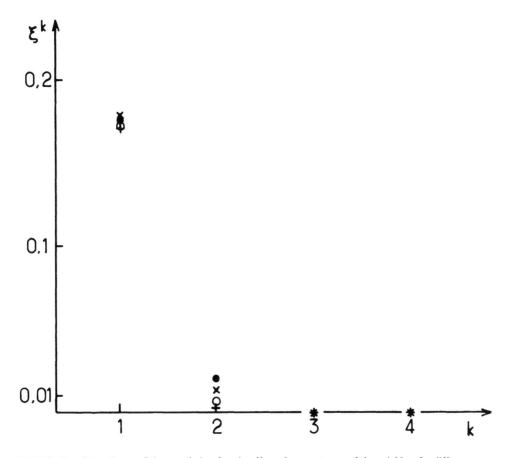

FIGURE 21. Dependence of the correlation function ξ^k on the remoteness of the neighbor for different mean areas per chain: ($\bullet$), $s = 26$ Å²; ($+$), $s = 28$ Å²; ($\times$), $s = 31$ Å²; ($\circ$), $s = 35$ Å².

energy per unit area equal to γ. Then, the full free energy per chain $\mathcal{F}_1^{tot}(s)$ will be equal to:

$$\mathcal{F}_1^{tot}(s) = \mathcal{F}_1(s) + \gamma \cdot s \tag{65}$$

The total lateral pressure Π_1^{tot} is

$$\Pi_1^{tot}(s) = -\frac{\partial \mathcal{F}_1^{tot}(s)}{\partial s} - \gamma \tag{66}$$

An equilibrium area per chain s_0 can be introduced through the equation:

$$\Pi_1^{tot}(s_0) = 0 \tag{67}$$

For $\gamma = 50 \pm 5$ dyn/cm, the predicted by our calculations value of s_0 lies in the interval:

$$28.5\text{Å}^2 \leq s_0 \leq 30.5\text{Å}^2 \tag{68}$$

It is in very good agreement with the experimentally measured values of this quantity for lecithin bilayers. The value of the stretching elastic modulus k_s for $s = s_0$, defined by

$$k_s = -s_0 \left.\frac{\partial^2 \mathcal{F}_1^{tot}(s)}{\partial s^2}\right|_{s=s_0}$$

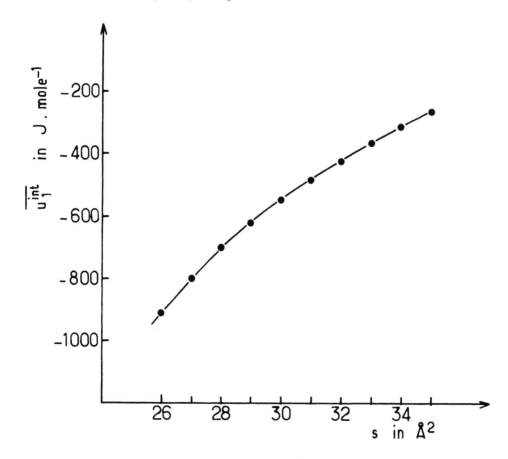

FIGURE 22. Dependence of the mean internal energy $\overline{u_1^{int}}$ per chain on the mean area per chain.

can be predicted to be in the interval:

$$100 \text{ dyn/cm} \leq k_s \leq 200 \text{ dyn/cm} \tag{69}$$

It is much closer to the experimentally measured one[30] for egg yolk lecithin bilayers, than the predicted by the preceeding models. All the numerical calculations were carried out on the VAX 8600 of the Centre de Recherche Paul Pascal and have taken about 1000 h of CPU time.

VII. PERSPECTIVES

The reported results show that the Monte Carlo simulations give important and reliable results for systems of biological interest. We envisage possibilities to enlarge the investigations of this type in the following directions:

1. Studying the dependence of the free energy vs. a larger range of surfaces
2. Carrying out the simulations described in Section VI. for cylindrically and spherically curved interface (The difference between the free energies of flat and curved monolayers will give the contribution of the hydrophobic core to the curvature elastic moduli of the monolayer.)
3. Simulations of bilayer consisting of two monolayers of the type described (The interactions between the monolayers of the bilayer will be taken into account in this way.)
4. Examining of systems containing not only hydrophobic chains, but hydrophilic heads, too

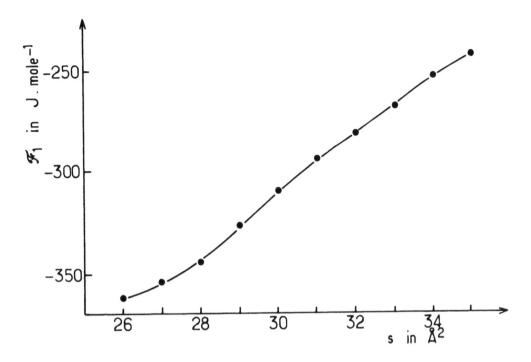

FIGURE 23.   Dependence of the free energy $\mathscr{F}_1$ per chain on the mean area per chain.

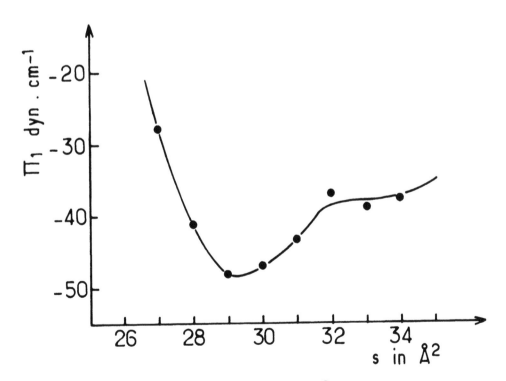

FIGURE 24.   Dependence of the lateral pressure $\Pi_1 = -\dfrac{\partial \mathscr{F}_1}{\partial_s}$ on the mean area per chain.

The first steps in this direction are already done.[30-32] The essential problem in dealing with the hydrophilic parts of the amphiphilic molecule is the interaction with the water molecules. The solution of this problem will help to make a step to the description of more realistic objects and to introduce proteins, nucleic acids, etc. in order to approach the real biological membrane.

ACKNOWLEDGMENTS

We should like to express our gratitude to Mr. Moineau for technical assistance in the preparation of the manuscript. One of us (I.B.) uses this opportunity to thank Professor Bothorel and all the colleagues of the Centre de Recherche Paul Pascal, Talence, France, where part of the work was done, with a grant of the Centre National de la Recherche Scientifique, for the hospitality during his stay there. This work is supported financially by the Centre National de la Recherche Scientifique in France and the Bulgarian Ministry of Culture, Science, and Education through Contract 587/15.07.1987.

REFERENCES

1. **Bothorel, P. and Lussan, C.,** Sur un modele de membrane biologique base sur les interactions lipides-proteines, *C. R. Acad. Sci.,* 266, 2492, 1968.
2. **Lussan, C. and Bothorel, P.** Quelques aspects nouveaux d'un modele de membrane biologique, *C. R. Acad. Sci.,* 268, 1118, 1969.
3. **Bothorel, P. and Lussan, C.,** Quelques aspects nouveaux d'un modele dynamique de membrane biologique, *C. R. Acad. Sci.,* 271, 680, 1970.
4. **Vanderkooi, G.,** Organization of proteins in membranes with special reference to the cytochrome oxidase system, *Biochim. Biophys. Acta,* 344, 307, 1974.
5. **Singer, S. J. and Nicolson, G. L.,** Fluid mosaic model of the structure of cell membrane, *Science,* 175, 720, 1972.
6. **Lennard-Jones, J. E.,** *Trans Faraday Soc.,* 28, 333, 1932.
7. **Lifson, S. and Warshel, A.,** Consistent force field for calculations of conformations, vibrational spectra, and enthalpies of cycloalkane and *n*-alkane molecules, *J. Chem. Phys.,* 49, 5116, 1968.
8. **van der Ploeg, P. and Berendsen, H. J. C.,** Molecular dynamics simulation of a bilayer membrane, *J. Chem. Phys.,* 76, 3271, 1982.
9. **Edholm, O., Berendsen, H. J. C., and van der Ploeg, P.,** Conformational entropy of a bilayer membrane derived from a molecular dynamics simulation, *Mol. Phys.,* 48, 379, 1983.
10. **van der Ploeg, P. and Berendsen, H. J. C.,** Molecular dynamics of a bilayer, *Mol. Phys.,* 49, 233, 1983.
11. **Ryckaert, J. P. and Bellemans, A.,** Molecular dynamics of liquid alkanes, *Faraday Discuss. Chem. Soc.,* 66, 95, 1978.
12. **Volkenstein, M. V.,** *Configurational Statistics of Polymeric Chains,* John Wiley & Sons, New York, 1963.
13. **Bothorel, P., Lussan, C., Lemaire, B., and Belle, J.,** Analyse conformationnelle des chaines aliphatiques de lecithines synthetiques en couches bimoleculaires, *C. R. Acad. Sci.,* 274, 1541, 1972.
14. **Phillips, M. C., Williams, R. M., and Chapman, D.,** On the nature of hydrocarbon chain motions in lipid liquid crystals, *Chem. Phys. Lipids,* 3, 234, 1969.
15. **Bothorel, P., Belle, J., and Lemaire, B.,** Theoretical study of aliphatic chain structure in mono- and bilayers, *Chem. Phys. Lipids,* 12, 96, 1974.
16. **Belle, J., Bothorel, P., and Lemaire, B.,** Melting entropy and structure of aliphatic chains in mono- and bilayers, *FEBS Lett.,* 39, 115, 1974.
17. **Bothorel, P.,** Sur quelques proprietes structurales interessantes des chaines aliphatiques, *J. Chim. Phys.,* 7-8, 1133, 1974.
18. **Belle, J.,** Birefringence, in De l'Etude Theorique des Proprietes Structurales des Chaines Aliphatiques dans les Milieux Modeles de Membranes: Mono et Bicouches Moleculaires, These de Docteur Ingenieur, Universite de Bordeaux, 1973, chap. 7.
19. **Metropolis, N., Rosenbluth, A. W., Rosenbluth, M. N., Teller, A. M., and Teller, E.,** Equation of state calculations by fast computing machines, *J. Chem. Phys.,* 21, 1087, 1953.

20. **Bothorel, P. and Belle, J.,** De l'influence de la flexibilite des chaines aliphatiques sur les proprietes thermodynamiques des couches monomoleculaires amphiphiles, *C. R. Acad. Sci.,* 282, 437, 1976.
21. **Belle, J. and Bothorel, P.,** Thermodynamical study of the phospholipid chain structure in mono- and bilayers, *Nouv. J. Chim.,* 1, 265, 1977.
22. **Bothorel, P.,** Conformations moleculaires aux interfaces, *Collol. nationaux C.N.R.S.,* 938, 91, 1978.
23. **Lemaire, B. and Bothorel, P.,** Conformational analysis of aliphatic chains at interfaces. Influence of the radius of curvature, *Macromolecules,* 13, 311, 1980.
24. **Lemaire, B. and Bothorel, P.,** Statistical mechanics of aliphatic chain layers, influence of chain length mixing, *J. Polym. Sci. Polym. Phys. Ed.,* 20, 867, 1982.
25. **Fourche, G. and Bothorel, P.,** *J. Chim. Phys.,* 66, 54, 1969.
26. **Hill, T. L.,** *Statistical Mechanics,* McGraw-Hill, New York, 1956.
27. **Kwok, R. and Evans, E. A.,** Thermoelasticity of large lecithin bilayer vesicles, *Biophys. J.,* 35, 637, 1981.
28. **Bivas, I., Lemaire, B., and Bothorel, P.,** to be published.
29. **Bivas, I., Lemaire, B., and Bothorel, P.,** to be published.
30. **Kreissler, M. and Bothorel, P.,** Theoretical conformational analysis of phospholipids: influence of the parallelism of the β and γ alkyl chains on the glycerol moeity conformations. Anchoring of the aliphatic chains at the hydrophobic-hydrophilic interface, *Chem. Phys. Lipids,* 22, 261, 1978.
31. **Kreissler, M., Lemaire, B., and Bothorel, P.,** Theoretical conformational analysis of phospholipids. I. Study of the interactions between phospholipid molecules by use of semi-empirical methods with the explicit introduction of polar headgroup interactions, *Biochim. Biophys. Acta,* 735, 12, 1983.
32. **Kreissler, M., Lemaire, B., and Bothorel, P.,** Theoretical conformational analysis of phospholipids. II. Role of the hydration in the gel to liquid crystal transition of phospholipids, *Biochim. Biophys. Acta,* 735, 23, 1983.

Chapter 1.A.3

COMPUTER AIDED METHODS FOR THE STUDY OF LIPID CHAIN PACKING IN MODEL BIOMEMBRANES AND MICELLES

H. L. Scott

TABLE OF CONTENTS

I. INTRODUCTION: LIPID CHAIN PACKING IN BILAYERS AND MICELLES

A. THE CHAIN PACKING PROBLEM IN LIPID AGGREGATES IN AQUEOUS SOLUTION

The distinguishing characteristic of all molecules with which this volume is concerned is their amphipathic nature, i.e., they contain both water-soluble (hydrophilic) and water-insoluble (hydrophobic) parts. It is well known that whenever molecules such as these are added to water in sufficient quantity, they self-associate into aggregates in order to minimize contact between the water and the hydrocarbon portion of each molecule. When this happens, the hydrocarbon chains of the surfactants are forced into close contact and each chain is limited in its conformational freedom by the close presence of neighboring chains. Aggregates of amphiphilic molecules in solution therefore can be said to contain two strongly interacting parts. The first is the interface with the aqueous solvent. In this region, the polar groups of the amphiphiles interact with water molecules electrostatically, via van der Waals or 6- to 12-type forces and via hydrogen bonding. The second strongly interacting part of an aggregate in solution occurs in the interior of the structure, where hydrocarbon chains translate, rotate, and change shape within the confined interior volume.

The purpose of this article is to describe methods by which high-speed computers have been used to generate and study models for the hydrocarbon interiors of surfactant aggregates in solution. This article will not address the very complex interfacial interactions directly. Rather, it will be assumed that these interactions effectively provide a geometrical constraint on the volume accessible to the hydrocarbon interior. The "chain packing problem" can then be stated as the problem of determining the optimum packing of hydrocarbon chains in the given volume. This is both a static and a dynamic problem. The static aspects involve average overall chain conformations and interaction strengths. The dynamic aspects involve the rotational, translational, and conformational mobility of the chains in the restricted volume. Both aspects of the chain packing problem are important for two reasons. Firstly, along with the interactions at the aqueous interface, the packing of the chains plays a major role in the determination of the ultimate overall shape of the aggregate. Secondly, the chain packing governs the physical state of the hydrocarbon interior of the structure. Of all the possible types of aggregates of surfactants in solution, the scope of this article will be limited to spherical and cylindrical micelles and planar bilayers.

In the next section, the nature of the information available from experimental and analytical theoretical studies of chain packing in bilayers and micelles will be described in order to point out the need for a detailed picture of the hydrocarbon region at the molecular level. The experimental data shed much light on this picture, but do not yet present an unambiguous picture at the microscopic level. Also, purely analytical theories are not yet capable of directly addressing microscopic behavior in such complex systems or do so only in very approximate ways. This leads naturally to the discussion in Sections II and III on the use of high-speed computers to add insights to the chain packing problem. Section II describes the numerical generation of hydrocarbon chains in various geometries, and Section III describes the application of these methods to the packing problem.

B. EXPERIMENTAL AND THEORETICAL STUDIES OF CHAIN PACKING

Experimental studies of the structure of the hydrocarbon region of bilayers[1-5] and micelles[6,7] have been described thoroughly in earlier reviews. Of all experimental tools available, the most detailed information related to the hydrocarbon interior of micelles and bilayers comes from magnetic resonance experiments[1,2] and for bilayers, information comes X-ray diffraction studies.[8] In order to introduce the reader to the physical properties of micelles and bilayer, the overall picture of the hydrocarbon interiors of these systems which has emerged from experiments will be described. Then a description of current analytical theoretical models for the same systems will be presented.

From the X-ray diffraction experiments which began in the 1960s,[8] it is known that the primary structure formed by double chain amphiphiles such as phospholipids is a single or multiple stack of bimolecular layers, each with the chains in the central region and the polar groups on the two outer surfaces. Within these layers the X-ray data further reveal that the chains are, at sufficiently high temperature, in a state resembling liquid hydrocarbon. As the temperature is lowered, the chains undergo one or more ordering phase transitions in which the packing becomes crystalline in nature, with interchain spacing (in a typical phospholipid, dipalmitoylphosphatidylcholine) of 4.85 Å and all chains aligned parallel to each other in extended (all-*trans*) conformations. At temperatures of biological interest, the hydrocarbon interior of most lipid bilayers is in its fluid state, and the detailed nature of the chain interactions has been probed using magnetic resonance methods.[1-3] By incorporating a small number of probe molecules which resemble the lipid molecules but contain an additional chemical group with an excess free electron such as a nitroxide radical to act as a spin label, the motional state of the hydrocarbon interior may be measured using electron spin resonance.[2,9] In general it is found that the lipid molecules diffuse laterally very rapidly and undergo rapid axial rotation. Nuclear magnetic resonance studies of the hydrocarbon region of lipid bilayers are possible using a variety of nuclei, including ^{13}C, ^{1}H, ^{2}H, and ^{19}F.[1,3,10] Collectively, these experiments reveal complex motions on fast and slow time scales. The fast motions (relaxation times $\sim 10^{-8}$ s or faster) include *trans-gauche* segmental rotations and lateral molecular diffusion. Slower motions include collective chain tilting, molecular long axis rotation, and diffusion near barriers such as proteins or cholesterol.[11]

The equilibrium picture of lipid chain packing in bilayers is best described by the segmental order parameter profile:

$$S_n = \tfrac{1}{2} <3\cos^2\theta_n -1> \tag{1}$$

where θ_n is the deviation of the nth C–C or C–H bond from its orientation in the *trans* configuration. This profile is important because segmental rotation is a major mechanism by which surfactant hydrocarbon chains fill available volume. One need only look at the chain melting phase transition in lipid bilayers to see the impact the segmental isomeric degrees of freedom have upon the chain states.[12] If θ_n is always zero, as in an ordered state, then S_n is identically 1. However, if θ_n varies freely, then S_n averages to zero. Values of S_n intermediate between 0 and 1 indicate intermediate states of isomeric disorder. The ^{2}H NMR experiments on bilayers composed of chains specifically deuterated at one segment provide the best order parameter data because the quadrupolar splitting in the spectrum is directly proportional to $P_2(\cos\beta_n)$, where $P_2(\cos\theta)$ is the second Legendre polynomial described in Equation 1 and β_n is the angle between C–^{2}H bond number n and the applied field. If β_n is substituted for θ_n in Equation 1, a perfectly ordered chain with axial symmetry will have order parameter -0.5 for each carbon position. An additional factor of -2 then converts the data to molecular long-axis order parameters and these fit the definition of the true segmental order parameter given in Equation 1.[3] Collective chain tilting reduces this value by roughly the same scale factor for each n^1 so that the experimental S_n's have maximum values of ~ 0.5. For a comparison between the order parameter data and calculations which do not include the effects of chain tilting, a scale factor of 0.5 is appropriate, as dividing all of the experimental order parameters by 0.5 normalizes the data so that the S_n are close to unity for n close to the upper end of the chain. In bilayers after normalization, the S_n are near unity for bonds within about 4 from the polar region and then gradually decrease in magnitude until the terminal bonds are reached, where $S_n \sim 0.4$. A graphical comparison between experimental and calculated order parameters for bilayers will be shown later in Section III.

While double-chain amphiphiles such as phospholipids generally form bilayers, the primary structure formed by amphiphiles with a single hydrocarbon chain is that of a spherical or cylindrical micelle, with polar groups roughly defining the outer surface. The same experimental techniques discussed above have been applied to the hydrocarbon interior of micelles, with qualitatively similar results.[7] Namely, the interior of micelles consists of hydrocarbon in a very liquid-like state. On an quantitative level, there are differences between chain packing in lamellar and micellar systems. Order parameters for the segments in micelles are found to be close to unity (after normalization) for the first one or two segments (as compared to four to six segments in bilayers). Then the S_n decrease more sharply with increasing n, reflecting a more highly disordered state than was found in the interiors of bilayers.[7] This is undoubtedly a consequence of the more-or-less spherical constraint on the overall micellar shape as opposed to the lamellar geometry of bilayers. It is difficult to directly compare the interiors of micelles and bilayers using such experimental data as relaxation times because of the contribution from tumbling of the micelles. A very rough picture of the hydrocarbon interior of both micelles and bilayers which emerges is one of an oily liquid, with some restrictions on orientational disordering and by implication fluidity, close to the polar group/water interface. In order to obtain deeper insights into the molecular properties responsible for the observed states, it is necessary to construct theoretical models for the systems under consideration.

Lipid bilayers have been the focus of numerous theoretical investigations,[13] with primary emphasis on the hydrocarbon region and in particular the chain melting phase transition in this region. In general the statistical mechanics of a system as complicated as a lipid bilayer or a micelle are far too complex to permit exact calculations of the properties of realistic models. Therefore two approaches to the problem have evolved. On the one hand, it is possible to design simple models which contain some of the salient properties of the lipid systems and which are amenable to exact statistical mechanical calculation. This approach was pioneered by Nagle.[14] However, the paucity of even simple models which are exactly solvable in statistical mechanics[15] severely limits the scope of this sort of effort. On the other hand, it is possible to devise more complex theoretical models and use various approximation techniques to assess the predictions of the theory. This latter approach is by far the most common and many different theoretical models and approximation schemes have been presented.[13] The model of Marcelja[16] is a very successful example of the use of well-conceived approximation schemes to study the equilibrium properties of the hydrocarbon region of bilayers and micelles. Marcelja's model[16] is an extension of the well-known mean field approximation of statistical mechanics. The theory considers a single hydrocarbon chain in a self-consistent mean field which represents the net interaction of the chain in question with all other chains. In order to include all contributions from the many different single-chain conformations, a computer is used to sequentially generate all single-chain conformations, and the mean field, which depends upon these conformations, is obtained through a nonlinear algebraic equation. What emerges from this procedure is the average segmental order parameters which may then be directly compared with experiment. With only two adjustable parameters, the agreement between theory and experiment is striking. This is very surprising because one suspects that the order parameter profiles should be the direct consequence of hard core excluded volume interactions between neighboring chains. The mean field approach does not incorporate these interactions, opting to consider a single isolated chain in a uniform interaction field. Marcelja's method has been further refined and applied to micelles by Gruen,[17,18] with equal success in matching the experimental order parameter profiles. A further assumption in Gruen's approach is that the density of the hydrocarbon core of amphiphilic aggregates is uniformly that of liquid hydrocarbon. Attempts to explicitly include the effects of the excluded volume interactions between hydrocarbon chain segments have been made by Dill and Flory[19] and more recently by Szleifer et al.[20-22] However, the formidable difficulties encountered in geometric molecular packing calculations have forced these authors to incorporate approximation schemes in order to derive properties of their models. It is again beyond the scope of the present article to describe the methods of these authors, but a simple synopsis is that in all cases single-chain mean field calculations are used. Realistic excluded volume calculations are simply not possible for such complex systems.

The experimental data provide a wealth of information concerning the motions and segmental rotations of the chains in the hydrocarbon region of bilayers and micelles, and the mean field theories provide a description of the systems. What is still missing, however, is detailed microscopic information. For instance, it is still unclear how many and what type of *gauche* rotations occur in the chains. The average chain shape and the interactions which affect chain packing are not yet clear. This is because no experimental technique is yet sufficiently sensitive to probe at the single-molecule level, and the mean field theories enclose all the interchain interactions in the mean field from which little or no microscopic information can be obtained. In the past decade, rapid advances in computer technology have made it possible to use high-speed machines to generate and examine molecular interactions at the molecular level. This has opened a new approach to complex scientific problems which is neither purely theoretical nor purely experimental and which makes it possible to examine static and dynamic properties of individual molecules in model systems. The high speed and storage capacity of modern computers makes it possible to use models which are very complex and realistic and to simulate systems which are sufficiently large that finite size effects are generally minimal. As will be discussed in subsequent sections, the use of computers for molecular simulation is not without drawbacks. However, the potential gains from simulations are sufficiently great that many scientists now regularly perform large-scale simulations in order to better interpret experimental data or in order to gain new theoretical insights. In the following sections, the methods used for the computer generation of molecular states of the hydrocarbon interior of amphiphilic aggregates will be described, and in Section III, the simulation techniques and the results will be detailed.

II. THE NUMERICAL GENERATION OF LIPID CHAIN CONFORMATIONAL STATES

A. METHODS INVOLVING LATTICE MODELS FOR LIPID AGGREGATES

The numerical generation of a polymeric chain or chains may be accomplished by a variety of means, but all methods are necessarily either lattice based or continuum based. The focus of this section is the lattice-based techniques. The earliest attempt to generate configurations of hydrocarbon-like chains on a lattice to this writer's knowledge is that of Whittington and Chapman[23] in which a line of chains was generated on a two-dimensional lattice with the constraint that one end of every chain was fixed on the top row of the lattice, simulating a one-dimensional monolayer. Chains were then generated segment by segment using a random walk procedure which disallowed overlaps. By varying the distance between the topmost carbons, Whittington and Chapman[23] obtained a qualitative picture of the effect of chain density on chain packing.

It is now possible, using faster computers with greater storage capabilities, to generate larger numbers of chains on full three-dimensional lattices. Pratt and co-workers[24,25] used a diamond lattice, which closely models the tetrahedral geometry of polymethylene chains, to study bilayers consisting of up to 336 chains of 6 carbons each and micelles of up to 50 chains of 4 segments each. Chain segments interact with other segments on neighboring lattice sites in this method, and the Monte Carlo method (to be discussed below) is used to both move chains laterally and perpendicular to the bilayer plane and to generate different chain conformations within the constraints of the underlying lattice. In both cases, 10^6 to

10^8 configurations were generated, and density profiles and order parameter profiles were calculated as averages over all the configurations. In all cases, the lattice spacing parameter was set equal to the average interchain spacing. This is, of course, larger than the bond length between adjacent carbons on any one chain, so Pratt et al. are forced to assume each lattice point represents not a single methylene, but an n-CH_2 group, where $n \sim 3$.[24,25] This places a severe constraint on the number of accessible configurations for each molecule, since molecular conformations may be generated by rotations about any C–C bond. In the micelle simulations, Haan and Pratt[24] begin with a spherical arrangement of chains on the underlying lattice and at each Monte Carlo step a chain configuration is changed to another by moving one or more of the subunits to adjacent lattice points. Since the chain density in the simulation is close to the experimental density, it is not surprising that $\sim$95% of the moves are rejected. It is also not surprising that the resulting picture of micelle structure differs substantially from that described in the theories discussed above. The main difference is that the simulation obtains highly nonuniform aggregates with uneven density profiles, while the theories assume uniformity. Unfortunately, it is unclear whether the discrepancy is due to a fault in the theoretical assumption or to oversimplification in the numerical model. At the densities of interest in micelles, one expects most lattice sites to be filled, so the rejection rate should indeed be very high for such a coarse-grained lattice. A finer lattice scale would allow smaller moves and fewer rejections. It would also allow lattice points to be sites for single molecules in the chains so that a far greater set of configurations would then be available. The effect of these improvements upon the simulations may be substantial. In the bilayer simulation, Owenson and Pratt[25] study a much larger system beginning in an ordered lamellar arrangement, and they are able to generate many more configurations. However, for the same reasons as in the micelle calculations, the rejection rate is very high. Order parameter profiles calculated in the simulations are in qualitative agreement with theoretical calculations, but quantitative comparison reveals differences which the authors attribute to interactions between the two monolayers in the bilayer. Clearly, the finer the lattice scale, the more accurate the simulation for lattice models such as these. A simulation of monomolecular layer of amphiphiles in which the underlying lattice constant is the C–C bond length was carried out by Harris and Rice.[26] Here the goal was to describe a monolayer of surfactant at an air-water interface under conditions of partial coverage, i.e., low hydrocarbon density. Densities were small compared to those found in the interiors of bilayers and micelles, although they were sufficiently high in some of the simulations to force chain alignment more or less perpendicular to the interface. This underscores the point that the major difficulty in the computer generation of chain configurations in dense surfactant aggregates is that it is extremely difficult to find free volume for any chain to utilize in changing conformations. This limitation is more severe for coarse-grained lattice simulations, but is a problem for any computer modeling effort. In the next section, continuum efforts will be discussed.

There is one type of lattice model for surfactant bilayers for which the excluded volume problem is avoided entirely in computer simulations. In this class of models, each point of the underlying lattice contains not some portion of the hydrocarbon chain of a amphiphile, but the entire chain,[27,28] i.e., the underlying lattice is now two dimensional for models of bilayers and the hydrocarbon chains are point particles occupying the lattice sites. In order to accommodate the large number of degrees of freedom associated with chain conformations, each lattice site is assigned a state variable which may take on a number of discrete values and may have a large degeneracy to accommodate multiple chain conformations. It is then possible to make an association between the state variable and a subset of chain conformations and to assign such chain properties as energy or lateral area to each state. One then has a statistical model which may be studied analytically or numerically. A ten-state version of this model has been used as a basis for Monte Carlo simulations to study phase equilibria, among other things, in lipid bilayers.[27] Models such as this have the advantage that many properties of the model system are accessible to calculations since they are so simple. It is further possible to construct the state properties of the models so that many of the calculated properties agree well with experiment. However, this class of models totally masks the underlying mechanisms which are in large part responsible for the behavior which they predict, namely, the detailed excluded volume interactions between chain segments. This class of models, like the mean field models, does not contribute to an understanding of the microscopic picture of chain interactions in surfactant aggregates.

B. METHODS INVOLVING CONTINUUM MODELS FOR LIPID AGGREGATES

If forcing hydrocarbon chains onto a lattice limits the number and type of chain conformations which one can generate by computer, then an attractive option is to simply abandon the lattice and to allow free placement of chain subunits with only the constraints imposed by the basic molecular geometry of the chains. In the continuum approach, the critical question is how does one numerically produce a set of coordinates which represents the molecules on the chain and which must satisfy the constraints imposed by the length and orientation of the bonds between molecules? Some of the standard methods include[29] the bead-rod model, in which the chain is represented by a "string of beads" with freely jointed bonds connecting the beads, and the bead-spring model, in which the inflexible rods are replaced by harmonic springs. (For a review of these methods and lattice techniques, see Reference 29.) The disadvantage of the string of beads method is that the tetrahedral bonding angles and *trans-gauche* isomerism are not included. For very long chains or for dilute polymer fluids, this approximation may not be severe, but for surfactant chain aggregates in solution, where chain density is relatively high due to hydrophobic pressures, the chain bonding geometry and the bond rotational degrees of freedom must play significant roles in the chain packing problem.

It is possible to generate arbitrarily long chains of hydrocarbon molecules with fixed bond angles and in a variety of conformations produced by *gauche* rotations about any of the bonds. This technique, introduced by Curro[30] for the simulation of polymer fluids, has been extensively refined and applied to the generation and analysis of chain configurations in lipid bilayers and micelles by Scott and co-workers.[30-34] The method faithfully reproduces chains with proper bond angles and allows for the insertion of *gauche* rotations at any desired bond location. It may be applied to planar, cylindrical, spherical, or three-dimensional arrays of chains. It is therefore a powerful tool for the study of these configurations. In the following paragraphs, this method will be described in detail.

The method for generation of a single chain in several conformational states will first be described. This method may be directly applied to chain coordinate calculations in a planar system. Later, modifications to allow for the study of chains in cylindrical or spherical geometries will be presented. Consider the Cartesian coordinate system shown in Figure 1. Place the first carbon of the chain at the origin. Supposing that the chain will propagate along the x-axis, place the second carbon at the point $(l\ 0\ 0)$, where l is the bond length. The position of the third carbon is then calculated by first relocating the origin of the coordinates at the position of the second carbon and then rotating the coordinate axes about the y or z-axis so that the new x-axis is inclined at an angle θ with the original x-axis, where θ is related to the bond angle α by $\theta = \pi - \alpha$. After placing the third carbon at the point $(l\ 0\ 0)$ in the new coordinate system, the fourth carbon position is determined by locating the origin of the coordinates at the third carbon position and rotating the axes about the same axis as used in the previous step, but now by the angle $-\theta$. After $N - 1$ successive translation and rotation steps, the coordinates of a chain of N carbons are calculated. The orientation of the chain may be changed by rotation of all C–C bonds about any axis. The entire operation is expressed mathematically by successive translations plus rotations so that

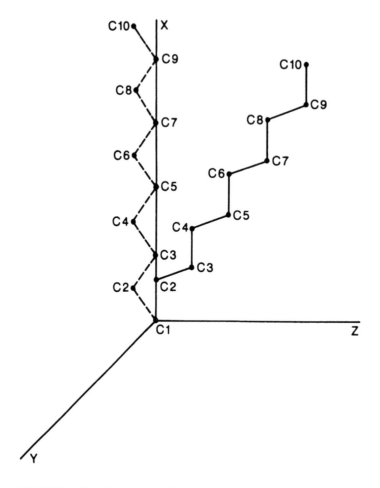

FIGURE 1.   Coordinate axes used in the algorithm for the generation of hydrocarbon chain coordinates of the carbon atoms: solid line, chain as generated by
the matrix $\vec{O}$; dashed line, chain after application of matrix $\vec{T}$. Matrices are defined
in text.

the position of carbon number $i + 1$ is obtained from the position of carbon number i by
the algorithm:[30]

$$\vec{R}_{i+1} = \vec{R}_i + \vec{T} \cdot \vec{O}_i \cdot \begin{pmatrix} 1 \\ 0 \\ 0 \end{pmatrix} \qquad (2a)$$

where the operator $\vec{O}_i$ has the form of a rotation operator about the z-axis:

$$\vec{O} = \begin{bmatrix} \cos\theta & \sin\theta & 0 \\ \sin\theta & -\cos\theta & 0 \\ 0 & 0 & 1 \end{bmatrix} \qquad (2b)$$

and the operator $\vec{T}$ performs the task of aligning the entire chain by rotating each bond by
the desired chain orientation angle about the same axis used in $\vec{O}$.

$$\overset{\Rightarrow}{T} = \begin{bmatrix} \cos\alpha & -\sin\alpha & 0 \\ \sin\alpha & \cos\alpha & 0 \\ 0 & 0 & 1 \end{bmatrix} \tag{3}$$

It should be noted that, while $\overset{\Rightarrow}{T}$ is a standard rotation operator,[35] $\overset{\Rightarrow}{O}$ is not. In order to achieve a zig-zag chain structure in the y direction as Figure 1 shows, the signs of the elements in the second column of $\overset{\Rightarrow}{O}$ are reversed from those of a standard uniaxial rotation operator. For poly-CH_2 chains, the bond angle is the tetrahedral angle 109.5°, so θ in Equation 2 is 70.5°. If α in Equation 3 is zero, the procedure produces the chain drawn in a solid line in Figure 1. In order to produce a chain which propagates along the positive *x*-axis, the angle α in Equation 3 is set at 35.25°, as shown by the dashed chain in Figure 1. Rotation of the entire chain about its long axis may be done by replacing $\overset{\Rightarrow}{T}$ by a matrix which, using the coordinate axes of Figure 1, produces rotations about the y-axis and following this with the chain orientation operator $\overset{\Rightarrow}{T}$. If β is the desired long-axis angle of rotation, then the operator $\overset{\Rightarrow}{T}$ becomes

$$\overset{\Rightarrow}{T} = \begin{bmatrix} \cos\alpha & -\sin\alpha\,\cos\beta\,\sin\alpha\,\sin\beta \\ \sin\alpha & \cos\alpha\,\cos\beta\,-\cos\alpha\,\sin\beta \\ 0 & \sin\beta & \cos\beta \end{bmatrix} \tag{4}$$

The above procedure produces chains in all-*trans* conformations which may be oriented in any direction. In order to obtain non-*trans* chain conformations, dihedral angle rotations must be included in the rotation operations. In the geometry of Figure 1, the dihedral axis of rotation is the *x*-axis. Thus, a *gauche* bond at bond number *n* requires that the entire chain below bond *n* be rotated about the *x*-axis by the *gauche* rotation angle. In the rotational-isomerism approximation, the allowed angles for this rotation are ± 120°. At the appropriate point in the operation given in Equation 2, one inserts a rotation operator about the *x*-axis with the desired *gauche* angle. This requires some care because of the alternating nature of the chains. The operator $\overset{\Rightarrow}{O}$ is actually a product of a standard rotation operator and an operator which reflects through the y axis. The *gauche* rotation operator does not commute with this operation, so the chain generation procedure must be modified when *gauche* rotations are included. The procedure is as follows:

1. Pick a bond, *k*, about which to perform the *gauche* rotation. Let$\overset{\Rightarrow}{R_k}'$ be the vector coordinate of the end point of bond k in the system in which the origin is at the beginning of bond k. $\overset{\Rightarrow}{R_k}$ is the vector coordinate of the end point of bond k when the origin is at the beginning of bond one.

2. Define the *gauche* rotation operator $\overset{\Rightarrow}{G}$ by

$$\overset{\Rightarrow}{G} = \begin{bmatrix} 1 & 0 & 0 \\ 0 & \cos\phi & \sin\phi \\ 0 & -\sin\phi & \cos\phi \end{bmatrix} \tag{5}$$

where ϕ is the *gauche* rotation angle.

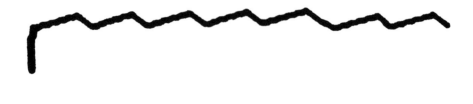

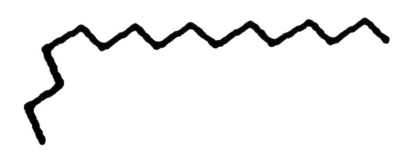

FIGURE 2.   Two chains produced by the matrix method described in the text, with *gauche* rotations. The chain on the left has a *gauche-trans-gauche* kink.

3.   If k is an even number, then

$$\vec{R}_{k+1} = \vec{\vec{T}} \cdot \vec{\vec{G}} \cdot \vec{\vec{O}} \cdot \vec{R}_k + \vec{R}_k \tag{6}$$

4.   If k is an odd number, then define the z-axis rotation operator $\vec{\vec{Z}}$ as

$$\vec{\vec{Z}} = \begin{bmatrix} \cos\theta & \sin\theta & 0 \\ -\sin\theta & \cos\theta & 0 \\ 0 & 0 & 1 \end{bmatrix} \tag{7}$$

where θ is 70.5° and calculate R_{k+1} as

$$\vec{R}_{k+1} = \vec{\vec{T}} \cdot \vec{\vec{Z}}^{-1} \cdot \vec{\vec{G}} \cdot \vec{\vec{Z}} \cdot \vec{\vec{O}} \cdot \vec{R}_k + \vec{R}_k \tag{8}$$

Figure 2 shows a chain with a single *gauche* bond and a chain with a *gauche⁺ trans-gauche⁻* kink sequence, both generated by the above procedure. It is evident that this procedure is capable of generating a hydrocarbon chain or a number of chains of any length, with any set of bond angles and dihedral angles, at any location in the space assigned to the model system. In the next section, application of the above and other numerical chain generation methods will be described.

III. APPLICATION OF NUMERICAL CHAIN GENERATION METHODS TO THE STUDY OF CHAIN PACKING

A. FEW CHAIN STUDIES

The method described above for the generation of coordinates for the carbon atoms on hydrocarbon chains can be used to investigate interactions between aggregates of many amphiphiles or to investigate interactions between pairs of triplets of molecules. In this section, the latter application will be presented. Figure 3 shows two phospholipid molecules in three pair configurations typical of a lipid bilayer. The method described in the previous section was used to produce the chains, while the head group atomic coordinates were entered by hand.[36,37] Once relative coordinates of a pair of chains are known, one may easily calculate the interaction energy between the pair. Knowledge of the magnitudes of the pair interaction energies is vital for the construction of analytical theoretical models for amphiphile aggregates. This is because thermodynamic predictions of statistical mechanical theories are derived from the partition function, Z, which is a sum over all configurations of the model system having the form:

$$E_{pair} = \sum_{i,j} \epsilon \left[\left(\frac{\sigma}{r_{i,j}}\right)^{12} - \left(\frac{\sigma}{r_{i,j}}\right)^6 \right] + \frac{qq'}{r_{i,j}} \tag{9}$$

where $\beta = 1/kT$, k is Boltzmann's constant, T is the absolute temperature, and E(C) is the energy of configuration C. In most cases of interest, E(C) is expressed as a sum over all the members of the system of microscopic interactions between (usually) pairs of molecules or atoms. While this is still a very arduous task for realistic systems due to the enormous number of configurations, in many cases only a few configurations dominate the sum in Equation 9, making computer enumeration of all the relevant pair configurations a possibility.

As an example of the use of pair configuration energies to form the basis of a statistical mechanical model, Scott and Pearce[38] have used the procedure described in Equations 6 and 8 to formulate a model for lipid bilayers in low-temperature condensed phases. In the low-temperature phases, *gauche* rotations are nearly nonexistent, so only straight chains need be considered, greatly reducing the number of relevant configurations. Figure 3 shows examples of closely packed pairs of double chain C-16 phospholipid molecules (dipalmitoylphosphstidylcholine or DPPC). It is evident from this figure that the protruding head group interferes with the chain packing. In order to pack the chains as closely as possible, several alternatives must be considered. The basic packing problem is illustrated in Figure 3A, where the head groups prevent the chains from achieving close-packing densities. Figures 3B and 3C, illustrate possible solutions to the problem. In order to describe the packing via a statistical mechanical model, it is necessary to determine the energies of all the important configurations. Since the configurations of the system are built from individual molecules, the task is to denumerate all important configurations of pairs of molecules and calculate the intermolecular energies. These energies are then used to construct the configuration energies needed in Equation 9. The energies are calculated directly from the atomic coordinates of the molecules as sums of 1-6-12 potential energies:

$$Z = \sum_C e^{-\beta E(C)} \tag{10}$$

where $r_{i,j}$ is the distance between atoms on neighboring molecules and the sum runs over all atoms on both molecules. The interaction strength ϵ and the van der Waals' radius σ were taken from optimized potential functions constructed by Jorgensen and co-workers[39] where possible. It is to be emphasized that no curve fitting is involved here. All parameters in Equation 10 are fixed before calculations are begun. The effective charges q are nonzero only for head group phosphate and choline groups, where $-0.5e$ and $+0.5e$, respectively, are used, e being the fundamental electronic charge.[36] The procedure used by Scott and Pearce[38] was to calculate pair interaction energies for DPPC molecules which were characterized by:

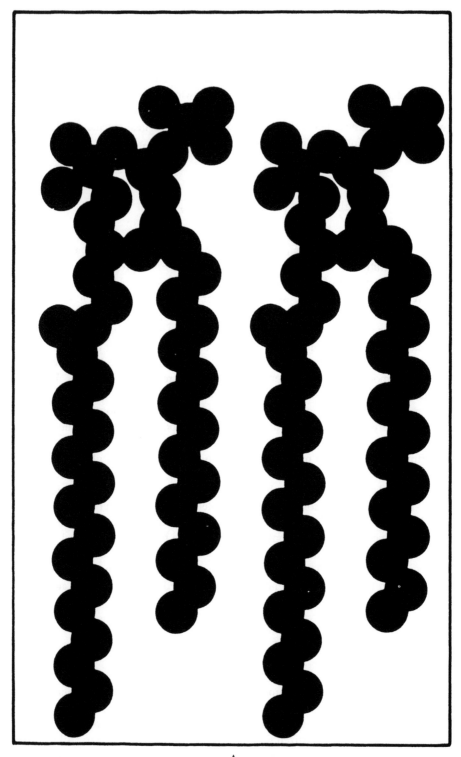

A

FIGURE 3.   Three illustrations of possible close packing configurations of two DPPC phospholipid molecules in one half of a bilayer in all-*trans* conformations. (A) Both molecules are at the same level relative to the bilayer plane. The protruding head groups make optimal chain packing impossible in this arrangement; (B) both molecules are at the same level, but the chains of the molecules tilt in order to pack more closely than in (A); (C) one chain is displaced 3 Å perpendicular to the bilayer plane with respect to the other to accommodate the head groups and to allow the chains to pack optimally.

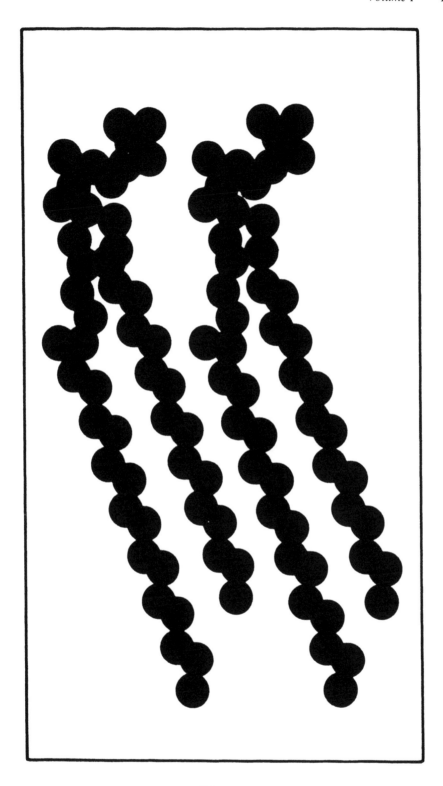

FIGURE 3B.

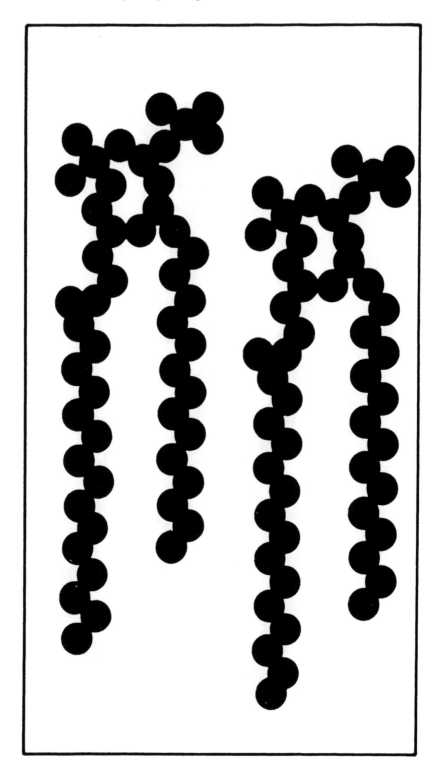

FIGURE 3C.

1. Parallel head groups, chain separation of 5.60 Å, chain tilt of 30°
2. Parallel head groups, chain separation 4.85 Å, no chain tilt, one chain displaced along chain long direction by varying amounts relative to the other
3. Antiparallel head groups, chain separation 4.85 and 5.60 Å, one chain displaced along long direction by varying amounts relative to the other

The data assembled from the above calculations provide a set of relative interaction strengths upon which to base the construction of a theoretical model. Clearly, no attempt was made to sample all possible pair configurations or perform a true energy minimization calculation. However, rigid large assymetrical molecules like DPPC can pack closely only in a limited number of ways. The two ways most commonly considered are those of (1) and (2) above. By tilting chains separated by 5.6 Å by 30°, one avoids head group overlap and allows close chain packing at the optimal separation of 4.85 Å (5.60 Å × cos30°). The alternative close chain packing scheme has chains displaced vertically relative to their neighbors and separated by 4.85 Å. The vertical separation avoids head group overlap and allows for optimal chain packing.[40] Both types of packing produce an ordered lipid phase with chains inclined by ~30° to the normal to the layer plane, but they are fundamentally different in that (1) requires cooperative long-range cooperative chain tilting, while (2) requires only single-molecule displacements by small amounts perpendicular to the layer plane. Scott and Pearce[38] used the pair interaction calculations to show that the perpendicular displacement packing mechanism (2) is slightly energetically favored over the direct chain tilting mechanism (1). They went on to use the relative energies calculated from the computer-generated conformations via Equation 10 to construct a lattice model for condensed phases in phospholipid bilayers.[38] The model not only predicts the correct type of chain tilted gel phase, but also exhibits a phase transition to a phase in which the molecular perpendicular displacements are trigonometrically modulated. Analysis of the model clearly shows a strong similarity between the modulations and the rippled $P_{\beta'}$ phase in DPPC and similar bilayers.

It is important to state precisely what the pair energies calculated above represent and what they do not represent. They do not represent the total interaction energies of the lipid molecules. Other contributions to the total energy include interactions with the aqueous solvent and interactions with chains in the other half of the bilayer. What the energies do represent are relative strengths of various packing configurations of pairs of isolated lipids. These may be used to construct a model for the lipid bilayer system under the assumption that all other contributions to the total energy are constant background terms in the temperature range of interest. Under this assumption, the technique of using a computer to generate the coordinates of atoms in lipid molecules and calculating interaction energies from these coordinates provides a powerful tool for the construction of theoretical models. Armed with the numerical data, a theoretical model may be constructed with fewer arbitrary assumptions about the nature of these interactions. Then, if the theoretical model fails to make predictions which are in accordance with experiment, the fault is more likely to lie in the analysis of the model than in the assumptions upon which it is built. Brasseur and Ruysschaert[41] have performed similar few-chain conformational analyses which are described elsewhere in this volume. The focus of this article will now shift to the computer generation of amphiphiles in larger numbers in aggregates and to the study of their properties by large-scale numerical simulation.

B. MONTE CARLO STUDIES OF MICELLES AND BILAYERS

In this section, computer simulation of amphiphilic aggregates will be discussed. There are two major classes of techniques most commonly utilized for large-scale simulations at this time, namely, Monte Carlo methods and molecular dynamics methods. The literature on both these techniques and their many applications is vast and beyond the scope of this report. Here the methods will be briefly outlined in this and the subsequent section and the applications relevant to amphiphilic aggregates will be discussed. In this section, the Monte Carlo method and its applications will be discussed. In the following section, the molecular dynamics method and its applications will be considered.

The Monte Carlo method for the study of many-particle systems is basically a method for numerically sampling the configuration space of the model system under consideration in order to estimate sums such as that in Equation 9 or averages based upon similar sums. The problem is that the number of configurations for even simple systems of modest size is astronomical, and so sampling algorithms must be devised to ensure sampling of the important configurations.[41] The procedure is simple to describe. First, it is necessary to define a model system consisting of a fixed number of objects (atoms or molecules) with well-defined constraints on their behavior interacting with each other via known potentials. Then a computer code must be written to carry out the sampling of the configuration space of the model in the following order:

1. Define and initialize all relevant physical properties of all constitiuents of the system
2. Pick a single member of the system (either by random choice or by sequentially moving through the system)
3. Change the state of the chosen member by a small random amount
4. Calculate the change in energy associated with the move and calculate the transition probability[42] associated with the change in state
5. Accept or reject the move according to how the transition probability compares with a random number
6. Calculate the contribution to any sums or averages of interest of the new configuration (In case of rejection, the old configuration becomes the new configuration)
7. Go to Step 2 until the desired number of configurations is generated

The above technique was first applied to a continuum model of lipid chains in half of a lipid bilayer by Scott.[31] The early work by Scott and Kalaskar has in recent years been improved and run on much larger and faster machines[33,34] and subsequently applied to nonlamellar systems. Here the application to lamellae will be described first and then the application to chains in spherical and cylindrical micellar systems will be presented. The model used consists of a number of chains, each of fixed length (between 10 and 18 carbons). The top carbons are positioned and constrained to remain on a flat plane representing the layer interface. In the early simulations, the chains interacted by hard sphere interactions only and the chain packing density was maintained by the fixed volume of the sample cell. In more recent work,[33,34] the interaction of Equation 10 is used. Chain configurations were generated by the method described in the previous section and the formation of kinks and jogs (pairs of *gauche* rotations separated by one or more *trans* bonds) were explicitly considered in each move. Because there are more degrees of freedom in an assembly of hydrocarbon chains, the configuration sampling algorithm must consider all of the following when a move is attempted: whole chain translation, long axis rotation, and one or more *gauche* rotations. Figure 4 shows a flowchart for a standard Monte Carlo simulation. The system size was limited to only six chains in the early work by available computing facilities, so the fluctuations in the data due to finite size effects were large. Nonetheless, it was possible to show definitively that the dominant mechanism by which lipid chains arrange themselves is the short range hard core repulsive interactions. In spite of the finite size effects, order parameter profiles produced during the Monte Carlo runs showed the same qualitative features as the experimental data. In the more recent work systems of 36 chains[33] and 100 chains,[34] the latter using a Cray supercomputer have been studied. It is interesting that for the larger systems, for which many more configurations were generated, the same

MONTE CARLO STUDY OF HYDROCARBON CHAINS

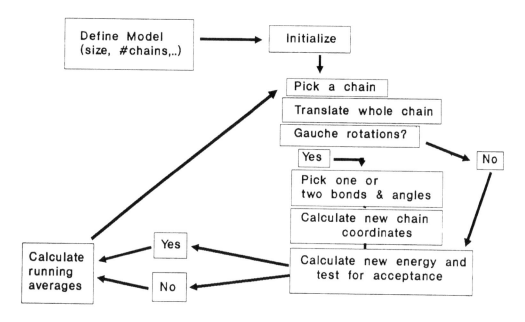

FIGURE 4.   Flow diagram of the Monte Carlo procedure for simulation of hydrocarbon chains in a continuum as described in the text.

basic trend in the order parameter profiles is reproduced, indicating that the conclusion drawn from the analysis of the smaller systems regarding the role of the repulsive excluded volume interactions is unchanged. Figure 5 is a plot of the order parameter profiles generated for bulk lipid chains, along with data from ^{2}H-NMR experiments on selectivity deuterated chains, with the latter data divided by 0.5 for reasons discussed earlier in this chapter. The objective of the recent work was, in addition to stimulating larger systems with more realistic interactions, to introduce a nonlipid membrane molecule into the simulation model cell in order to microscopically study the effect of this molecule on the lipid chain packing. This is important because perturbation of the lipid chains by proteins, cholesterol, or other nonlipid molecules could lead to indirect interactions between the nonlipid molecules in membranes which could be of biological significance.[43]

The first effort[33] in this direction considered an array of 35 lipid chains plus 1 immovable hard rod with rigid lumps representing a crude model membrane protein. It was found that the lipid chain conformations for chains adjacent to the model protein were only very slightly different from the lipids far away from the perturbant. However, this was a very simple model. When supercomputer time became available at the U.S. National Center for Supercomputing Applications, a system of 99 chains plus a cholesterol molecule was studied. The model for the cholesterol molecule consisted of the atomic coordinates of all nonhydrogen atoms, and the tail chain was allowed to change its conformation during the Monte Carlo moves. Figure 6 shows the cholesterol molecule and two of its near-neighbor chains. The major conclusion of this work was that the chains nearest the cholesterol are not forced into all-*trans* conformations, but their rotational freedom is restricted. This result represents the first microscopic picture of lipid-cholesterol interactions. It must be interpreted solely within the context of the model system used in the simulations, and it must be understood that the picture is not a dynamic one because the Monte Carlo method produces equilibrium results

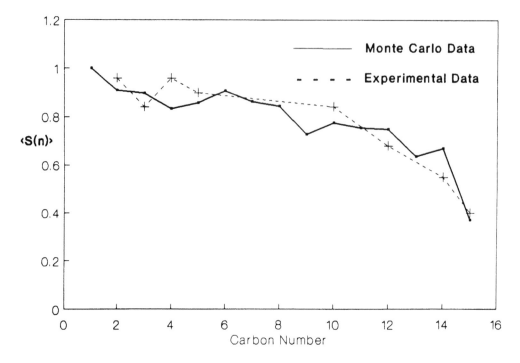

FIGURE 5.   Order parameter profiles for DPPC chains. Plot of $<S_n>$ vs. carbon number, n: solid line, Monte Carlo data from Reference 34; dashed line, experimental data from Reference 3 divided by 0.5 for reasons described in text.

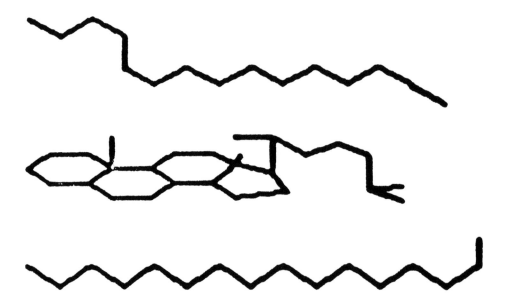

FIGURE 6.   A typical configuration, from the data of Reference 34, of a cholesterol molecule and two neighboring chains. Some folding of the lipid chains under the rigid portion of the cholesterol molecule is evident.

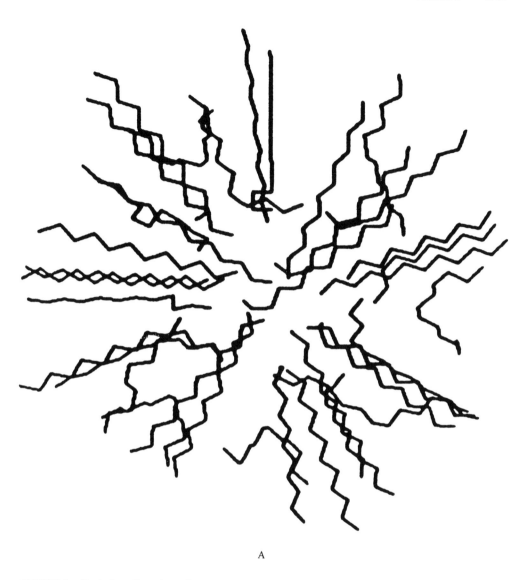

A

FIGURE 7. Typical configurations of a cylindrical micelle as produced by the technique described in the text. The micelle consists of 36 C-12 chains and has a radius of 15.65 Å. Views along a cross section (A) and along a long axis (B) are given.

only. With these limitations, there is still insight to be gained from the picture the numerical calculations provide. Efforts are currently underway to replace the cholesterol molecule with a gramicidin A polypeptide chain, complete with all side chains, to consider the effect of this larger and more complex membrane molecule on the lipid chains.

In very recent work, the method described above and in the flowchart of Figure 4 has been applied to chains in spherical and cylindrical micelles. In these systems, excluded volume problems are more severe than in bilayers because of the crowding near the center of the aggregate. If one starts the simulation with all chains packed in the smallest possible volume, the excluded volume effect will lead to the rejection of all Monte Carlo moves. The solution to this problem is to start the system at a larger radius and gradually shrink the aggregate until an optimum packing state is achieved. Figures 7 and 8 show chain configurations in spherical and cylindrical geometries, respectively. Figure 9 shows the order parameter profiles for the two geometries as calculated by the simulations. As might be

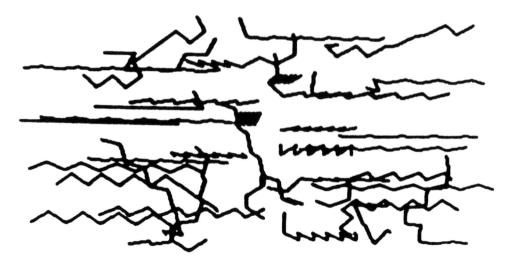

FIGURE 7B.

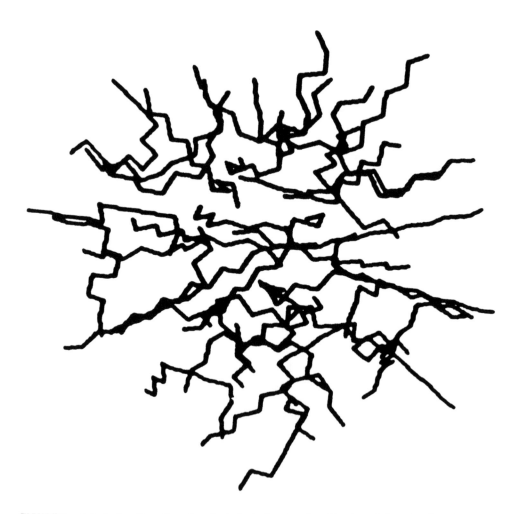

FIGURE 8.   A typical configuration of a spherical micelle as produced by the technique described in the text. The micelle consists of 36 C-12 chains the radius of the sphere is 18.55 Å.

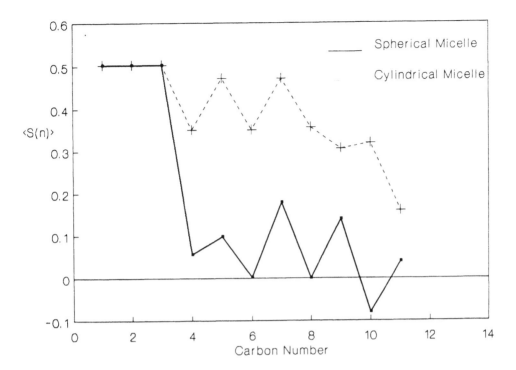

FIGURE 9. Order parameter profiles for cylindrical and spherical micelles. Plots of $<S_n>$ vs. bond number, n: dashed line, cylindrical micelle data; solid line, spherical micelle data. Data were based upon averages over 4000 Monte Carlo steps per chain (1.44×10^5 total steps) after equilibration for a like number of steps, all at 300 K.

expected, the calculated order parameter profiles are highly sensitive to the initial state of the model. If the simulations begin with a closely packed array of straight chains, then the profiles will reflect this order even after many Monte Carlo steps because there is little room for disordering. If the simulation begins with an expanded micelle and allows the chains to rotate as the micelle shrinks, the order parameter profiles of Figure 9 are obtained. This latter procedure is probably closer to the natural assembly process at room temperature. Another important consideration in the study of nonlamellar aggregates is the locations in the aggregate of the various carbon atoms, i.e., are carbons from the tail of the chains likely to migrate to the surface of the micelle, and vice versa, and how uniform is the hydrocarbon density within the micelle (as required by many of the theories discussed earlier)? Figure 10 shows the probability distribution of the various chain carbons in a spherical micelle as a function of the distance from the center of the micelle. The data and the pictures suggest that, beyond the two to three carbons closest to the surface, chain folding allows the carbon atoms to reside almost anywhere in the aggregate and the density does indeed appear fairly uniform, especially in the spherical systems. Comparison of the micelle densities produced by the above simulation and those used in the theoretical model of Gruen[18] reveals that the simulations produce model micelles with densities much lower than the theory. The simulations equilibrate at densities which correspond to methylene groups separated on average by ~3.9 Å, approximately the van der Waals radius, σ in Equation 1, for the intermethylene interaction. After this the interaction, energy grows so rapidly that further attempts at micelle shrinkage in the Monte Carlo calculations are rejected. By contrast, the theoretical model assumes nearly close-packed amphiphile densities, with little or no free volume between atoms. The correct density appears to be closer to the simulation than to Gruen's models.[18] In 0.15 NaCl solution, sodium dodecyl sulfate (SDS) forms micelles of hydrodynamic radius ~25 Å and aggregation number ~60.[7] This gives a volume per SDS molecule of 1091 Å³,

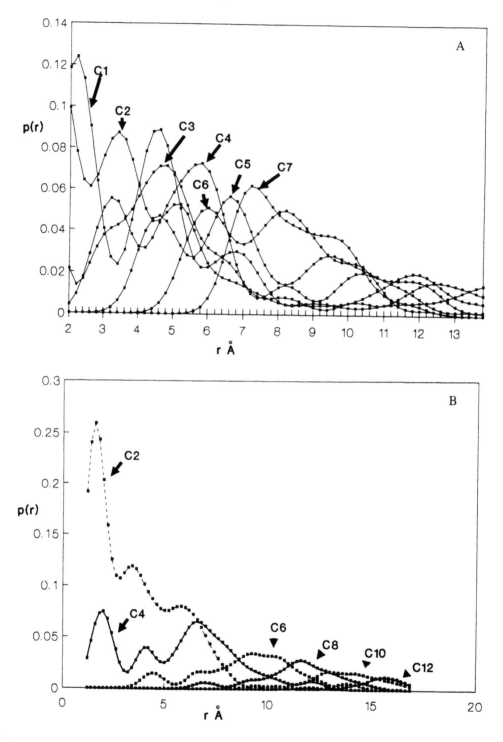

FIGURE 10.   Plots of normalized radial probability distribution function, p(r), vs. r, the distance from the center or axis of the micelle, for carbons at varying positions on the chains. The numbering is defined so that C1 is the carbon on the chain end which is initially closest to the micelle center. (A) Cylindrical micelle; (B) spherical micelle. The data were obtained by dividing the micelles into concentric spherical or cylindrical shells of thickness 2 Å and monitoring the bins in which all the carbon atoms were located at each Monte Carlo step. The number of steps is the same as that used to produce Figure 9.

while the micelle of Figure 8 has a volume of about 800 $Å^3$ per chain. Some of the SDS volume must be attributed to the ionic surface, but it is unlikely that the chains are as closely packed as Gruen[18] assumes in his theory.

Monte Carlo simulations of a continuum model for hydrocarbon chains in a lipid bilayer have been carried out by Vacatello and co-workers[44,45] using a method very different from the one described above. Vacatello et al. start with a two-dimensional array of carbon atoms, representing the topmost layer of a bilayer.[44,45] They then use a Monte Carlo algorithm to "grow" the configuration carbon by carbon. When a full chain configuration was finally generated, average properties were calculated over that configuration. While the model used is realistic, and the intermolecular potential function is adequate, the technique of step-by-step growing of the system is extremely inefficient, and, as the authors point out, rejection rates are very high. Thus, the averages reported are based only upon a few configurations, and so are subject to large uncertainties.

C. MOLECULAR DYNAMICS STUDIES OF MICELLES AND BILAYERS

The alternative to the Monte Carlo method for the computer calculation of the properties of systems of molecules is the molecular dynamics approach. In this approach, one begins, as in the Monte Carlo method, with a model system which has a fixed number of atoms or molecules and a postulated interaction function between them. The molecular dynamics method consists simply of solving Newton's equations of motion numerically for the system, starting from a specific initial state and following the temporal evolution of the system as long as available computer time allows. In order to simulate a system at a constant temperature, it is necessary to periodically rescale the velocities of all the particles in the system so that the average kinetic energy is consistent with the given temperature (usually via the equipartition theorem of statistical mechanics). In addition, when studying long chain molecules by molecular dynamics, the force will in general not be the same at different parts of the chain, and steps must be taken to ensure that the molecules do not fly apart.

The earliest molecular dynamics simulation of a lamellar array of amphiphiles was carried out by Kox et al.[46] The model used in this simulation is a system of 90 molecules. Each consists of a head group which was confined to a plane and a chain of seven CH_2 groups. The head groups interact through a 6 to 12 potential of the same form as the first part of Equation 9, and the chains are held together and bond angle constraints satisfied by strong harmonic forces. CH_2's on different chains interact through strong short-range repulsive forces only. Although the energy associated with the formation of a *gauche* bond in a chain was not included in the simulation, the order parameter profile calculated from the data has the same qualitative features as found in the Monte Carlo data[31-34] and the experimental plots.[1] This indicates again that the hard core repulsive force plays the crucial role in the determination of the chain ordering. More recently, Berendsen and co-workers have performed molecular dynamics simulation of models for lipid bilayers[47-49] containing 2 layers of up to 64 chains each. The molecular bonding constraints were enforced by an algorithm, SHAKE, written by this group. Also included were 6 to 12 potentials between CH_2's and a dihedral potential function for *gauche* rotations. In addition to order parameter profiles, the authors studied the dynamic properties of the system over the time scale of the runs (usually about 80 ps). It is of interest that the order parameter profiles are somewhat flatter in these simulations than the experimental profiles or the Monte Carlo profiles. This suggests than, while *trans-gauche* isomerization occurs on a fast time scale, 80 ps is not quite enough time to obtain a reasonable sampling of all accessible molecular conformations. The chief advantage of the molecular dynamics method is that dynamical properties of the system may be studied, while the Monte Carlo method yields only equilibrium, long-time averages. Berendsen et al.[47-49] obtain translational diffusion rates from their data which are about an order of magnitude larger than the experimental values. Also, simulation of an entire bilayer allows for calculation of the pressure as a function of depth within the bilayer. The resulting profile shows large pressures at the two aqueous interfaces and in the bilayer center, but with regions of negative pressure in between. In general, large-scale dynamics simulations of this type complement the equilibrium Monte Carlo simulations by providing a short time scale picture of the system, as contrasted with an equilibrium picture.

Other molecular dynamics calculations of models for lipid bilayers have been carried out by Khalatur and co-workers.[50,51] The model used by this group is simpler than that of Berendsen et al.[47-49] in that the potential for the dihedral bond rotations is not included, and the number of chains in the system is considerably smaller (10 chains per layer), although the chains themselves are longer (16 carbons). The order parameter profiles in this work are in better agreement with experiment than the profiles of Berendsen et al., but without dihedral rotational energies, this agreement may very well be fortuitous.[47-49] In a more recent simulation of a flat monolayer of 36 chains of 16 carbons per chain, Northrup and Curvin[52] employ an umbrella sampling technique, requiring two sets of molecular dynamics calculations, to extract detailed information about chain rotational states. The chains are initially placed in the layer with interchain spacing of 4.6 Å, smaller than the 4.85-Å spacing found in the ordered phase of lipid bilayers, but closer to the spacing in closely packed *n*-alkanes. One of the major conclusions of Northrup and Curvin[52] is that cooperative chain tilting plays an important role on the chain disordering mechanism. This is at odds with the argument given in Section I for a displacive mechanism as the mechanism for the tilted chains in bilayers, rather than long-range cooperativity. The chain tilting in the simulation is not long ranged, since the system is a 6 × 6 array of chains, and the chain density is higher than that found in bilayers, so the conclusions may not apply to lipid bilayers. However, Cardini et al.[53] also observe chain tilting in a molecular dynamics simulation of 90 chains of 20 carbons each packed in a monolayer with an interchain separation of 4.9 Å. In this model, there are no head groups to compete with the chains in packing considerations, so again the conclusions do not necessarily carry over to membranes.

There have also been a number of molecular dynamics simulations of hydrocarbon chains in spherical micelles.[54-56] The general goal of these simulations is to determine the distribution of chain segments within the micelle and to analyze chain motion in the severely confined interior of the micelle. The calculation of Haile and O'Connell[54] uses a model with chains anchored at a spherical surface, while the calculations of Jonsson et al.[55] and Watanabe et al[56] allow the chains to move freely and also to include water molecules. Since there are no current experimental data available with which to compare the results of the calculations, the alternative is to compare the calculations to each other. There is at best rough qualitative agreement that the initial chain segments are more likely to be found near the micelle surface while the chain terminii are spread out over much of the micelle interior. This is indicative of many highly folded chains and is in qualitative agreement with the Monte Carlo results discussed earlier. However, quantitative agreement between the various calculations is lacking. This is certainly due to the greater difficulty of the chain packing problem in a spherical volume compared to a monolayer. The optimal packing arrangement is likely to be far more complex in the spherical case so that computer simulations which run over only a few tens of picoseconds cannot sample enough of the possible arrangements, and the results of the simulations depend strongly on the assumptions which are input into the models.

IV. CONCLUSIONS

In this article, a number of different theoretical methods for studying lipid chain configurations in lamellae and micelles have been described. In all the cases considered, chain coordinates have been produced and chain states have been changed and monitored according to well-known simulation methods. The methods for calculating the chain coordinates vary between models and computational procedures, so the choice of methods depends mainly upon the goals of the calculation. This means that interpretation of the results of all of the simulations must be made in the light of the methods used. Although supercomputer speeds allow for far more realistic systems to be simulated now than a decade ago, the systems are still much simplified in comparison to real systems. Thus, the computational results are compromised by both finite size effects and computer time limitations on the number of configurations that can be generated. In general, it is also true that the more complex the system under simulation, the greater is the chance for errors.

Having said the above, it can also be said that in spite of the inherent limitations, computer generated studies of lipid aggregates are providing an unprecedented microscopic view of how molecules may be interacting in lipid aggregates. This new viewpoint can only aid in the design of future experimental and analytical theoretical efforts to understand these systems.

ACKNOWLEDGMENTS

The author wishes to thank A. H. Chowdhury for important contributions to the computer code, D. W. Magee for assistance in the analysis of some of the numerical results, and W. Scott McCullough for a critical reading of the manuscript. This work was partially supported by the U.S. National Science Foundation under Grant No. DMB 8703644.

REFERENCES

1. **Davis, J. H.**, The description of membrane lipid conformation, order, and dynamics by ^{2}H-NMR, *Biochim. Biophys. Acta,* 737, 117, 1983.
2. **McConnell, H. M.**, Molecular motion in biological membranes, in *Spin Labeling Theory and Applications,* Academic Press, New York, 1976, 525.
3. **Seelig, J. and Seelig, A.**, Lipid conformation in model membranes and biological membranes, *Q. Rev. Biophys.,* 13, 19, 1980.
4. **Israelachvili, J., Marcelja, S., and Horn, R. G.**, Physical properties of membrane organization, *Q. Rev. Biophys.,* 13, 121, 1980.
5. **Nagle, J. F. and Scott, H. L.**, Biomembrane phase transitions, *Phys. Today,* 31, 38, 1978.
6. **Menger, F. M.**, On the structure of micelles, *Acc. Chem. Res.,* 12, 111, 1979.
7. **Wennerstrom, H. and Lindman, B.**, Micelles. Physical chemistry of surfactant association, *Phys. Rep.,* 52, 1, 1979.
8. See the Chapter by T. J. McIntosh, this Volume.
9. **Marsh, D.**, ESR probes for structure and dynamics of membranes, *Spectroscop. Dyn. Mol. Biol. Syst.,* Bayley, P. and Dale, R. E., Eds., Academic, London, 1985, 209.
10. **Peng, Z.-Y., Simplaceanu, V., Lowe, I. J., and Ho, C.**, Rotating frame relaxation studies of slow motions in flourinated phospholipid model membranes, *Biophys. J.,* 54, 81, 1988.
11. **Davis, J. H.**, The influence of membrane proteins on lipid dynamics, *Chem. Phys. Lipids,* 40, 223, 1986.
12. **Nagle, J. F. and Wilkinson, A.**, Lecithin bilayers, density measurements and molecular interactions, *Biophys. J.,* 23, 159, 1978.
13. **Nagle, J. F.**, Theory of the main lipid bilayer phase transition, *Annu. Rev. Phys. Chem.,* 31, 157, 1980.
14. **Nagle, J. F.**, Theory of biomembrane phase transitions, *J. Chem. Phys.,* 58, 252, 1973.
15. **Baxter, R. J.**, *Exactly Solved Models in Statistical Mechanics,* Academic Press, New York, 1982.
16. **Marcelja, S.**, Chain ordering in liquid crystals. II. Structure of bilayer membranes, *Biochim. Biophys. Acta,* 367, 165, 1974.
17. **Gruen, D. W. R.**, A model for the chains in amphiphilic aggregates. I. Comparison with a molecular dynamics simulation of a bilayer, *J. Phys. Chem.,* 89, 146, 1985.
18. **Gruen, D. W. R.**, A model for the chains in amphiphilic aggregates. II. Thermodynamic and experimental comparisons for aggregates of different shape and size, *J. Phys. Chem.,* 89, 153, 1985.
19. **Dill, K. A. and Flory, P. J.**, Molecular organization in micelles and vesicles, *Pro. Nat. Acad. Sci. U.S.A.,* 78, 676, 1981.

20. **Ben-Shaul, A., Szleifer, I., and Gelbart, W. M.,** Chain organization in micelles and bilayers. I. Theory, *J. Chem. Phys.,* 83, 3597, 1985.
21. **Szleifer, I., Ben-Shaul, A., and Gelbart, W. M.,** Chain organization and thermodynamics in micelles and bilayers. II. Model calculations, *J. Chem. Phys.,* 83, 3612, 1985.
22. **Szleifer, I., Ben-Shaul, A., and Gelbart, W. M.,** Chain statistics in micelles and bilayers: effect of surface roughness and internal energy, *J. Chem. Phys.,* 85, 5345, 1986.
23. **Whittington, S. and Chapman, D.,** Effect of density on configurational properties of long chain molecules using a Monte Carlo method, *Trans. Faraday Soc.,* 62, 3319, 1966.
24. **Haan, S. W. and Pratt, L. R.,** Monte Carlo study of a simple model for micelle structure, *Chem. Phys. Lett.,* 79, 436, 1981.
25. **Owenson, B. and Pratt, L. R.,** Monte Carlo calculation of the molecular structure of surfactant bilayers, *J. Phys. Chem.,* 88, 6048, 1984.
26. **Harris, J. and Rice, S. A.,** A lattice model of a supported monolayer of amphiphile molecules: Monte Carlo simulations, *J. Chem. Phys.,* 88, 1298, 1988.
27. **Caillé, A., Pink, D. A., de Verteuil, F., and Zuckerman, M. J.,** Theoretical models for quasi two-dimensional mesomorphic monolayers and membrane bilayers, *Can. J. Phys.,* 58, 582,
28. **Mouritsen, O. G.,** *Computer Studies of Phase Transitions and Critical Phenomena,* Springer-Verlag, Berlin, 1984.
29. **Buamgartner, A.,** Simulations of polymer models, in *Monte Carlo Methods in Statistical Physics,* 2nd ed., Binder, K., Springer-Verlag, Berlin, 1984.
30. **Curro, J. G.,** Computer simulation of multiple chain systems — the effect of density on the average chain dimensions, *J. Chem. Phys.,* 61, 1203, 1974.
31. **Scott, H. L.,** Monte Carlo studies of the hydrocarbon region of lipid bilayers, *Biochim. Biophys. Acta,* 469, 264, 1977.
32. **Scott, H. L. and Cherng, S.-L.,** Monte Carlo studies of phospholipid lamellae. Effects of proteins, cholesterol, bilayer curvature, and lateral mobility on order parameters, *Biochim. Biophys. Acta,* 510, 209, 1978.
33. **Scott, H. L.,** Monte Carlo calculations of order parameter profiles in models of lipid-protein interactions in bilayers, *Biochemistry,* 25, 6122, 1986.
34. **Scott, H. L. and Kalaskar, S.,** Lipid chains and cholesterol in model membranes: a Monte Carlo study, *Biochemistry,* in press.
35. **Arfken, G.,** *Mathematical Methods for Physicists,* Academic Press, New York, 1970.
36. **Hauser, H., Pascher, I., Pearson, R. H., and Sundell, S.,** Preferred conformation and molecular packing of phosphatidylethanolamine and phosphatidylcholine, *Biochim. Biophys. Acta,* 650, 21, 1981.
37. **Hussin, A. and Scott, H. L.,** Density and bonding profiles of interbilayer water as functions of bilayer separation: a Monte Carlo study, *Biochim. Biophys. Acta,* 897, 423, 1987.
38. **Scott, H. L., Pearce, P. A., and McCullough, W. J.,** Calculation of intermolecular interaction strengths in the $P_{\beta'}$ phase in lipid bilayers: implications for theoretical models, *Biophys. J.,* in press, 1990.
39. **Jorgensen, W.,** Revised TIPS for simulations of liquid water and aqueous solutions, *J. Chem. Phys.,* 77, 4156, 1982.
40. **Pearce, P. A. and Scott, H. L.,** Statistical mechanics of the ripple phase in lipid bilayers, *J. Chem. Phys.,* 77, 951, 1982.
41. **Brasseur, R. and Ruysschaert, J.-M.,** Conformation and mode of organization of amphiphilic membrane components: a conformational analysis, *Biochem. J.,* 238, 1, 1986.
42. **Binder, K.,** in *Monte Carlo Methods in Statistical Physics,* Binder, K., Ed., Springer-Verlag, Berlin, 1978.
43. **Marcelja, S.,** Lipid-mediated protein interaction in membranes, *Biochim. Biophys. Acta,* 455, 1, 1976.
44. **Vacatello, M., Busico, V., and Corradini, C.,** The conformation of hydrocarbon chains in disordered layer systems, *J. Chem. Phys.,* 78, 590, 1983.
45. **Vacatello, M. and Busico, V.,** The structure and conformation of *n*-hydrocarbon chains in bilayer systems in the fluid phase, *Mol. Cryst. Liq. Cryst.,* 107, 341, 1984.
46. **Kox, A. J., Michels, J. P. J., and Wiegel, F. W.,** Simulation of a lipid monolayer using molecular dynamics, *Nature (London),* 287, 317, 1980.
47. **van der Ploeg, P. and Berendsen, H. J. C.,** Molecular dynamics simulation of a bilayer membrane, *J. Chem. Phys.,* 76, 3271, 1982.
48. **Edholm, O., Berendsen, H. J. C., and van der Ploeg, P.,** Conformational entropy of a bilayer membrane derived from a molecular dynamics simulation, *Mol. Phys.,* 48, 379, 1983.
49. **van der Ploeg, P. and Berendsen, H. J. C.,** Molecular dynamics of a bilayer membrane, *Mol. Phys.,* 49, 233, 1983.
50. **Khalatur, P. G., Balabaev, N. K., and Pavlov, A. S.,** Molecular dynamics study of a lipid bilayer and a polymer liquid, *Mol. Phys.,* 59, 753, 1986.

51. **Khalatur, P. G. and Pavlov, A. S.,** Molecular motions in a liquid-crystalline lipid bilayer. Molecular dynamics simulation, *Makromol. Chem.,* 188, 3029, 1987.
52. **Northrup, S. H. and Curvin, M. S.,** Molecular dynamics simulation of disorder transitions in lipid monolayers, *J. Phys. Chem.,* 89, 4704, 1985.
53. **Cardini, G., Bareman, J., and Klein, M. L.,** Characterization of a Langmuir-Blodgett monolayer using molecular dynamics calculations, *Chem. Phys. Lett.,* 145, 493, 1987.
54. **Haile, J. M. and O'Connell, J. P.,** Internal structure of a model micelle via computer simulation, *J. Phys. Chem.,* 88, 6363, 1984.
55. **Jonsson, B., Edholm, O., and Teleman, O.,** Molecular dynamics of a sodium octanoate micelle in aqueous solution, *J. Chem. Phys.,* 85, 2259, 1986.
56. **Watanabe, K., Ferrario, M., and Klein, M. L.,** Molecular dynamics study of a sodium octanoate micelle in aqueous solution, *J. Phys. Chem.,* 92, 819, 1988.

Chapter 1.A.4

COMPUTER SIMULATION OF BIOLOGICAL MEMBRANES

David A. Pink

TABLE OF CONTENTS

I. INTRODUCTION

In the last 25 years, computer simulation has been used increasingly in order to understand the statics and dynamics of physical systems. This method has been used because the Hamiltonians which describe the systems of interest are sufficiently complicated so that the free energy cannot be written down in terms of known functions or functions whose behavior is understood over a sufficiently wide range of the parameters. There are essentially two kinds of systems of interest: (1) systems which are idealizations or simple models of real systems, such as the Ising model in three-dimensions or the Potts model, and (2) systems which are as close as possible to "real life", such as a model of two molecules interacting via van der Waals' and electrostatic forces and hydrogen bonding. In the second case, if one uses molecular dynamics, one is almost carrying out a "computer experiment" on the system. One may want to simulate a system and get the correct (numerical) result for functions of interest in order to compare the results of approximations for which analytical results can be obtained.

In this review of computer simulation of biological and model biological membranes, an outline of the principle techniques will first be given. In the third section, recent studies in this field shall be described. This section shall describe the simulation of the statics and dynamics of lipid bilayers with or without intrinsic molecules such as proteins, the dynamics of intrinsic molecules in membranes, the packing of proteins in membranes, and what factors affect the lateral diffusion of integral proteins in membranes. Although this review will concentrate on computer simulation of aspects of biological membranes, it is desirable to set these studies in the context of other theoretical calculations on these systems. Thus, where appropriate, mention will be made of analytical calculations so as to compare their results to those of computer simulation. A number of reviews have appeared which describe theoretical work done before 1984.[1-3] This review will therefore concentrate on work done since then.

II. MODELING AND COMPUTER SIMULATION METHODS

In order to model molecules in and around a membrane, one must decide two things: (1) how the molecules are going to be represented, i.e., whether all the molecules will be represented by discrete objects or whether some aspect will be represented as belonging to a continuum, and (2) how the statics and dynamics of the molecules are going to be modeled.

In (1), these are two extreme ways in which molecules have been modeled, either by including all the details of molecular structure on a resolution of ≤ 0.1 Å with the details of electrostatic, van der Waals', and hydrogen bonding interactions included or else by making a judgment about what aspect of the molecular properties are most important, including them and ignoring all the rest. Thus, for example, if one wants to calculate hydrocarbon chain "order parameters", one can use a model in which the space-filling structures of hydrocarbon chains attached to glyceride backbones are included. A 6 to 12 potential interaction can be included as well as the kinetic energy of the hydrocarbon chains. A potential can be applied to keep the molecules approximately in a plane, thus forming one half of a bilayer as well as to possess some average nearest neighbor distance in the plane of the membrane. Starting from, say, an all-*trans* state for each chain, the simulation can use molecular dynamics at various temperatures in order to calculate both the (static) averages associated with hydrocarbon chain order as well as the (dynamic) lateral diffusion coefficient or relaxation times. If, on the other hand, one wishes to study, for example, protein adsorption at membrane surfaces, it may be useful to first map this problem onto a lattice-gas type of model in order to establish the general properties of the phase diagram. In this case, one may represent proteins by disks or some other simple geometrical shape which impinge upon a plane and interact via some short-range force. The proteins can also interact with each other and possess various internal conformational states described by an energy and density of states distribution. The thermodynamics of this model is easier to study than that of a model which includes the details of the protein structure, the surrounding water which contains ions, and the details of the polar region of the membrane.

In (2), two methods have been predominantly used to calculate static and dynamic quantities at finite temperatures: These are the molecular dynamics method[4,5] and the Monte Carlo method.[6] The molecular dynamics method involves numerically integrating the classical equations of motion for the system and corresponds to the use of the microcanonical ensemble in statistical mechanics. An initial configuration is assigned a definite total energy made up of kinetic and potential energy which is conserved during the motion of the system. The acceleration of any part of the total system is defined by the force on it which is obtained from the gradient of the potential in which that part finds itself. Numerically integrating the equations of motion yields the velocities and positions at the end of each time step. Because of round-off errors in the numerical integration methods, the total energy drifts as the calculation proceeds and must be reset at appropriate intervals. In order to obtain a sufficiently good phase space sampling, it is necessary to average over $\sim 10^4$ time steps. Thus, if each time step has to be as small as, say, 10^{-15} s in order to obtain reliable results for the numerical integration of the equations of motion, then a total elapsed time of $\sim 10^{-11}$ s is obtained. Comments will be made below about calculations of a lateral diffusion coefficient in this time interval. The Monte Carlo method makes use of the Metropolis algorithm[7] to generate a sequence of microstates of the system. It simulates the differential equation satisfied by $P(\alpha, t)$, the probability for finding the system in state α at time t,

$$\frac{dP(\alpha,t)}{dt} = -\sum_{\alpha'} W_{\alpha\alpha'} P(\alpha,t) + \sum_{\alpha'} W_{\alpha'\alpha} P(\alpha',t) \tag{1}$$

where $W_{\alpha\alpha'}$ is the probability per unit time of the system making a transition from state α to state α'. In principle, the set $\{W_{\alpha\alpha'}\}$ can be any set that yields desired conditions on $P(\alpha, t)$. In order to calculate averages that reflect thermodynamic equilibrium, however, one requires that

$$\lim_{t \to \infty} P(\alpha, t) \propto e^{-\beta E(\alpha)} \tag{2}$$

where $E(\alpha)$ is the energy of state α and $\beta = 1/k_B T$, where k_B is Boltzmann's constant. The Metropolis algorithm can be realized by the following procedure.[3,6] If the system is in state α, then choose randomly another state, α' with energy $E(\alpha')$. If $E(\alpha') \leq E(\alpha)$, then the system makes a transition from α to α'. If $E(\alpha') > E(\alpha)$, then define $\Delta E = E(\alpha') - E(\alpha)$. Choose a number, r, randomly from the set (0, 1). Then if $r \leq e^{-\beta \Delta E}$, the system makes the transition from state α to α'. Otherwise, it remains in state α. The Glauber realization of the Metropolis algorithm concerns itself with attempting to change the internal states of a system, e.g., the change of a lipid hydrocarbon chain from one conformational state to another. The Kawasaki realization involves the exchange, in spatial position, of two parts of a system, e.g., the hopping of a particle to fill a vacancy involves the spatial exchange of the particle and vacancy. In both methods, periodic boundary conditions are generally used, but this introduces a perferred scale into the system which may manifest itself as a static or dynamic wavelength. Alternative boundary conditions have been proposed.[6]

Finally, one can ask what is the difference between the physics of the two methods. The physics of the molecular dynamics method is clear. It is classical mechanics applied to an atomic system, in which quantum effects are either ignored or else included in a phenomenological fashion. Thus, hydrogen bonding is taken into account by a 10 to 12 potential together with rules concerning O-OH or O-NH distances and the angles between the various atoms.[8] When simulating spatial movement, the Monte Carlo method involves translations in randomly chosen directions by random distances (within some limits) with no correlation between successive translations. This corresponds to Brownian motion of a molecule in a solute which is subject to random forces. Some aspects of simulating kinetics using Monte Carlo methods, however, should be borne in mind. The Monte Carlo method generates a sequence of microstates of the model. It can be proven that use of the Metropolis algorithm will lead to thermodynamic equilibrium averages after a sufficiently long sequence, though discussions related to finite size effects, the thermodynamic limit, and broken ergodicity should be taken into account when reporting results.[2,6] There is no prior reason why the sequence of microstates generated should represent the kinetics of the system which is being modeled, i.e., although both the molecular dynamics method, say, and the Monte Carlo method will lead to thermodynamic equilibrium, they may arrive there via different paths through phase space. If, however, random forces are dominant in the system of interest and if sequential microstates differ from each other by a sufficiently small amount, then it is possible that the path through phase space generated by the Monte Carlo method is sufficiently close to the path that the system would follow. This interpretation should be borne in mind when we discuss Monte Carlo methods applied to kinetic studies. A second reason why Monte Carlo simulations of kinetics should be treated with caution is the ambiguity in choices for $W_{\alpha\alpha'}$ in Equation 1. If the conditions imposed on $W_{\alpha\alpha'}$ are those of Equation 2, for example, then there are a number of different choices of $W_{\alpha\alpha'}$ that yield the Boltzmann distribution as $t \to \infty$. It is not obvious, however, that one will obtain essentially the same kinetics irrespective of the choice of $W_{\alpha\alpha'}$ that satisfies only Equation 2. A third reason for caution is that one does not have a recipe for identifying Monte Carlo steps with time intervals. Although it may seem intuitively reasonable that far-from-phase transitions each Monte Carlo step is equivalent to the same time interval, it would be happier to be in the possession of a theorem which says under what conditions this is so.

III. THERMODYNAMICS OF BILAYER MEMBRANES

In this section, the thermodynamics of models of lipid bilayers containing integral proteins will be reviewed. The behavior of such systems depends, in part, upon the thermodynamics of the lipids in which the proteins are embedded. Accordingly, a review will be given of recent work done on computer simulation of models of pure lipid bilayers. As before, the section will concentrate on work done in the last 5 years since substantial reviews exist of work prior to 1983.[1,5,9,10] In addition to these, there are several general reviews of protein dynamics, protein interactions, and computer simulation of proteins.[4,11,12]

A. MONTE CARLO SIMULATION OF LATTICE MODELS OF PURE LIPID BILAYERS

Lattice models have been widely used to study different aspects of lipid bilayer phase transitions. Before models of lipid-protein bilayers are described, recent studies of pure lipid bilayers phase transitions will be described. Most of the recent work on lattice models originated with the ten-state model introduced by Pink et al.[13] to model the main lipid melting transition at $T = T_m$ in saturated phosphatidylcholines and its observation via raman scattering. The plane of the membrane was represented by a triangular lattice each site of which was occupied by a lipid hydrocarbon chain which could be in one of ten states: nine low-energy states, in which the hydrocarbon chain possesses a low number of *gauche* bonds and therefore a small internal energy, E_n, a low degeneracy, D_n, and a small cross section area, A_n, projected onto the bilayer plane (n = 1, . . . 9), and one "excited" state, possessing a larger number of *gauche* bonds, a large internal energy, E_e, a large degeneracy, D_e, and a larger area, A_e. Polar interactions which bring the bilayer into existence were represented by a lateral pressure, Π, which couples to the cross section areas. Hydrocarbon chains interact via an attractive van der Waals' interaction and the Hamiltonian is

$$\mathcal{H}_c = \frac{-J_o}{2} \sum_{<ij>} \sum_{nm} J(nm)\mathcal{L}_{in}\mathcal{L}_{jm} + \sum_i \sum_n \epsilon_n \mathcal{L}_{in} \qquad (3)$$

Here $-J_o J$ (nm) represents the van der Waals' interaction between hydrocarbon chains at sites i and j, $\epsilon_n = E_n + \Pi A_n$ $\mathcal{L}_{in}$ is a projection operator for state n at site i, and $<ij>$ indicates a summation over site i and its nearest neighbors j.

Mouritsen[14] performed Monte Carlo simulations on q-state models (q = 2, . . . , 10) using the Hamiltonian Equation 3. These models were obtained from the ten-state model by simply deleting various states and studying their phase transitions. In a series of very careful simulations, it was shown that for $q \leq 5$, hysteresis is manifested in the melting transition at $T = T_m$, but that for $q \geq 6$, a continuous transition is obtained, indicating that the system is relaxing slowly in the transition region. Inspection of instantaneous states of the lattice showed that for $|T - T_m| \leq 0.3°C$, huge clusters are formed which alternate between fluid-like and gel-like characteristics as the simulation proceeds so that the phase of the system appears to be ill-defined. This cannot be true thermodynamic equilibrium and therefore implies the very slow relaxation mentioned above. Although nucleation and the growth of nucleation centers proceeds rapidly, the fusion of clusters is very much slowed down by the low cluster surface energies due to the ability of the variety of states available to produce soft domain walls. Subsequent studies of the q = 6 case showed that relaxation following a quench from above T_m to below T_m proceeds via a staircase of metastable states.[2] It was suggested that the "continuous" melting observed experimentally for pure wet lipid bilayers is understandable in terms of the large number of lipid states which gives rise to soft domain walls. In a subsequent paper,[15] quantitative cluster analysis was carried out for q-state models ($2 \leq q \leq 10$) to determine the relative importance of intermediate states. Monte Carlo simulations were performed on triangular lattices with 900, 1600, and 3600 sites with toroidal boundary conditions. An α-cluster was defined as a set of sites all in state α connected by nearest neighbor bonds. Average cluster sizes as well as probabilities of occurrence of clusters containing ℓ^α sites each in state α were calculated. It was found that the thermal density fluctuations together with the observed slow relaxation in the transition region near T_m, indicated that the lipid bilayer softens at T_m and that this is due to the presence of several intermediate conformations at the interfaces between the clusters for $q \geq 6$. The cluster sizes observed in $q \geq 6$ state models is in accord with calorimetric data which shows the existence of clusters containing between 100 and 1000 molecules. The model presented here is the only one from which this picture of clusters has been derived. The q = 10 state model displays a specific heat that shows critical-like behavior. The agreement between the cluster results and those observed from electron microscopy of lipid monolayers suggests that the large variety of intermediate states stabilize the fluctuating distribution of clusters.

Zuckermann and Mouritsen[16] extended the ten-state model in order to study both the freezing of the lipid hydrocarbon chains and the onset of crystallization of the lipid bilayer. They defined a Hamiltonian, $\mathcal{H}_p$, to consider in-plane orientation of lipid crystallites. This Hamiltonian is a modification of one for a q-state Potts model which was used to study grain growth.[17] The Potts states represent orientational states of the lipids, and $\mathcal{H}_p$ is written as

$$\mathcal{H}_p = J_p \sum_{<ij>} \sum_{nn'} \sum_{pp'} (1 - \delta_{pp'}) \mathcal{L}_{ipn}\mathcal{L}_{jp'n'}$$

$$\mathcal{H} = \mathcal{H}_c + \mathcal{H}_p \qquad (4)$$

where $\mathcal{H}$ is the total Hamiltonian and $\mathcal{L}_{ipn}$ is the projection operator for a lipid at site i in state n and with orientation state p. It should be noted that $\mathcal{L}_{ipn}$ can be factored (though Zuckermann and Mouritsen did not make use of it),

$$\mathcal{L}_{ipn} = \mathcal{L}_{in}\mathcal{L}_{ip} \tag{5}$$

where $\mathcal{L}_{in}$ are the projection operators of Equation 3 and $\mathcal{L}_{ip}$ is a projection operator for a lipid at site i in orientation state p. The sum over n and n′ ranges from 1 to 9 under the reasonable assumption that the melted state e will not display crystalline orientation. The sum over the orientation labels, pp′, ranges from 1 to q and the authors took q = 30 which was found to adequately describe the q → ∞ limit.[18] The model studied was solved by using a mean field approximation[1] as well as by Monte Carlo simulation. The $(T - J_p)$ phase diagram displayed three phase boundaries, separating a fluid phase, a disordered gel phase, and a crystalline gel phase, which meet at a triple point at J_p^*. Lattices with 900 and 10,000 sites were used. It was observed that the melting of grains of crystalline gel phase occurred via interfacial melting at the grain boundaries. Previous work[14] found that the ten-state model displayed a continuous transition near T_m. The addition of $\mathcal{H}_p$ sharpens this transition and causes the total system to exhibit a wide hysteresis cycle.

Pink et al.[19] constructed a model of hydrogen bonding in *N*-palmitoylgalactosylsphingosine (NPGS) by restricting the number of lipid hydrocarbon chain states to two: an effective ground state, g, and the excited state, e. The effective ground state is obtained by performing a mean field average over the nine low-energy states. Equation 3 was reinterpreted so that each site of the triangular lattice was occupied by a lipid molecule, made up of two chains, which could be in one of three states: G madeup of each chain being in their g state, (g,g); I madeup of (g,e) and (e,g); and E madeup of (e,e). The sum over n,m in Equation 3 ranges over G, I, and E. The J(nm), E_n, D_n, and A_n are redefined so that they refer to properties of molecules. To this form of Equation 3 was added a Hamiltonian describing hydrogen bond formation:

$$\mathcal{H}_{HB} = J_o \sum_{<ik>} \sum_{nm} K(nm) \, \mathcal{L}_{in}\mathcal{L}_{i+km}(\mathcal{B}_{ik}\mathcal{B}_{i+kk}$$
$$+ \, \mathcal{B}_{i-k}\mathcal{B}_{i+k-k}) + \sum_i \left(\Delta(b) \sum_k \mathcal{B}_{ik} + \Delta(u)\mathcal{U}_i \right) \tag{6}$$

Here $\mathcal{B}_{ik}$ is the projection operator for a collinear donor-acceptor group pointing in direction k, on a lipid molecule located at site i. $-J_o K$ (nm) is the energy of a hydrogen bond formed when the donor-acceptor groups on adjacent lipid molecule sites line up in the same direction as the vector from one site to the other. Monte Carlo simulations studied the thermodynamics of this system which was found to display a hysteresis loop $\sim 20°C$ wide even though the system corresponding to DPPC (by choosing all K(nm) = 0) displayed a hysteresis loop $\sim 1°C$ wide. The main phase transition temperature, at $T_m = 68°C$, agreed with measurements on NPGs, as did the 20°C hysteresis loop. Relaxation studies were carried out by computer simulation and predictions were made about the relaxation of the spectrum of the amide I and II bands, as well as about the phenomena to be observed when the system was heated or cooled in different ways. Cruzeiro-Hansson and Mouritsen[20] used the ten-state model to perform computer simulation studies on ion permeability through bilayer membranes. By assuming that this takes place preferentially at the interfaces between the dynamic domains observed in other simulation studies[14] and using the approach of Kanehisa and Tsong,[21] they calculate the relative permeability of Na$^+$ ions in liposomes. The fundamental difference between this work and others[22] is that the former takes account of local permeability via the correlation between local fluctuations (largest at interfaces) and permeability and obtains the global permeability by averaging over the local values, while the latter performs global averages to obtain an area fluctuation characteristic of the membrane and deduces the permeability via an Eyring rate formula. Because the ions probably have only local interactions of finite range it seems, a priori that the theory of Cruzeiro-Hansson and Mouritsen[20] must be preferred.

Further computer simulation work using the ten-state model has been by Mouritsen et al.[23] on calculating equilibrium and nonequilibrium isotherms of a monolayer model and lateral density fluctuations, deducing indications of a critical point, and the accumulation of cholesterol at interfaces[24] which thereby enhances the interfacial area and lateral density fluctuations. The concentration of cholesterol at interfaces is about twice that elsewhere in the bilayer. The effect of this upon passive ionic permeability is studied and found to be in accord with experiments. This simulation and that of Cruzeiro-Hansson and Mouritsen[20] have important implications for understanding the passive permeability of the lipid-protein bilayers to small ions and work is under way on this subject.

Tevlin et al.[25] calculated the density of states of a single lipid chain. This calculation is important for it establishes whether the single chain degeneracies of the ten-state model are sufficiently accurate. Using simulation algorithms, they find that there is qualitative agreement between their result and the degeneracies of the ten-state model.

B. MONTE CARLO SIMULATION OF LATTICE MODELS OF PROTEIN-LIPID BILAYERS

Pink[3] modeled integral proteins in a lipid bilayer by representing the cross section of a bilayer-spanning protein by a hexagon, the center and six vertices of which occupied lattice sites. The size of a hexagon was defined by the number of lattice constants from the hexagon center out to one of the vertices. This number is denoted by R. Two hexagons could not occupy the same site. This "lattice-hexagon" model was used to calculate a phase diagram, together with specific heats and transition enthalpies. The hexagons were constrained to lie on a superlattice composed of hexagon-size unit cells and could move from one superlattice cell to another. A two-state model of lipid hydrocarbon chains was used, an effective temperature-dependent ground state g obtained via a mean field average over the nine low-energy states as described before and the excited state e. Each lattice site could be occupied by one such chain. Accordingly, to the hydrocarbon chain Hamiltonian (Equation 3), where n and m range over g and e, was added a lipid-protein Hamiltonian.

$$\mathcal{H}_{LP} = -J_o \sum_{<i\ell>} \sum_n K(n) \mathcal{L}_{in} \mathcal{P}_\ell - \frac{J_o}{2} J_p \sum_{<k\ell>} \mathcal{P}_k \mathcal{P}_\ell$$

$$\mathcal{H} = \mathcal{H}_c + \mathcal{H}_{LP} \tag{7}$$

Here $\mathcal{P}_\ell$ is a projection operator for a protein in cell ℓ, $<i\ell>$ indicates a summation of all cells ℓ and their nearest neighbor sites, i, which are occupied by lipid chains, and $-J_o K(n)$ and $-J_o J_p$ are the protein-lipid (in state n) and protein-protein interactions. It was assumed that $K(e) \approx 0$ and that $J_p = 0$ for simplicity. It was necessary to choose $K(g)$ to be small and attractive in order to obtain results consistent with ^2H NMR measurements on lipid chain "order parameters" in a lipid-protein bilayers for $T > T_m$. This approach to protein-lipid interactions can be criticized on the grounds that in the absence of a specific interaction between lipids and proteins, the effect of a protein might be to change the degeneracies of the states of the lipids adjacent to them. The physics of this is that the proximity of the protein to a lipid chain removes ΔD_g and ΔD_e of the available states because of steric effects. In keeping the degeneracies unchanged, however, and treating this entropic effect as an interaction, one identifies:

$$\ell n\left(\frac{D_g - \Delta D_g}{D_e - \Delta D_e}\right) = -\beta K(g) - \ell n\left(\frac{D_g}{D_e}\right) \tag{8}$$

If $(D_g - \Delta D_g)/(D_e - \Delta D_e) > D_g/D_e$, then $K(g) > 0$. This means that if the fractional decrease in the effective ground state degeneracy is less than that in the excited state degeneracy, then $K(g) > 0$. Of course, $K(g)$ should be temperature dependent. The assumption that it is a constant keeps the model simple by avoiding having to choose two degeneracy changes, ΔD_g and ΔD_e. In the range of temperatures studied, $15°C < T < 50°C$, $K(g)$ will be approximately constant. If we define the fractional area of the membrane "covered" by the proteins to be f_A and the protein concentration to be c, then

$$f_A = n_H N_H/N$$

$$c = N_H/(N - (n_H - 1)N_H) \tag{9}$$

where N, N_H, and n_H are the number of lattice sites, the number of hexagons, and the number of lattice sites per hexagon, respectively. If R is the size of the hexagon, then $n_H = 3R(R + 1) + 1$. When $f_A = 0.36$, it was found that $T_m(c)$, the temperature at which hydrocarbon chains undergo a transition between their g and e states, with $T_m(0) = T_m$, decreased by $\leq 2°C$. The results of the simulation showed that for $T < T_m(c)$, there is an essentially pure lipid phase in a gel-like state coexisting with a protein-rich phase and lipids in their melted states if T is not too low below $T_m(c)$. There also appears to exist a temperature $T_K \leq T_m(c)$ at which the protein-rich phase achieves a closest packing of proteins. The results of the thermodynamic calculations appeared to be in accord with experiments on a variety of integral proteins for which the protein polar group does not take part in the bilayer thermodynamics in the neighborhood of T_m. Some of these calculations have been repeated for cases where the hexagons do not occupy cells of a superlattice, but can move between adjacent sites, and the results are the same as summarized here.[81]

MacDonald and Pink[26] extended the lattice-hexagon model of a lipid-protein bilayer to model the thermodynamics of glycophorin in a phospholipid bilayer. This glycoprotein exhibited a phase diagram and transition enthalpy, $\Delta H(c)$, quite unlike proteins or polypeptides which have a polar group smaller than the transmembrane segment,[27] and there was evidence that other glycoproteins behaved in similar ways.[28]

In the case of glycophorin, the polar segments are much larger than the single α-helical transmembrane core. Each site of a triangular lattice could be occupied by a lipid chain or the "α-helical core" of a model "glycophorin" molecule. The polar group of the protein was assumed either to project out of the membrane and so project an area onto the surface of the membrane that could be represented by a hexagon, centered on the α-helix site, of size R_U, or to lie in a "pancake" conformation on the membrane which was represented by a hexagon of size $R_D > R_U$. The Hamiltonian of the lipids was taken to be Equation 3 with $n = g,e$, g being the effective temperature-dependent ground state. The protein Hamiltonian was assumed to be

$$\mathcal{H}_{pp} = \frac{-J_o}{2} \sum_{kk'} \sum_{aa'} H(|\vec{r}_a(k) - \vec{r}_{a'}(k')| - R_a - R_{a'} - 1)\mathcal{P}_{ka}\mathcal{P}_{k'a'} + \sum_k \sum_a \epsilon_a \mathcal{P}_{ka} \tag{10}$$

where $\vec{r}_a(k)$ is the position of the α-helix at site k when its polar group is in state a, and a,a' range over U,D. $\mathcal{P}_{ka}$ is a protein projection operator for an α-helix located at site k with polar group in state a. $H(x) = 0$ when $x > 0$ and $H(x) = \infty$ when $x \leq 0$ and describes a hard-core repulsion between polar groups. $\epsilon_a = E_a - k_B T \ell n D_a$ describes the internal energy, E_a, and degeneracy, D_a, of a protein polar group in state a. Finally, the interaction of lipids and proteins was represented by

$$\mathcal{H}_{LP} = -J_o \sum_{<ki>} \sum_n K(n)\mathcal{L}_{in}(\mathcal{P}_{kU} + \mathcal{P}_{kD}) +$$

$$\sum_k \sum_a \left[\frac{-J_o}{2} \sum_{[ij]_{ka}} \sum_{nm} \Delta I_a(nm)\mathcal{L}_{in}\mathcal{L}_{jm} + \sum_{[i]_{ka}} \sum_n \Delta\epsilon_a(n)\mathcal{L}_{in} \right]\mathcal{P}_{ka} \quad (11)$$

where the first term describes the interaction between a lipid chain at site i and an α-helical core at site k and the second describes the effect upon lipids due to their position "underneath" a glycophorin polar group. The key aspect of the model was the assumption that lipids under a glycophorin polar "umbrella" in its U state but not adjacent to an α-helical core were considered to be unperturbed ($\mathcal{H}_{LP} = 0$), but that those under a D polar group experienced a reduction in their effective lateral pressure, Π, because of a postulated perturbation of the interfacial layer between the water and the membrane. These restricted sums over these sets of lipids are indicated by $[ij]_{ka}$ and $[i]_{ka}$.

It was found that this model reproduced details of the studies of Ruppel et al.[27] The specific heat peak broadened and its temperature decreased by $\sim 2°C$ as c increases from 0 to c_1. Its temperature remained constant for a further increase in c and the specific heat peak narrowed. Thereafter, as c increased, the peak broadened and its temperature decreased. The transition enthalpy, $\Delta H(c)$, decreased between $c = 0$ and $c = c_1$ and then remained constant, after which it continued to decrease. The phase diagram showed that for $c < c_1$, all proteins are in their D ("pancake") conformation when $T > T_m(c)$ and $\sim 80\%$ of them are in their D state when $T \approx T_m(c) - 5°C$. When $c > c_2$, all protein polar groups are in their U state due to the packing term in $\mathcal{H}_{pp}$ which constrains them to be out of the membrane plane at sufficiently high concentrations. It was found that a decrease in the effective lateral pressure from 30 to ~ 27 dyn/cm accounted for the results. Some measurements were proposed to test this model.

C. MONTE CARLO STUDIES OF CONTINUUM MODELS

By a continuum model is meant one in which the lipids and other molecules are not constrained to be spatially located at lattice sites. Before introducing computer simulation of these models, it is worth studying a system, which may be a good model, but for which the thermodynamic calculations have not obviously been done correctly.

Scott and Coe[29] made use of a model that describes the main and pretransitions, at temperatures T_m and T_p, of phosphatidylcholine bilayers.[30] Although this calculation does not make use of computer simulations, it is useful to discuss the approach. The bilayer is represented by a plane surface on which proteins are represented as disks and lipid molecules are represented as shapes of various sizes representing the different cross sections of states of different energy. Scaled particle theory is applied to obtain a free energy functional and a discontinuous phase transition at $T = T_m(c)$ and protein concentration c is identified. For various assumptions as to the state of the lipids adjacent to the protein, $T_m(c)$ decreases far more than experimental results show. The transition enthalpy, $\Delta H(c)$, also decreases. Only if there are many "rings" of lipid molecules constrained to prefer their all-*trans* state can $T_m(c)$ remain constant with c over some range. This result which appears to be approximately in accord with experiment is, in fact, in disagreement with studies using Fourier transform infrared (FTIR) techniques.[31] Despite their claim to the contrary, their result, that lipids adjacent to proteins are highly ordered, is not in agreement with the results of Pink et al.[32] In fact, the calculation[29] makes the unwarranted assumption that the system is in a single phase, whereas, in general, two-component mixtures of this kind may be in two co-existing phases for some range of temperature. This is possibly the cause of the substantial difficulties arising from the results and probably invalidates the conclusions.

Fraser et al.[33] modified the model of Scott[30] and represented the projection of a DPPC molecule on the plane of membrane by a "triple" constructed from three overlapping disks. The length to breadth ratio describes the conformational state of the molecule and seven such states were identified as the most important. These were classified by the number of *gauche* bonds, g_n, which defines the internal energy, $\epsilon_g g_n$, where ϵ_g is the energy of a *gauche* rotation, the degeneracy, ω_n, and the cross section area, A_n. The model thus combines hydrocarbon chain ordering with the packing of anisotropic lipid molecules as was simulated by Zuckerman and Mouritsen.[16] The Monte Carlo method was used in both constant NVT and constant NPT simulations. The setting up of the system in order to achieve sufficiently high densities of lipids was discussed. The simulations made use of the Metropolis method and involved between 100 and 900 triples. No phase transition was observed and neither was any long-range orientational ordering exhibited. The reason for this was discussed and various possibilities were raised, the system being compared to the case of a hard-disk system which exhibits a discontinuous transition near packing density, $\eta \approx 0.7$, while the lipid model appears to freeze at $\eta \approx 0.71$ to 0.76. Various correlation functions were calculated together with free energy and the lateral pressure. It would be interesting to study whether the absence of a phase transition is intrinsic to the system or whether it is an artifact of the simulation. Once this is established, the use of this system to model a lipid-protein bilayer would be of interest.

Work has been done on the calculation of conformations of some glycosphingolipids using the SIMPLEX routine to search for deep meta-stable-type energy minima.[34] This approach, which searches for minima of the potential energy, is not a Metropolis Monte Carlo routine which calculates average values at definite temperature. The minimization of the potential energy ignores contributions to the free energy from entropic effects, which the Metropolis algorithm includes, and therefore is useful to study conformational states in, say, a crystal or at sufficiently low temperatures, but may not be sufficient to calculate thermodynamic averages appropriate to biological membranes at physiological temperatures.

D. MOLECULAR DYNAMICS STUDIES

van der Ploeg and Berendsen[35,36] studied the statics and dynamics of one half of decanoate bilayer membrane. They retained the molecular structure only of the hydrocarbon chains and ignored the polar groups of the lipids together with water and ions. They introduced a harmonic interaction between the CH_2 end of the hydrocarbon chain and a plane representing the interface between the hydrophobic and water regions which is defined by the average position of all the head groups. Edholm and Johansson[37] used this model to study the effect of the α-helical segment of polyglycine and glycophorin upon the statics and dynamics of surrounding hydrocarbon chains. The included both halves of the bilayer since the α-helices span a bilayer. They integrated the classical equations of motion numerically, using a time step of 5.10^{-15} s, for 64 hydrocarbon chains in each half of the bilayer and performed simulations for 75.10^{-12} s. In the case of glycophorin, they considered both the case in which the α-helix is constrained or in which it is free to move. They found that polyglycine induced some static ordering compared to ordering in the absence of the α-helix, by increasing the magnitude of S_{chain}.

$$S_{chain} = (3<\cos^2\theta> - 1)/2 \qquad (12)$$

where θ is the angle between the normal to the bilayer and the normal to the H-C-H plane. Glycophorin had a similar but very much smaller effect, though close to the α-helix, the groups at the end of the hydrocarbon chain displayed pronounced ordering. No immobilized lipids were found near the α-helices so that there is no evidence for an immobilized boundary layer of lipids close to the α-helix. The dynamics of the system gave a lateral diffusion coefficient for the lipids which is ~80 times larger than observed experimentally. Below it is suggested that 10^{-11} s, the time over which a diffusion coefficient was calculated, is too short a time for comparison with fluorescent recovery after photobleaching (FRAP) measurements. The decay times for orientational reorientation of CH_2 groups was found to be ~ 10^{-11} s which gave values of T_1 that are too slow by over an order of magnitude. The movement of the glycophorin α-helix showed that the groups at the two ends undergo considerable reorientation. It was suggested that the very fast lipid dynamics obtained may be due to ignoring the water region. It is possible, however, that the lipid diffusion coefficient and decay times obtained from the simulation are characteristic only of very short-time motion and that measurements of lateral diffusion coefficients and ^{2}H NMR may reflect longer-time dynamics. One, possibly important, omission is the exclusion of the glycophorin polar group. This segment accounts for ~ 80% of the mass of the molecule and its presence might change the observed deviations at the ends of the α-helix. Work on glycophorin[26] using a lattice model and Monte Carlo simulation suggested that its polar group may interact nontrivially with the lipid polar groups and thus affect the statics of the hydrocarbon chains. A molecular dynamics simulation would be able to see whether such an interaction would affect the dynamics.

IV. LATERAL DIFFUSION

The calculation of lateral diffusion coefficients in lipid bilayer membranes has, on the whole, followed three approaches: the solution of appropriate equations, such as the Langevin equation, to calculate a velocity or conductivity or the use of effective medium theory; use of the free-volume model; and applications of percolation theory. The effective medium theory was developed to calculate the electrical conductivity of composite materials[38] and yields an equation for the conductivity based on a requirement about average values.[39] It is thus a mean-field type of calculation and will incorrectly reproduce percolation behavior in two dimensions. Its advantage is that it relates a macroscopic quantity, the conductivity or current of diffusing species, in the membrane containing the two regions, to the value of the conductivity in each region. It thus does not assume any particular mechanism for diffusion which more microscopic theories have to assume.

The free-volume model of diffusion[40-42] involves a three-step microscopic process to describe a molecule moving in a solvent of other, possibly similar, molecules: the creation of a hole of a minimum size, adjacent to the diffusing molecule, in the solvent via density fluctuations; the movement of the molecule into this hole; and the filling of the void left by the diffusing molecule by solvent molecules.

Percolation theory,[43-45] as applied to diffusion in membranes, assumes that one of two types of region of the plane of the membrane is impermeable to the diffusing molecule. This molecule executes a walk on the membrane with the proviso that it may not step onto the impermeable regions. These regions may be other individual molecules or much larger areas representing clusters of molecules. Rules are set up which specify how the direction of a given step of some size is to be selected. It is found that the mean square distance, $<R^2>$, that the molecule travels either increases with time t like $t^{2/d}$ or remains finite as t increases. The fraction of the area of the membrane covered by all of the impermeable regions, f_A (Equation 9), plays an important role in deciding whether $<R^2>$ diverges with t or not. If f_A is less than some critical area, f_{Ac}, then $<R^2>$ diverges, while if it is greater, then $<R^2>$ remains finite; f_{Ac} defines the percolation limit. Percolation theory includes the correlations between different parts of the impermeable regions, once the rules for defining the impermeable regions have been given. It is thus not an approximation and, accordingly, it has not been possible to obtain closed analytical expression for diffusion coefficients in many cases of interest.

Saxton[46] assumed that a diffusing molecule moved in the plane of the membrane which may be divided into two regions: one through which movement is relatively easy and represents regions of lipid molecules in a fluid state and one through which movement is either relatively slow or impossible representing regions of solid-domain lipids or proteins. He used effective medium theory to obtain results for cases where the fractional area of the less permeable region, f_A, is small and percolation theory where f_A is larger. Saxton[46] fitted the results of both approaches to a phenomenological expression for the conductivity written in integral powers of x, where $x = 1 - f_A$ is the fractional area of the membrane on which diffusion can take place. Saxton's model[46] is applicable not only to molecules diffusing in a fluid lipid bilayer which contains proteins, but also to a bilayer which is composed of regions of fluid-like and gel-like lipids. The constraint is that the impermeable areas are essentially static on a time scale of the motion of the diffusing molecule. Saxton[46] points out that in such a system, there will be an abrupt change of the diffusion coefficient at the percolation limit, when $x = x_c$ ($f_A = f_{Ac}$), and that these effects can be seen as functions of temperature or relative concentration of two species in a two-component membrane.

Eisinger et al.[47] studied the diffusion of lipid-analogue monomers and excimers in membranes containing proteins. Their model represents the plane of the membrane by a lattice, each site of which is occupied either by a lipid molecule or an excimeric probe. Probes move by moving to nearest neighbor sites at an exchange rate of v, and if two such probes are adjacent with one of them excited, then p_E is the probability that they will form an excimer in the time interval v^{-1}. The excimer formation rate is then proportional to $n(p_E, x)^{-1}$, where $n(p_E, x)$ is the average number of nearest neighbor moves that leads to the formation of an excimer and x is the fraction of sites occupied by probes. Simulations were performed to calculate $n(p_E, x)$ numerically and the results were compared to the predictions of a diffusion limited model and to the results of Galla et al.[48] who took $p_E = 1$. They calculated how a model of proteins in a membrane influenced $n(p_E, x)$ and represented the proteins by fixed hexagons on a triangular lattice. The hexagons can share edge sites in common, unlike the models used by Saxton[46] and by Pink (below), where two hexagons may not have any sites in common. Eisinger et al.[47] also considered the cases in which the sites at the edge of a hexagon can either represent exchangeable lipids or represent parts of the protein. The essence of this model is, however, (1) the time scale defined by v^{-1} and the excimer formation probability defined by P_E; (2) the nearest neighbor jump method of movement by probes; and (3) the representation of proteins by unmoving hexagons. Not surprisingly, the diffusion coefficient appears to go to zero at a fractional area coverage by hexagons characteristic of a percolation limit. In a subsequent paper,[49] analytical solutions were given to a formulation of a model of the diffusion of membrane components toward certain regions of a membrane such as occurs in the formation of coated pits and "patch" and "cap" formation in connection with which one should note the work of Goldstein et al.[50] Nadler et al.[51] modeled diffusion of lipid probes in a bilayer membrane in the cases where the probe spanned one half of, or all of, the bilayer. They proposed that each segment of a bilayer-spanning lipid probe located in each half of the bilayer carries out a walk which is random, subject to the restriction that the location of the two ends must be within a given lateral distance. They successfully accounted for the observed ratio of diffusion constants (bilayer-spanning to half-bilayer) of ~2/3. O'Leary[52] used the free-volume model together with a removal of the requirement that the semiempirical set of constants $\{\gamma_i\}$, which appear in the expression, obtained from scaled-particle theory, for the work required to create a hole of a given radius, are each equated $\gamma_i = 1$. Good agreement was obtained for lipid diffusion in a pure lipid bilayer and in a bilayer containing bacteriorhodopsin.[53]

Pink[54,55] studied the movement of hexagons on a triangular lattice in order to establish the effect of the blocking of diffusion pathways by integral proteins upon their self-diffusion coefficient $D^s(f_A)$, as a function of the fractional area of the lattice, f_A, covered by the hexagons. Hexagons of size R = 4 were used. Hexagons were not allowed to occupy sites in common, but otherwise did not interact. It was found that $D^s(f_A)$ decreased as

$$D^s(0.55) \cong 0.12 \, D^s_0$$

$$D^s(0.82) \cong 0.05 \, D^s_0 \qquad (13)$$

where D^s_0 is the diffusion coefficient when $f_A = 0$. This result, that even at such large values of f_A D^s appears to be relatively large, is understandable when it is realized that in two dimensions random close packing occurs at $f_A \approx 0.81$ and ordered close packing occurs at $f_A \approx 0.86$.[56,57] Subsequently, the effect of an additional attractive interaction between proteins, upon protein self-diffusion, and the question of aggregation was studied,[58] using the Metropolis algorithm. It was found that as the effective protein-protein interaction $K = J_p/k_BT$ ranged from 0 to ~ 4, D^s decreased by a factor of ~ 1000 when $f_A \cong 0.51$, a concentration typical of biological membranes. For a fixed value of $f_A = 0.1$, as K decreased from 0 to -4, aggregation ranged from almost nonexistent (K = 0 to ~ -2) to very long-lived compact aggregates (K = -4). For $f_A = 0.51$, however, long-lived aggregation was apparent at K = -1.5. The self-diffusion coefficient of bacteriorhodopsin in DMPC bilayers at 30°C was calculated for a range of protein concentration from $f_A = 0$ to $f_A \cong 0.5$ using a value of K = -1.7 which yielded the observed decrease of nearly two orders of magnitude.[53] It was predicted that at lipid to protein ratios of $\sim$90 to 100, dynamic clusters with lifetimes of ≥ 1 to 10 ms should be observed and that cluster size and lifetime should increase with f_A.

Saxton[59] extended his calculations to cases of hexagons moving on a lattice to complements the results obtained by Pink.[54,55] The new results of this paper are a comparison of the self-diffusion coefficients of hexagons of a variety of sizes excluding the size treated earlier by Pink,[58] together with a phenomenological expression for D^s in terms of a power series in integral powers of f_A. The results of D^s for hexagon sizes ranging from R = 1 to R = 4 are not in agreement with measurements on bacteriorhodopsin and rhodopsin. This is not surprising because earlier studies by Pink[58] for size R = 3 showed that hexagons interacting only via a hard-core repulsive interaction gave results not in accord with experimental data, but that a small attractive interaction between hexagons reduced D^s by over one order of magnitude at higher hexagon concentrations in agreement with measurements on bacteriorhodopsin.[53]

Recently, Scalettar et al.[60] compared self-diffusion, as measured by FRAP, and mutual diffusion measured by postelectrophoresis relaxation. They adapted the work of Ohtsuki and Okano[61] to write the self-diffusion, $D^s(\rho)$, or mutual diffusion, $D^m(\rho)$, coefficients for a dilute system of proteins in a membrane as:

$$D^s(\rho) = D_o\left[1 + \rho\beta \frac{\pi}{2} \int_o \frac{du(r)p(r)g(r)rdr}{dr}\right]$$

$$D^m(\rho) = D_o\left[1 - \rho\beta\pi \int_o \frac{du(r)r^2g(r)dr}{dr}\right] \qquad (14)$$

where ρ is the protein density assumed to be sufficiently small, u(r) is a pairwise additive potential, g(r) is the equilibrium radial distribution function, and p(r) is the radial component of the perturbed distribution. In applications they took u(r) to be either a 6-4 potential or a hard-core potential. In subsequent work,[62] they extended their theory to higher densities and showed that their calculations of D^s and the computer simulation studies of Pink[55] and Saxton[59] are all in excellent agreement.

In Section II, on Modeling and Computer Simulation Methods, comments were made concerning the use of the Monte Carlo method to study kinetics. There it was argued that if sequential microstates differ by a sufficiently small amount and that if random forces are dominant, then the Monte Carlo path through phase spaces might coincide with the path that the system would actually follow.

It is for this reason that results deduced from models in which tracers can move, at each Monte Carlo step, a distance equivalent to the diameter of its cross section (a lattice constant in lattice models) should be treated with caution. In cases of hexagon movement, if the lattice constant is a small fraction of the hexagon size (given by R), then one might have more confidence in the results. In cases, too, when hexagons interact very strongly, random forces may not be dominant and again the kinetics may not represent those of the models.

The advantage of the Monte Carlo method is that it permits relatively long "times" to be averaged over. Typical times for molecular dynamics simulations are of the order of 10^{-10} s which is a very short time in which to deduce a value of D^s to compare with the results of a FRAP experiment. If, for example, $D^s = 5.10^{-9}$ cm^2/s and t $= 10^{-10}$ s, then $<R^2> = 2Dt$ gives $<R^2> \approx 10^{-2}$ Å^2. It is unlikely that over this distance a protein would experience any aspect of protein packing unless f_A was near the close packing limits, so that any agreement with the results of a FRAP measurement might be purely fortuitous. Recent work on lipid hydrocarbon chain dynamics and polypeptide conformations,[37] using molecular dynamics, was described in the previous section. From their results over a simulation time of 10^{-11} s, a value of D^s for lipid diffusion was found to be ~ 80 times larger than relevant experimental results. Although the authors suggest that the damping influence of the water, which was ignored, may be important, it is possible that the simulation time has been too short in order to get reliable values for D^s.

V. PROTEIN DISTRIBUTION AS MEASURED BY PERTURBING PROBES IN MEMBRANES

In this section, computer simulation methods which have been used to model the distribution of proteins in membranes in a fluid-like phase will be described. The experimental data are all obtained from studies using perturbing probes such as nitroxide spin labels attached to lipid hydrocarbon chains or the fluorescent probe 1,6-diphenyl-1,3,5-hexatriene (DPH). Work on computer simulation of probe motion will also be described.

The question of protein lateral distribution in membranes and how it is measured has been of interest since early measurements via electron paramagnetic (or spin) resonance (EPR or ESR) using nitroxide spin labels were interpreted as showing that some membrane proteins in a fluid-like lipid phase (T > T$_m$) were surrounded by an unbroken ring (or "annulus") of "motion-restricted" lipid molecules.[63,64] This interpretation depended upon the assumption that, on a time scale of $\sim 10^{-8}$ s, characteristic of EPR measurements, the EPR spectrum is approximately a linear combination of two independent components.[65,66] One spectral component, $S_f(\omega)$, is characteristic of "free" fluid-like lipid hydrocarbon chains, while the other, $S_i(\omega)$, is characteristic of "motion-restricted" hydrocarbon chains and ω is the angular frequency. The total spectrum per probe molecule at protein concentration c is then

$$S(\omega,c) = S_f(\omega)(1 - f_i(c)) + S_i(\omega)f_i(c) \qquad (15)$$

where $f_i(c)$ is the probability of finding a labeled lipid molecule to be in a "motion-restricted" environment. Calculations have shown, however, that if the exchange rate between lipids adjacent to the protein and those further away takes $\sim 10^{-8}$ s, then a spectrum which could be interpreted as indicating a "motion-restricted" component would be obtained.[67] ^{2}H NMR measurements[68] appear to indicate, however, that such exchange takes place in 10^{-7} s so that the assumption of two sufficiently independent spectral components may be sufficiently good.

Apart from the work of Davoust and Devaux,[67] attempts to understand the observed results have concentrated on calculating $f_i(c)$, the fraction of spin-labeled lipids which contribute to the "motion-restricted" EPR spectral component. In these calculations, it has always been assumed that the spin-labeled probes are distributed like the unlabeled lipids. The "annulus model", which assumes that each protein gives rise to M "motion-restricted" lipid molecules independent of protein concentration, can obtain $f_i(c)$ trivially. It is

$$f_i^A(c) = Mc/(1 - c) \qquad (16)$$

Hoffmann et al.,[69] in a paper largely devoted to fluorescence polarization, pointed out that their theory could be applied to EPR measurements. They assumed that the plane of the bilayer could be represented by a triangular lattice with a protein cross section represented by a hexagon on this lattice. Each site represented a lipid hydrocarbon chain, and the number of such chains around an isolated hexagon is M. If the size of the hexagon is given by R (above), then $M = 6(R + 1)$. Hoffmann et al.[69] assumed that a spin-labeled lipid hydrocarbon chain would report a "motion-restricted" spectrum if it were adjacent to at least one protein. They thus wanted to calculate $p(M,c)$, the probability that a lipid hydrocarbon chain is adjacent to at least one hexagon. They argued that if the hexagons are randomly distributed, then

$$f_i^H(c) = 1 - (1 - c)^M + \Delta f_i(c) \qquad (17)$$

where $\Delta f_i(c) \approx 0$ and can be ignored. Some discussion ensued concerning the validity of putting $\Delta f_i(c) = 0$ and in a subsequent paper,[70] computer simulations were performed to check it. Monte Carlo simulations were carried out on triangular lattices with up to 40,000 sites for values of $M = 6, 12, 18, 30$, and 48 and for fractional coverage of the lattice by hexagons, f_A, from $f_A \approx 0.1$ to $f_A \leq 0.8$. In all cases, it was found that the simulation gave results in very good agreement with Equation 17 with $\Delta f_i(c) = 0$. The results of these calculations showed that the existing EPR data on lipid-protein bilayer membranes[71] were in accord with a model in which the proteins are randomly distributed so that protein-protein "contacts" could occur. However, because EPR data has not been obtained at sufficiently low protein concentration, c, it has not been possible to obtain M from experimental data as $c \to 0$ and then to deduce the protein lateral distribution by finding a model which fits the data for higher values of c. All the data must be used in deducing both M and the correct protein distribution model. It is for this reason that it has not yet been able to demonstrate unambiguously which model of protein distribution is the correct one. Subsequent work was concerned with protein distribution when there is an interaction, apart from the hard-core repulsion forbidding two hexagons to cover any lattice sites in common. Studies were carried out for hexagons with $M = 24$ $(R = 3)$ and the effects of attractive or repulsive nearest neighbor interactions upon $f_i(c)$ were calculated.[72] The results of the simulations were compared to experiments and it was found that weak interactions (which might be zero) may exist between the proteins studied. Studies were also done to show that the Monte Carlo simulations carried out on this problem were done correctly and gave quite different results to a model in which hexagons were allowed to occupy any number of lattice sites in common.

The question can be raised as to how realistic are models which represent the (three-dimensional) lipid bilayer membrane by a two-dimensional surface in which a protein is represented by a shape, appropriate to its cross section projected onto this surface and moving in a "sea" of lipids. The validity of representing the "lipid sea" of a bilayer by a triangular lattice and the protein cross section by a hexagon was raised implicitly by Mountain et al.[73]

They represented the cross sections of lipid molecules by nearly hard disks and those of proteins by nearly hard disks of a bigger radius. Mountain et al.[73] thus represent the lipid sea, treated as surface-filling (except for protein hexagons) areas in the "lattice-hexagon" model, by a set of disks moving in the plane. They defined, in various ways, what they considered to be lipid molecules which are adjacent to at least one protein and carried out a molecular dynamics simulation to obtain $f_i^{TD}(c)$ for the "two-disk" model. They found that the results showed that $f_i^{TD}(c) \leqq f_i^H(c)$, with the disagreement becoming substantial at achievable protein concentrations in membranes. The implication of this result is that if the two-disk model is a better representation of the plane of a bilayer than the lattice-hexagon model, then results deduced from calculations based upon the latter are irrelevant. Pink et al.[57] performed Monte Carlo simulations to compare the results of lattice hexagon models with a "disk" model in which protein cross sections are represented by hard disks moving on a continuum representing the "lipid sea". They defined lipids adjacent to proteins to be the area of a region around a disk. This region can be an unbroken ring, in the case of an isolated disk, or not, when disks are closely packed. They found that for the disk model, $f_i^D(c) \geqq f_i^H(c)$, which is not surprising because such a model assumes that all of the space, not filled by protein disks, can be filled by lipids or fractions thereof. They modified this model to exclude certain regions to lipids where proteins packed together very closely, and in this "modified disk" model, they found that $f_i^{MD}(c) \approx f_i^H(c)$ up to fractional area coverage by proteins of $f_A \cong 0.78$. Pink et al.[57] also showed that the lattice-hexagon model underwent a transition, probably to a random close-packed structure at $f_A \cong 0.805$ and probably to an ordered close-packed structure at $f_A \cong 0.86$. These results agree with simulations on hard disks in a plane.[56]

It was concluded that a model which projects the three-dimensional lipid hydrocarbon chains onto a two-dimensional surface should represent the lipid regions as being a continuum with no holes in it. The reason is that in a more realistic three-dimensional model, the hydrocarbon chains should be to some extent intertwined and that if such a structure is projected onto a surface then that surface will be covered except possibly in the neighborhood of proteins. The two-disk model, which can give rise to areas not covered by lipids may thus not be a good model for a bilayer membrane, especially with proteins in it, and a better model is a lattice model of the bilayer in which protein cross sections are represented by appropriate shapes.

Pink et al.[74] modified the lattice models described here to include the effects of protein polar regions which, because of their size and shape, can affect protein lateral packing. The effect of various isotropic and anisotropic shapes were studied and results were obtained for spin-labeled lipids covalently bonded to polar regions which "overhang" the hydrophobic region to a greater or lesser extent. Monte Carlo simulations were performed to obtain $f_i(c)$, the probability that a "free" spin-labeled lipid is adjacent to the hydrophobic core of at least one protein, and $g_i(c)$, the probability that a labeled lipid, covalently bonded to a protein, is adjacent to the hydrophobic core of at least one protein (which may, in certain cases, be its "own" protein). The results were compared with measurements reported on cytochrome *c* oxidase[75] and good agreement between theory and data was obtained.

Although most of the applications of these protein packing studies have been to EPR measurements, the original study was applied to fluorescence polarization measurements using the probe DPH.[69,70] There has been much work done on the dynamics of DPH, and similar fluorescent probes, in membranes, All models have represented this molecule as moving in a potential $V(\hat{r},\phi,\eta)$, where $\hat{r}$ is a unit vector along the long axis of the molecule, ϕ defines the angle of rotation around $\hat{r}$, and η represents a set of variables describing the state of the membrane with which the probe is interacting. The wobbling-in-the-cone model,[76,77] for example, chooses

$$V = \begin{array}{ll} 0 & \text{if} \quad \theta < \theta_c \\ \infty & \text{if} \quad \theta > \theta_c \end{array}$$

$$\theta = \cos^{-1}(\hat{r} \cdot \hat{z}) \qquad (18)$$

where $\hat{z}$ is a unit vector perpendicular to the membrane and θ_c is the "cone angle" defined by the state of the membrane within which the probe is free to sample all angles. From this, the "order parameter" of the probe $\langle S_D \rangle = (3\langle\cos^2\theta\rangle - 1)/2$ can be calculated, where $\langle \ldots \rangle$ denotes the thermal average, and this, in turn, yields an expression for the anisotropy at infinite times.[76]

$$r = r_o \langle S_D \rangle^2 \qquad (19)$$

where r_o is the value of the anisotropy at $t = 0$.

Martinez and de la Torre[78] used computer simulation methods to calculate the time dependent of $\langle S_D \rangle$, assuming three forms of the potential:

$$V(1) = \tfrac{1}{2}K\theta^2$$

$$V(2) = Q(1 - \cos\theta)$$

$$V(3) = C\sin^2\theta \qquad (20)$$

They modeled a DPH molecule as a sphere tethered to a fixed point in space by a frictionless stiff spring and simulated Brownian dynamics via a Langevin equation containing the forces due to the spring and one of the potentials of Equation 20 together with random forces. Their results were in excellent agreement with the wobbling-in-the-cone model.[79]

VI. CONCLUSIONS

Computer simulation is a powerful technique which has enabled information to be obtained about the statics and dynamics of complex cooperative systems for which the classical equations of motion are too difficult to solve analytically and for which approximations, such as mean field approximations, are inadequate because of the importance of correlations. The molecular dynamics method can be used for any study as long as the system simulated encompasses all the structures that may be important and as long as sufficiently long time simulations are carried out. The Monte Carlo method, using, say, the Metropolis algorithm, should be used with caution in certain conditions to study dynamic phenomena. If its use is valid, then long time simulations can be obtained. Care should be taken, however, in ensuring that random forces do sufficiently dominate the dynamics of the system and that one can obtain a recipe to assign to each Monte Carlo step a time interval. Other cautionary comments were made in the second section of this review. One should note that there are various realizations of Monte Carlo procedures and care should be taken that the procedure used does indeed simulate the system which is being studied.[80]

Recent years have seen a consolidation of theoretical models of pure lipid bilayers and studies done on them to discover their properties. The discovery of the "soft" walls between dynamic domains of the ten-state model has thrown light on bilayer phase transitions. There has been a convergence of various models and the original simple models have been extended to study the packing of anisotropic lipid molecules or hydrogen-bonded lipid bilayers. Progress has been made on discovering the factors which determine protein diffusion in membranes, but the theoretical modeling of integral membrane proteins in lipid bilayer membranes is still at an early stage. This review has described the beginning of what will eventually develop into a field of interest to theoretical physicists and chemists with probable applications to studies of biocompatibility, cell-cell recognition, drug delivery, biosensors, and dynamic structures at interfaces and the diffusion of molecules through them.

ACKNOWLEDGMENTS

It is a pleasure to thank Martin Zuckermann for all the discussions that we have had over many years and Donna Osborne in St. John's, Newfoundland for her help. Ivy Green typed this with her usual calm competence. This work was supported in part by the Natural Sciences and Engineering Research Council of Canada.

REFERENCES

1. **Pink, D. A.,** Theoretical models of monolayers, bilayers and biological membranes, in *Biomembrane Structure and Function,* Chapman, D., Ed., MacMillan Press, London, 1983, chap. 6.
2. **Mouritsen, O. G.,** *Computer Studies of Phase Transitions and Critical Phenomena,* Springer-Verlag, Heidelberg, 1984.
3. **Pink, D. A.,** Theoretical studies of phospholipid bilayers and monolayers. Perturbing probes, monolayer phase transitions and computer simulations of lipid-protein bilayers, *Can. J. Biochem. Cell. Biol.,* 62, 760, 1984.
4. **Wodak, S. J., DeCrombrugghe, M., and Janin, J.,** Computer studies of interactions between macromolecules, *Prog. Biophys. Mol. Biol.,* 49, 29, 1987.
5. **Karplus, M. and McCammon, J. A.,** Dynamics of proteins: elements and function, *Annu. Rev. Biochem.,* 53, 263, 1983.
6. **Binder, D. and Stauffer, D.,** A simple introduction to Monte Carlo simulation and some specialized topics, in *Applications of the Monte Carlo Method in Statistical Physics,* Binder, K., Ed., Springer-Verlag, Heidelberg, 1984, chap. 1.
7. **Metropolis, N., Rosenbluth, A. W., Rosenbluth, M. N., Teller, A. H., and Teller, E.,** Equation of state calculations by fast computing machines, *J. Chem. Phys.,* 21, 1087, 1953.
8. **van Gunsteren, W. F. and Karplus, M.,** Effects of constraints on the dynamics of macromolecules, *Macromolecules,* 15, 1528, 1982.
9. **Karplus, M. and McCammon, J. A.,** The internal dynamics of globular proteins, *CRC Crit. Rev. Biochem.,* 9, 293, 1981.
10. **Nagle, J. F.,** Theory of the main lipid bilayer phase transition, *Annu. Rev. Phys. Chem.,* 31, 157, 1980.
11. **McCammon, J. A.,** Protein dynamics, *Rep. Prog. Phys.,* 47, 1, 1984.
12. **Rogers, N. K.,** The modelling of electrostatic interactions in the function of globular proteins, *Prog. Biophys. Mol. Biol.,* 48, 37, 1986.
13. **Pink, D. A., Green, T. J., and Chapman, D.,** Raman scattering in bilayers of saturated phosphatidylcholines. Experiment and theory, *Biochemistry,* 19, 349, 1980.
14. **Mouritsen, O. G.,** Studies on the lack of cooperativity in the melting of lipid bilayers, *Biochim. Biophys. Acta,* 731, 217, 1983.
15. **Mouritsen, O. G. and Zuckermann, M. J.,** Softening of lipid bilayers, *Eur. Biophys. J.,* 12, 75, 1985.
16. **Zuckermann, M. J. and Mouritsen, O. G.,** The effects of acyl chain ordering and crystallization on the main phase transition of wet lipid bilayers, *Eur. Biophys. J.,* 15, 77, 1987.
17. **Sahni, P. S., Grest, G. S., Anderson, M. P., and Srolovitz, D. J.,** Kinetics of the q-state Potts model in two dimensions, *Phys. Rev. Lett.,* 50, 263, 1983.
18. **Mouritsen, O. G., Fogedby, H. C., Sorensen, E. S., and Zuckermann, M. J.,** Pattern formation in lipid membranes, in *Time-Dependent Effects in Disordered Materials,* Pynn, R. and Riste, T., Eds., Plenum Press, New York, 1987, 457.
19. **Pink, D. A., MacDonald, A. L., and Quinn, B.,** Anisotropic interactions in hydrated cerebrosides. A theoretical model of stable and metastable states and hydrogen-bond formation, *Chem. Phys. Lipids,* 47, 83, 1988.
20. **Cruzeiro-Hansson, L. and Mouritsen, O. G.,** Passive ion permeability of lipid membranes modelled via lipid-domain interfacial area, *Biochim. Biophys. Acta,* 944, 63, 1988.
21. **Kanehisa, M. I. and Tsong, T. Y.,** Cluster model of lipid phase transitions with application to passive permeation of molecules and structure relaxations in lipid bilayers, *J. Am. Chem. Soc.,* 100, 424, 1978.

22. **Caille, A., Pink, D. A., de Verteuil, F., and Zuckermann, M. J.,** Theoretical models for quasi-two-dimensional mesomorphic monolayers and membrane bilayers, *Can. J. Phys.,* 58, 581, 1980.

23. **Mouritsen, O. G., Ipsen, J. H., and Zuckermann, M. J.,** Lateral density fluctuations in the chain-melting phase transition of lipid monolayers, *J. Colloid Interface Sci.,* in press.

24. **Cruzeiro-Hansson, L., Ipsen, J. H., and Mouritsen, O. G.,** Intrinsic molecules in lipid membranes change the lipid-domain interfacial area: cholesterol at domain interfaces, *Biochim. Biophys. Acta,* in press.

25. **Tevlin, P., Jones, F. P., and Trainor, L. E. H.,** Phase transitions of lipid bilayers. I. Density of states calculation, *J. Chem. Phys.,* 87, 5483, 1987.

26. **MacDonald, A. L. and Pink, D. A.,** Thermodynamics of glycophorin in phospholipid bilayer membranes, *Biochemistry,* 26, 1909, 1987.

27. **Ruppel, D., Kapitza, H. G., Galla, H.-J., Sixl, F., and Sackmann, E.,** On the microstructure and phase diagram of dimyristoylphosphatidylcholine-glycophorin bilayers. The role of defects and the hydrophilic lipid-protein interaction, *Biochim. Biophys. Acta,* 692, 1, 1982.

28. **Chicken, C. and Sharom, F.,** Lipid-protein interactions of the human erythrocyte concanavalin. A receptor in phospholipid bilayers, *Biochim. Biophys. Acta,* 774, 110, 1984.

29. **Scott, H. L., Jr. and Coe, T. J.,** A theoretical study of lipid-protein interactions in bilayers, *Biophys. J.,* 42, 219, 1983.

30. **Scott, H. L.,** Phosphatidylcholine bilayers. A theoretical model which describes the main and lower phase transition, *Biochim. Biophys. Acta,* 643, 161, 1981.

31. **Cortijo, M., Alonso, A., Gomez-Fernandez, J. C., and Chapman, D.,** Intrinsic protein-lipid interactions. Infrared spectroscopic studies of gramicidin A, bacteriorhodopsin and calcium-ATPase in biomembranes and reconstituted systems, *J. Mol. Biol.,* 157, 597, 1982.

32. **Pink, D. A., Georgallas, A., and Chapman, D.,** Intrinsic proteins and their effect upon lipid hydrocarbon chain order, *Biochemistry,* 20, 7152, 1981.

33. **Fraser, D. P., Chantrell, R. W., Melville, D., and Tildesley, D. J.,** Two-dimensional Monte Carlo studies of lipid molecules in a bilayer membrane, *Liquid Cryst.,* 3, 423, 1988.

34. **Wynn, C. H. and Robson, B.,** Calculation of the conformation of glycosphingolipids. II. G_{M1}- and G_{M2}-gangliosides, *J. Theor. Biol.,* 123, 221, 1986.

35. **van der Ploeg, P. and Berendsen, H. J. C.,** Molecular dynamics simulation of a bilayer membrane, *J. Chem. Phys.,* 76, 3271, 1982.

36. **van der Ploeg, P. and Berendsen, H. J. C.,** Molecular dynamics of membranes, *Mol. Phys.,* 49, 233, 1983.

37. **Edholm, O. and Johansson, J.,** Lipid bilayer polypeptide interactions studied by molecular dynamics simulation, *Eur. Biophys. J.,* 14, 203, 1987.

38. **Landauer, R.,** Electrical conductivity in inhomogeneous media, in *Electrical Transport and Optical Properties of Inhomogeneous Media,* Garland, J. C. and Tanner, D. B., Eds., American Institute of Physics, New York, 1978, 2.

39. **Kirkpatrick, S.,** Classical Transport in disordered media: scaling and effective-medium theories, *Phys. Rev. Lett.,* 27, 1722, 1971.

40. **Turnbull, D. and Cohen, M. H.,** Free-volume model of the amorphous:glass transition, *J. Chem. Phys.,* 34, 120, 1961.

41. **MacCarthy, J. E. and Kozak, J. J.,** Lateral diffusion in fluid systems, *J. Chem. Phys.,* 77, 2214, 1982.

42. **Galla, H.-J., Hartmann, W., Theilen, U., and Sackmann, E.,** On two-dimensional passive random walk in lipid bilayers and fluid pathways in biomembranes, *J. Membrane Biol.,* 48, 215, 1979.

43. **Kehr, K. W. and Binder, K.,** Simulation of diffusion in lattice gases and related kinetic phenomena, in *Applications of the Monte Carlo Method in Statistical Physics,* Binder, K., Ed., Springer-Verlag, Heidelberg, 1984, chap. 6.

44. **Stauffer, D.,** *Introduction to Percolation Theory,* Taylor & Francis, London, 1985.

45. **Havlin, S. and Ben-Avraham, D.,** Diffusion in disordered media, *Adv. Phys.,* 36, 695, 1987.

46. **Saxton, M. J.,** Lateral diffusion in an archipelago. Effects of impermeable patches on diffusion in a cell membrane, *Biophys. J.,* 39, 165, 1982.

47. **Eisinger, J., Flores, J., and Petersen, W. P.,** A milling crowd model for local and long-range obstructed lateral diffusion. Mobility of excimeric probes in the membranes of intact erythrocytes, *Biophys. J.,* 49, 987, 1986.

48. **Galla, H.-J. and Hartmann, W.,** Excimer-forming lipids in membrane research, *Chem. Phys. Lipids,* 27, 199, 1980.

49. **Eisinger, J. and Halperin, B. I.,** Effects of spatial variation in membrane diffusibility and solubility on the lateral transport of membrane components, *Biophys. J.,* 50, 513, 1986.

50. **Goldstein, B., Wofsy, C., and Echavarria-Heras, H.,** Effect of membrane flow on the capture of receptors by coated pits, *Biophys. J.,* 53, 405, 1988.

51. **Nadler, J., Tavan, P., and Schulten, K.,** A model for the lateral diffusion of "stiff" chains in a lipid bilayer, *Eur. Biophys. J.,* 12, 25, 1985.

52. **O'Leary, T. J.,** Lateral diffusion of lipids in complex biological membranes, *Proc. Natl. Acad. Sci. U.S.A.,* 84, 429, 1987.

53. **Peters, R. and Cherry, R. J.,** Lateral and rotational diffusion of bacteriorhodopsin in lipid bilayers: experimental test of the Saffman-Delbruck equations, *Proc. Natl. Acad. Sci. U.S.A.,* 79, 4317, 1982.

54. **Pink, D. A.,** Constraints on protein lateral diffusion, *Trends Biochem. Sci.,* 10, 230, 1985.

55. **Pink, D. A.,** Protein lateral movement in lipid bilayers. Simulation studies of its dependence upon protein concentration, *Biochim. Biophys. Acta,* 818, 200, 1985.

56. **Berryman, J. G.,** Random close packing of hard spheres and disks, *Phys. Rev. A,* 27, 1053, 1983.

57. **Pink, D. A., Quinn, B., and Laidlaw, D. J.,** Deducing the lateral distribution of proteins in lipid bilayer membranes, *Eur. Biophys. J.,* 16, 31, 1988.

58. **Pink, D. A., Laidlaw, D. J., and Chisholm, D.,** Protein lateral movement in lipid bilayers. Monte Carlo simulation studies of its dependence upon attractive protein-protein interactions, *Biochim. Biophys. Acta,* 863, 9, 1986.

59. **Saxton, M. J.,** Lateral diffusion in an archipelago. The effect of mobile obstacles, *Biophys. J.,* 52, 989, 1987.

60. **Scalettar, B. A., Abney, J. R., and Owicki, J. C.,** Theoretical comparison of the self diffusion and mutual diffusion of interacting membrane proteins, *Proc. Natl. Acad. Sci. U.S.A.,* 85, 6726, 1988.

61. **Ohtsuki, T. and Okano, K.,** Diffusion coefficients of interacting Brownian particles, *J. Chem. Phys.,* 77, 1443, 1982.

62. **Abney, J. R.,** personal communication, 1988.

63. **Jost, P. C., Griffith, O. H., Capaldi, R. A., and Vanderkooj, G.,** Evidence for boundary lipid in membranes, *Proc. Natl. Acad. Sci. U.S.A.,* 70, 480, 1973.

64. **Jost, P. C. and Griffith, O. H.,** Lipid-protein interactions: influence of integral membrane proteins on bilayer lipids, in *Biomolecular Structure and Function,* Agris, P. F., Ed., Academic Press, New York, 1978.

65. **Devaux, P. F. and Seigneuret, M.,** Specificity of lipid-protein interactions as determined by spectroscopic techniques, *Biochim. Biophys. Acta,* 822, 63, 1985.

66. **Esmann, M., Watts, A., and Marsh, D.,** Spin-label studies of lipid-protein interactions in sodium-potassium ATPase membranes from rectal glands of *Squalus acanthius, Biochemistry,* 24, 1386, 1985.

67. **Davoust, J. and Devaux, P. F.,** Simulation of electron spin resonance spectra of spin-labelled fatty acids covalently attached to the boundary of an intrinsic membrane protein. A chemical exchange model, *J. Magn. Reson.,* 48, 475, 1982.

68. **Meier, R. P., Sachse, J.-H., Brophy, P. J., Marsh, D., and Kothe, G.,** Integral membrane proteins significantly decrease the molecular motion in lipid bilayers: a deuteron NMR relaxation study of membranes containing myelin proteolipid apoprotein, *Proc. Natl. Acad. Sci. U.S.A.,* 84, 3704, 1987.

69. **Hoffmann, W., Pink, D. A., Restall, C., and Chapman, D.,** Intrinsic molecules in fluid phospholipid bilayers. Fluorescence probe studies, *Eur. J. Biochem.,* 114, 585, 1981.

70. **Pink, D. A., Chapman, D., Laidlaw, D. J., and Wiedmer, T.,** Election spin resonance and steady-state fluorescence polarization studies of lipid bilayers containing integral proteins, *Biochemistry,* 23, 4051, 1984.

71. **Silvius, J. R., McMillen, D. A., Saley, N. D., Jost, P. C., and Griffith, O. H.,** Competition between cholesterol and phosphatidylcholine for the hydrophobic surface of sarcoplasmic reticulum Ca^{2+}-ATPase, *Biochemistry,* 23, 538, 1984.

72. **Laidlaw, D. J. and Pink, D. A.,** Protein lateral distribution in lipid bilayer membranes, *Eur. Biophys. J.,* 12, 143, 1985.

73. **Mountain, R. D., Mazo, R. M., and Volwerk, J. J.,** Molecular dynamics simulation study of a two-dimensional fluid mixture system: a model for biological membranes, *Chem. Phys. Lipid,* 40, 35, 1986.

74. **Pink, D. A., Chisholm, D. M., and Chapman, D.,** Models of protein lateral arrangements in lipid bilayer membranes. Application to electron spin resonance studies of cytochrome c oxidase, *Chem. Phys. Lipids,* 46, 267, 1988.

75. **Griffith, O. H., McMillen, D. A., Keana, J. F. W., and Jost, P. C.,** Lipid-protein interactions in cytochrome c oxidase. A comparison of covalently attached phospholipid photo-spin label with label free to diffuse in the bilayer, *Biochemistry,* 25, 574, 1986.

76. **Kinosita, K., Kawato, S., and Ikegami, A.,** A theory of fluorescence depolarization decay in membranes, *Biophys. J.,* 20, 289, 1977.

77. **Kinosita, K., Ikegami, A., and Kawato, S.,** On the wobbling-in-a-cone analysis of fluorescence anisotropy decay, *Biophys. J.,* 37, 461, 1982.

78. **Martinez, M. C. L. and de la Torre, J. G.,** Brownian dynamics simulation of restricted rotational diffusion, *Biophys. J.,* 52, 303, 1987.

79. **Lipari, G. and Szabo, A.,** Pade approximants to correlation functions for restricted rotational diffusion, *J. Chem. Phys.,* 75, 2971, 1981.

80. **Jan, N., Lookman, T., and Pink, D. A.,** On computer simulation methods used to study models of two-component lipid bilayers, *Biochemistry,* 23, 3227, 1984.

81. **Pink, D. A.,** unpublished calculations.

Chapter 1.A.5

DETERMINATION OF CHAIN CONFORMATIONS IN THE MEMBRANE INTERIOR BY BROWNIAN DYNAMICS SIMULATIONS

Richard W. Pastor

TABLE OF CONTENTS

I. INTRODUCTION

A realistic computer simulation of the membrane bilayer interior must deal with problems similar to those encountered in alkane melts and liquid crystals: the individual chains are highly flexible and interconvert between hundreds of thousand of configurations; the bilayer is oriented, thereby allowing an assortment of collective and noncollective motions. Consequently, it is important to consider carefully which of the three common simulation methods, molecular dynamics (MD), Monte Carlo (MC), or stochastic dynamics (SD), is most appropriate to apply to a particular problem. This chapter reviews how a stochastic approach, Brownian dynamics (BD), has been used to develop a new motional model for the bilayer, which, in turn, yields a detailed description of chain conformations.

The work described here was initially motivated by the dynamic behavior of the bilayer, namely, the unusual frequency dependence of the experimental ^{13}C NMR T_1 (longitudinal or spin-lattice) relaxation times in dipalmitoylphosphatidylcholine (DPPC) vesicles.[1-3] For this reason, MC methods were not considered, as an MC simulation does not yield time-dependent properties. In designing MD simulations, both the timing and the number of atoms are relevant. DPPC contains 50 heavy (i.e., nonhydrogen) atoms. Thus, even without solvent or explicit hydrogens, a bilayer simulation consisting of 12 lipid molecules of each face would include 1200 atoms. Timing results for MD on a Cray-IS (a supercomputer with a maximum processing speed of 100 million floating point operations per second) for a comparably sized system (lysozyme, 1264 atoms) are 0.39 per energy evaluation;[4] including a 10% overhead for the remainder of the algorithm and assuming a time step of 0.001 ps, a 1-ns trajectory would require approximately 125 h of (cpu)time. Is this sufficient for a simulation-based analysis of the T_1 in bilayers? Analyses of the relaxation data indicated the existence of at least one slow motion with a relaxation time of about a nanosecond; it was not clear whether its source was rigid body reorientation of the lipid[2,5] or collective motions of the entire bilayer.[2] Numerous previous studies[6-12] (cf. References 1 and 2) based on other data had failed to reach a consensus. Additionally, the *trans* to *gauche* isomerization rates of alkanes are in the range of 100 ps^{-1} to 1 ns^{-1},[13-21] making internal motions a possible source of the frequency dependence. Hence, multinanosecond simulations are required to obtain a statistically meaningful number of transitions and to properly sample the slow motion.

At the core of stochastic approaches is the replacement of an explicit solvent by a heat bath with suitable statistical properties. In this way, a smaller number of atoms can be explicitly simulated, enabling significantly longer simulations than are currently possible with molecular dynamics. In the case of a lipid bilayer, this involves the simulation of only one chain, or several chains, in the presence of forces that mimic the structural and dynamic properties of the rest of the bilayer. Because the application of stochastic dynamics to biopolymers is relatively new, Section II contains a fairly detailed discussion of the assumptions that go into any stochastic simulation.

The development of a new motional model, based on our simulation results[22] and fits to relaxation data[23] is reviewed in Section III. First, as described in Section III.B, BD simulations were carried out in the Marcelja mean field potential,[24] and calculated order parameters were shown to converge to values observed for DPPC multilayers. Next (Section III.C), time correlation functions for internal reorientation calculated from the trajectories were used in different models to calculate the ^{13}C T_1 relaxation times for DPPC vesicles. It was shown that a model consisting of internal motions with axial rotation and noncollective long axis rotation provided excellent agreement with experiment; models including only internal or axial motions were unsatisfactory. The validity of such a dynamic model with finite has important consequences for a structural description of the bilayer. It implies that the observed deuterium order parameter results from at least two factors: one associated with internal disorder of the chains and the other associated with orientational disorder, or tilt, of the lipid. Section III.D illustrates how the effects of tilt may be incorporated into the Marcelja model and thus in BD simulations. Selected results of the simulations follow in Section IV, including chain conformations and average dimensions; a comparison with the crankshaft model; and errors that arise from constraining the chain to a diamond lattice (i.e., the rotational isomeric model).

II. STOCHASTIC DYNAMICS

A. OVERVIEW

BD is a simulation technique based on the Langevin equation,[25-27] which we write for a particle of mass m and friction constant ζ:

$$m\, d^2x/dt^2 \;=\; F(t) - \zeta\, dx/dt + R(t) \tag{1}$$

where x is the position and F is the systematic force. As we show in Section III.B, the systematic force may include solvent effects on the structure of the solute, in this case the favoring of particular configurations of a chain molecule over and above the Boltzmann weighting arising from intrachain interactions. The dynamical influence of the solvent is modeled by the random force R(t) and a frictional proportional to the velocity. The random force is assumed to be uncorrelated with the positions and velocities of the particles, and by the fluctuation-dissipation theorem,[28] its statistical properties are related to the friction constant. It is convenient to define the collision frequency $\gamma = \zeta/m$; then,

$$< R(t) > \,= 0$$

$$< R(t)\, R(t') > \,= 2m\gamma kT\, \delta(t-t') \tag{2a}$$

where k is the Boltzmann's constant, T is the absolute temperature, and $\delta(t - t')$ is the Dirac delta function. On average, the random and frictional forces balance, and there is no net heating or cooling of the system. As $\gamma \rightarrow 0$, coupling to the heat bath vanishes, and Langevin's equation becomes Newton's equation, $m\, d^2 x/dt^2 = F(t)$. As γ becomes large, Equation 1 describes overdamped motion, and the dynamics becomes purely diffusive; it is in this limit that Brownian, or diffusive, algorithms are valid. Other models have been made for the stochastic properties of the solvent;[16,29-31] however, in the limit of high γ, diffusive motion also results for these models, and we restrict our discussion to the Langevin equation. The following subsections discuss parametrizing the friction constant and neglecting the effects of hydrodynamic interaction; choosing an algorithm and time step; estimating the validity of the diffusive approximation; and finally, some of the limitations of stochastic approaches.

B. HYDRODYNAMICS
1. Estimating the Friction Constant

The intrachain force is the same in both Langevin's and Newton's equations, so most of the force field used for MD can be carried over for an SD simulation. This subsection considers the friction constant, ζ. When a simulation is to be carried out on an individual particle (e.g., a protein) or a system of nonbonded particles (e.g., ions in solution), ζ may be obtained from the Stokes-Einstein relationship:[32]

$$D = kT/\zeta \tag{3}$$

where D is the experimental translational diffusion constant extrapolated to infinite dilution. If the particle is spherical and relatively large, the translational friction constant can be calculated from Stokes' law with *stick* boundary conditions:[33,34]

$$\zeta = 6\pi\eta a \tag{4}$$

where η is the viscosity of the medium and a is the effective hydrodynamic radius of the particle. In a water-soluble protein, for example, a includes a part of a shell of bound waters and is consequently larger than the radius of an unhydrated protein.[34-36] Perhaps surprisingly, a hydrodynamic approach can be extended to the level of small molecules with quite reasonable results. An important proviso is that *slip* boundary conditions appear to be operative:[37,38] for a sphere, the 6 in Equation 4 is replaced by a 4. As an example, the self-diffusion constant of water at 307.6 degrees is 2.85×10^{-5} cm^2/s.[39] Assuming a radius of 1.6 Å, the Stokes' law slip value is 2.89×10^{-5} cm^2/s; this corresponds to a collision frequency of 54.9 ps^{-1}.

Most applications of SD require knowledge of the friction constant for an individual subunit of a polymer, e.g., the methylene group of an alkane chain. Again, we turn to hydrodynamics, with the notion that it should be possible to derive the methylene friction constant from experimentally measured diffusion constants of alkanes. Consider a polymer represented by an array of N beads. Physically, as the polymer diffuses, some of the beads are shielded from the solvent, and we expect that the friction constant of the polymer is not simply the sum of the friction constants of the individual beads; conversely, the bead friction constant would not equal the polymer friction constant divided by N. To a good approximation, the friction force $\mathbf{F}_i$ exerted on the solvent by the ith bead can be written:[26,33]

$$\mathbf{F}_i + \zeta_i \sum_j' \mathbf{T}_{ij} \cdot \mathbf{F}_j = \zeta_i (\mathbf{u}_i - \mathbf{v}_i^\circ) \tag{5}$$

where ζ_i is the friction constant of the bead, $\mathbf{u}_i$ is its velocity, and $\mathbf{y}_i^\circ$ is the unperturbed solvent velocity at point i. The prime on the summation denotes omission of the $i = j$ terms. $\mathbf{T}_{ij}$ is the Oseen tensor which describes the hydrodynamic interaction between the point sources of friction in an incompressible fluid:[26,33]

$$\mathbf{T}_{ij} = \frac{1}{8\pi\eta r_{ij}} \left[\mathbf{I} + \frac{\mathbf{r}_{ij}\mathbf{r}_{ij}^\dagger}{r_{ij}^2} \right] \tag{6}$$

where η is the viscosity of the medium $\mathbf{I}$ is the identity matrix, $\mathbf{r}_{ij}$ is the vector from element i to element j, with $\mathbf{r}_{ij}^\dagger$ its adjoint. (Note that the outer product $\mathbf{r}_{ij}\mathbf{r}_{ij}^\dagger$ is a matrix.) Garcia de la Torre and Bloomfield[40] have developed expressions for the overall translational and rotational friction coefficients for a rigid array of beads with arbitrary friction and configuration in terms of the inverse of the following 3N $\times$ 3N matrix:

$$\mathbf{Q}_{ij} = \delta_{ij}\mathbf{I} + (1-\delta_{ij})\zeta_i\mathbf{T}_{ij} \tag{7}$$

where $\mathbf{I}$ is the identity matrix and δ_{ij} is the Kronecker delta.

The preceding method, however, is difficult to apply even to a moderately sized flexible chain, as a 3N $\times$ 3N matrix must be inverted for each configuration (a forbidding calculation even with modern computers). Kirkwood and Riseman[41] avoided this problem by preaveraging the Oseen tensor and derived the following expression for the translational friction, f_t, coefficient of N beads:

$$f_t = N\varsigma \left[1 + (\varsigma/6\pi\eta N) \sum_{ij}' <r_{ij}^{-1}> \right]^{-1} = N \varsigma/Z_t \tag{8}$$

The evaluation of the average $<r_{ij}^{-1}>$ for a series of normal alkanes was later carried out by Paul and Mazo,[42] who then obtained an estimate of the methylene friction constant by fitting Equation 8 to experimental diffusion constants. The fit was quite good, and it is convenient to express their results in terms of collision frequency (in ps^{-1}) and the viscosity (in centipoise)[22]

$$\gamma = 62.44\eta \tag{9}$$

A collision frequency of 150 ps^{-1}, therefore, corresponds to viscosity of approximately 2.4 cP.

Recent work[43-45] has shown that because of the preaveraging approximation, Equation 8 underestimates the molecular friction constant by about 10%. This is not a serious error given the scatter in the experimental data and the approximate character of the theory, and Equation 9 is suitable for the present purpose. Other approaches[36,46] have been developed recently to provide friction constants for proteins and other polymers.

2. Neglecting Hydrodynamic Interaction

Most Langevin and Brownian simulations of flexible molecules have neglected hydrodynamic interaction (HI); to include HI requires an evaluation of the Oseen interaction at each time step,[47] resulting in a large increase in computer time. Given that we have explicitly included HI in deducing a value of the friction constant, is it consistent to ignore it in the simulation?

This question can be answered by considering the free draining limit, where the particles are far apart and their hydrodynamic interaction is small. The denominator in Equation 8, Z_t, then approaches one, and the friction constant of the polymer is the simple sum of the friction constants of the monomer units. However, it has been shown for normal alkanes, that Z_t varies from 2 for butane to over 5 for a 40-carbon chain.[46] Consequently, neglect of HI results in a serious error for translational diffusion of alkane chains, assuming that Equation 9 is used to assign the methylene friction constants.

Similar estimates may be carried out for the effect of HI on rotation[46] and isomerization.[48,49] Here the effects are much smaller and partly cancel: HI tends to decrease the effective friction on rotation and increase the friction on isomerization. Thus, if a simulation primarily concerns overall and internal rotation, neglect of HI is a reasonable approximation, even though the translational motion found in such a simulation would not agree with experiment.

C. ALGORITHMS AND ERRORS

MD trajectories are commonly propagated by the Verlet three-step algorithm:[50]

$$x_{n+1} = 2x_n - x_{n-1} + (\Delta^2/m) F_n \tag{10}$$

where x_{n-1}, x_n, and x_{n+1} are the positions at successive time steps, Δ is the value of the timestep, and F_n is systematic force applied at step n. When numerically solving the Langevin equation, however, the stochastic properties of the random force must also be taken into account. Algorithms fall into three general classes,[51] depending on the product of the collision frequency and the time step.

1. $\gamma\Delta \ll 1$

The first class is valid at low friction. It is convenient to write these algorithms in a

Verlet-like form. One such example is the algorithm of Brunger et al.:[52]

$$x_{n+1} = x_n + (x_n - x_{n-1}) \frac{1 - \frac{1}{2}\gamma\Delta}{1 + \frac{1}{2}\gamma\Delta} + (\Delta^2/m)(F_n + R_n)(1 + \frac{1}{2}\gamma\Delta)^{-1} \qquad (11)$$

where R_n, the random force applied at step n, is taken from a Gaussian distribution of mean zero and variance:

$$< R_n^2 > = 2m\gamma kT/\Delta \qquad (12)$$

Note that when $\gamma = 0$, the Verlet algorithm is recovered.

An important consideration when carrying out a simulation is the time step. Too small a time step is inefficient; however, as with the numerical solution of any differential equation, errors propagate more rapidly as the time step is increased. In MD simulations, time step errors can be seen by nonconservation of energy and departures from the exact trajectory.[54] There is no "exact" trajectory in a stochastic simulation. Nevertheless, time averages can be readily calculated for simple cases. For example, consider the mean square displacement, $< x^2 >$, for a particle of mass m in a harmonic potential of frequency ω. By suitable averaging over the random force and positions, it can be shown[53] that a trajectory propagated by Equation 11 will yield the value:

$$< x^2 > = (kT/m\omega^2)(1 - \frac{1}{4}\omega^2\Delta^2)^{-1} \qquad (13)$$

Thus, as the time step approaches 0, the exact result for a harmonic oscillator, $kT/m\omega^2$, is recovered; however, at any nonzero time step, there is an error. The value of γ does not appear in the average in Equation 13, which is physically correct, although this is not the case for all low γ algorithms.[53] Finally, note that this estimate does not include statistical errors arising from the finite length of the trajectory.

2. $\gamma\Delta \gg 1$

The second class applies to the diffusive regime, where γ is large, and thus $\gamma\Delta \gg 1$. Two algorithms have been commonly used:

$$x_{n+1} = x_n + (\Delta/m\gamma) F_n + X_n \qquad (14)$$

$$x_{n+1} = x_n + (\Delta/m\gamma) F_n + (\Delta^2/2m\gamma) \dot{F}_n + X_n \qquad (15)$$

where

$$\dot{F}_n = (F_n - F_{n-1})/\Delta \qquad (16)$$

Equation 15, introduced by van Gunsteren and Berendsen,[51] includes the derivative of the systematic force for increased accuracy. In both of these equations, the stochastic term, X_n, represents a random displacement in the position. It is taken from a Gaussian distribution with zero mean and variance:

$$< X_n^2 > = 2kT\Delta/(m\gamma) \qquad (17)$$

As was the case with low-friction algorithm, it is straightforward to calculate the mean squared displacement for a harmonic potential:[53]

$$< x^2 > = (kT/m\omega^2)(1 - \xi)^{-1} \qquad \text{for Eq. (14)} \qquad (18)$$

$$= (kT/m\omega^2) \left[1 - \frac{2\xi^2}{(1-\xi)} \right]^{-1} \qquad \text{for Eq. (15)} \qquad (19)$$

where

$$\xi = \omega^2\Delta/2\gamma \qquad (20)$$

Thus, at the expense of including the derivative of the force, the error can be greatly reduced. For example, the values of Δ and γ used in the simulations presented in this chapter were 0.015 ps and 150 ps^{-1}, respectively, and the Ryckaert-Bellemans[55] parametrization was used to describe the threefold dihedral angle potential along the chain. The frequency of the *trans*-well of butane with the Ryckaert-Bellemans[55] potential is $\omega \approx 30$ ps^{-1}.[21] Hence, the simulated $< x^2 >$ for butane would be in error by 5% if the trajectory were propagated using Equation 14, but only by 0.5% if Equation 15 were used.

Note that for the diffusive algorithms the time step and the collision frequency always appear as a ratio. This is an important feature and is not the case for the low-friction Langevin algorithms. As a result, time-dependent quantities (e.g., isomerization rates and time constants from correlation functions) calculated from BD trajectories can be scaled to represent the dynamics at an arbitrary collision frequency. The collision frequency may be related to the effective viscosity of the solvent (as in Equation 9). This feature was critical for applying the method to membranes, where the experimental value of the viscosity is a matter of controversy.[56,57]

3. Arbitrary $\gamma\Delta$

A third class, which is valid for arbitrary $\gamma\Delta$, has been developed[51,58,59] using the analytic solution of the Langevin equation for a particle in a constant force. This makes it possible to increase the time step to where it is limited by the systematic force; however, sampling from a bivariate distribution is required to properly treat the random force, and these algorithms are correspondingly more complex than those discussed above. We restrict their use to systems where the assumptions necessary for either the low or high friction are violated.[21]

D. INERTIAL EFFECTS

Physically, for diffusive motion to occur, the momentum relaxation time, γ^{-1}, must be very small with respect to the time scale for the displacements of interest.[25] At lower collision frequencies, the motion of a particle is underdamped and is influenced by the inertia of the particle. These deviations from pure diffusive behavior are referred to as *inertial effects*. The magnitude of the inertial terms then limits the applicability of Brownian dynamics or, correspondingly, of a diffusion equation for certain systems.

An analytic estimate of the importance of inertial terms in isomerization reactions may be obtained from Kramers approximate high γ solution[60] for the rate constant k_{Kram} for passage out of a harmonic well over a barrier of height U_b:

$$k_{Kram}/k_{TST} = (\gamma/2\omega_b) \left[\{ 1 + (4\omega_b^2/\gamma^2)\}^{1/2} - 1 \right] \qquad (21)$$

where

$$k_{TST} = (\omega_a/2\pi) \exp(-U_b/kT) \qquad (22)$$

Here k_{TST} is the rate constant from classical transition state theory,[61] the frequency of the harmonic well is given by ω_a; and $i\omega_b$ is the imaginary frequency associated with the inverted parabola representing the barrier. Equation 21 is then expanded in powers of ω_b/γ.

$$k_{Kram}/k_{TST} = (\omega_b/\gamma)\left[1 - (\omega_b/\gamma)^2 + 2(\omega_b/\gamma)^4\right] + O(\gamma^{-7}) \qquad (23)$$

As in the preceding subsection, we use Ryckaert-Bellemans[55] potential; for butane the frequency of the *trans-gauche* barrier is 16.112 ps^{-1}. Thus, from Equation 23, the diffusive approximation overestimates the Kramers[60] rate by approximately 9.5% at $\gamma = 50$ and by 68.5% at $\gamma = 15$. These estimates agree with both simulations[21] and other theoretical estimates.[62] Consequently, when applying BD, it is important to note that as γ decreases, both errors in the algorithm become large (Equations 14 and 15) and the diffusive approximation begins to break down.

Similar analytic and numerical estimates for butane[21] have also shown that inertial effects are smaller at a given collision frequency for rotational motion than for isomerization. Additionally, inertial effects become less important as the length of the alkane increases.[21]

E. LIMITATIONS OF STOCHASTIC APPROACHES

All computer simulations of real physical systems are approximate. The intermolecular potentials are idealized, parametrized, and, for the most part, many body and quantum effects are neglected. Stochastic approaches introduce another level of approximation over and above molecular dynamics simulations: a model of the solvent.

We have tried to demonstrate that the model is plausible. A hydrodynamic approach for alkanes is consistent with a wide range of experiments, and the friction constants can be parametrized to these experiments. The neglect of hydrodynamic interaction is also justified in many cases where simulation of translational diffusion is not a primary object of the study.

Nevertheless, there are cases where important details of the solvent interaction with the solute may be lost. For example, in a SD simulation of a peptide in water, solvent binding increases the friction;[36] similar effects would be expected for lipid head groups.

In Langevin dynamics, it is assumed that the solvent responds instantaneously to the solute. For certain high-frequency motions such as barrier crossing in chemical reactions, this is not the case, and accurate stochastic description of these systems requires a generalized Langevin equation.[63] For the typical frequencies of alkane dynamics, this does not appear to be a serious problem. However, for diffusion of small molecules in alkane solvents[64] (which would include the interior of the bilayer[57]), the simple hydrodynamic model probably needs revision.

III. A SIMULATION-BASED MODEL

A. OVERVIEW

A description of chain conformations within the bilayer often begins with the deuterium order parameter, S_{CD}, which is experimentally measured from the NMR line shape of selectively deuterated lipids.[65,66] S_{CD} is related to the average orientation of the methylene groups in lipid chains as follows:

$$S_{CD} = (1/2) \langle 3\cos^2\theta - 1\rangle \qquad (24)$$

where θ is the angle made by the particular CD vector and the bilayer normal. A microscopic interpretation of S_{CD}, however, is highly model dependent because different motions can lead to very similar order parameters. For this reason, it is useful to include both structural

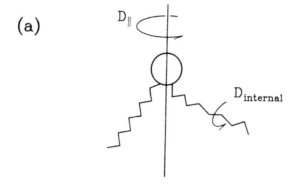

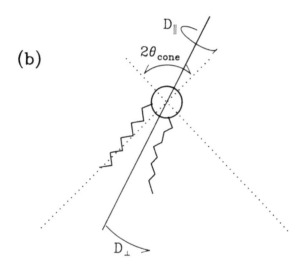

FIGURE 1. Schematic of lipid motions. (a) A model corresponding to zero chain tilt; only internal and axial motions contribute to the ^{13}C NMR relaxation; (b) wobbling in a cone resulting in nonzero chain tilt. Collective director fluctuations would also reduce the tilt order parameter. (From Pastor, R. W., Venable, R. M., Karplus, M., and Szabo, A., *J. Chem. Phys.*, 89, 1128, 1988. With permission.)

and dynamic data when developing a model and to generate configurations which are consistent with both. Such a model is the subject of this Section. Three classes of motion (sketched in Figure 1) and their associated order parameters are considered: internal (order parameter S_I), arising from isomerizations and oscillations of the chain dihedral angles; wobble (order parameter S_W) arising from noncollective long axis fluctuations; and axial rotation, which does not directly affect the deuterium order parameter. It will be assumed that wobble and internal reorientation are uncoupled; in this case,[10,65]

$$S_{CD} = (S_I)(S_W) \qquad (25)$$

Because the degree of wobble was not known at the onset of the study, simulations were first carried out assuming that $S_I = S_{CD}$; this work is reviewed in Section III.B. Fits to the ^{13}C NMR T_1 relaxation data (Section III.C) indicated that wobble cannot be ignored

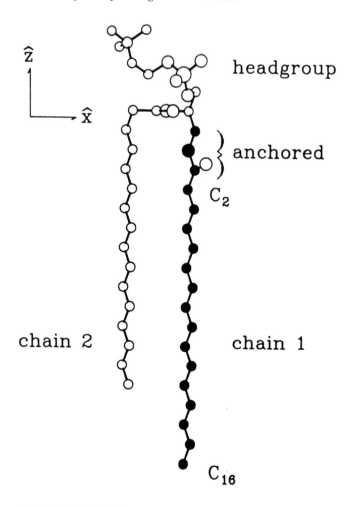

FIGURE 2.   1,2-Dipalmitoyl-3-sn-phosphatidylcholine on a tetrahedral lattice; chain 1 and the glycerol atoms included in the model are shown in black. (From Pastor, R. W., Venable, R. M., and Karplus, M., *J. Chem. Phys.*, 89, 1112, 1988. With permission.)

(i.e., $S_w < 1$). Finally, Section III.D presents simulations of internal motions consistent with the deduced value of S_w.

B. BROWNIAN DYNAMICS SIMULATIONS IN A POTENTIAL OF MEAN FORCE

1. Description of Chain Geometry and Parameters

The simulations reviewed in this chapter were all carried out on a model for chain 1 of DPPC, shown in solid in Figure 2. Extended atoms (i.e., hydrogens are not explicitly included, but their effect is parametrized) represent the glycerol carbon, 14 methylene groups, and 1 methyl group of the palmitoyl chain. Together with the glycerol oxygen, and the carbonyl carbon, a total of 18 atoms are represented. There are 15 dihedral angles, with ϕ_1 specified by the 2 glycerol atoms and carbons 1 and 2 of the chain. The all-*trans* state lies along the z-axis, which is normal to the plane of the bilayer. In order to mimic the tethered character of the chain, the first three atoms were anchored on the x-z plane; this accounts for the small differences in the anisotropic order parameters and in some of the distributions shown later.

The internal energy of the chain for the BD simulations was calculated with potentials commonly used in complete molecular dynamics of alkanes and in an earlier MD simulation of a bilayer:[67] the Ryckaert-Bellemans torsional potential,[55] harmonic bond angles,[67] constrained bond lengths,[68] and 6-12 Lennard-Jones potential.[67] Because only the hydrocarbon chain was considered, electrostatic interactions were not included.

We also discuss a series of calculations carried out on a lattice using the rotational isomeric approximation. Bond lengths and angles were fixed, and each dihedral angle was restricted to one of three states: *trans* (t = 0 degrees), *gauche*$_+$ (g$_+$ = 120 degrees), and *gauche*$_-$ (g$_-$ = -120 degrees). The energy difference between *gauche* and *trans* was 0.7 kcal/mol (as in the Ryckaert-Bellemans potential), and pairs consisting of g$_+$g$_-$ and g$_-$g$_+$ were excluded. Lennard-Jones interactions served to lower the effective *trans-gauche* energy difference to approximately to 0.5 kcal/mol[69] and eliminate configurations with intrachain overlap. Finally, all configurations of the chain were restricted to lie at or below the surface. With these restrictions, the rotational isomeric calculations included a total of 436,755 distinct configurations. These same configurations formed the basic space for the BD simulations: the dynamics consisted of oscillations in each torsional minimum and transitions between them. The detailed form and parameters for the torsional, angular, and constraining potentials and other technical points are described in Reference 22.

2. The Marcelja Model

If the systematic force in a stochastic simulation were only to contain intramolecular terms, the resulting dynamics and equilibrium distributions would be that of a neat liquid. The structural effects of the surrounding bilayer must be taken into account using a potential of mean force. The Marcelja model is used here, as it had been shown[70] to accurately predict many of the equilibrium properties of the membrane, including the deuterium NMR order parameters above the phase transition, the linear expansion coefficient, the change in bilayer thickness upon melting, and the gel to liquid crystal phase transition temperature. The potential energy for the lipid chain in a discrete configuration i is written in the Marcelja model as follows:

$$E^i = E^i_{int} + \Gamma /z^i_{16} - \Phi (n^i_{tr}/n) S^i \tag{26}$$

E^i_{int} is the internal energy of the isolated chain, and the latter two terms represent the contributions of the remainder of the bilayer to the energy of the individual chain in a computationally convenient though phenomenological manner. In the second term, z^i_{16} is the position of the last carbon on the chain, and Γ is a parameter that has been loosely associated with the effects of interfacial tension. The final term is analogous to the Maier-Saupe potential used in liquid crystals:[71] Φ is the mean field; n^i_{tr} is the number of *trans* dihedral angles in state i, and n is the total number of dihedral angles in the chain; and S^i is the order parameter for the chain given by

$$S^i = \sum_j (1/2) (3 \cos^2\beta_j - 1) = \sum_j (S_{mol})_j \tag{27}$$

where β_j is the angle between the bilayer normal and the vector normal to the plane spanned by the two C–H vectors of the jth carbon. The term $(S_{mol})_j$ in Equation 27 is called the molecular order parameter for carbon j.

The approximate nature of the Marcelja parameters has been noted,[72,73] and a number of workers have provided more detailed mean field models.[74-77] (Reference 78 provides a good review of bilayer models, including lattice approaches.[72,73]) From a simulator's point of view, however, the differentiable form of the Marcelja model is critical, and we simply

TABLE 1
Order Parameters for DPPC at T = 323 K

Carbon	S_{CD} (exp)	Calc ($\Phi = 161$; $\Gamma = -4900$)[a]		
		S_I	S_{mol}	$-2 S_I$
2	−0.215	−0.217	0.388	0.434
3	−0.195	−0.197	0.358	0.394
4	−0.215	−0.209	0.380	0.417
5	−0.205	−0.205	0.374	0.410
6	—	−0.209	0.384	0.419
7	—	−0.200	0.366	0.400
8	—	−0.196	0.357	0.391
9	−0.190	−0.183	0.334	0.367
10	−0.180	−0.174	0.317	0.348
11	—	−0.160	0.291	0.320
12	−0.140	−0.148	0.269	0.296
13	—	−0.132	0.239	0.264
14	−0.110	−0.115	0.207	0.230
15	−0.080	−0.088	0.156	0.176

Note: The internal (S_I) and molecular (S_{mol}) order parameters were calculated using the Marcelja model, where states were enumerated using the rotational isomeric approximation and assuming no contribution from tilt. Experimental values for the deuterium order parameters (S_{CD}) are from Seelig and Seelig.[66]

[a] Φ in cal/mol; Γ in cal-Å/mol.

consider Equation 26 a two-parameter potential of mean force which models both steric and attractive interactions between the hydrocarbon chain and its environment. As such, it is very useful for the sort of exploratory research described here.

The initial parametrizations[22,69] for the simulations were made in a manner similar to earlier work by Schindler and Seelig.[70] Φ and Γ were adjusted to provide the best fit of the internal order parameter to the experimental deuterium order parameter[66] upon Boltzmann averaging over all allowed rotational isomers. As shown in Table 1 for T = 323 K, the agreement with experiment is very good for the parameters $\Phi = 161$ cal/mol and $\Gamma = -4900$ cal-Å/mol. (For simplicity, we henceforth omit the units of Φ and Γ in the text.)

Before proceeding to the simulations, we comment briefly that the relation between the molecular order parameter and the deuterium order parameter,

$$(S_{mol})_j = -2 (S_{CD})_j \qquad (28)$$

is only true when axial averaging is complete.[65] This condition is not necessarily met in a lattice calculation, as the molecule is fixed in an initial orientation. The effect is generally small, as shown in the third column in Table 1, but it should not be ignored.

3. Calculation of S_I from Simulations

Recall the important assumptions implicit in the preceding fits: (1) that S_{CD} can be accurately described with the rotational isomeric model and (2) that internal motions alone contribute to S_{CD}. The first assumption can be easily tested by direct simulation of the internal motions with identical mean field parameters. The internal order parameters calculated from a time average of a 24 million step simulation (requiring approximately 50 h of cpu time on an IBM 3090) are compared with experiment in Figure 3. (This simulation was carried

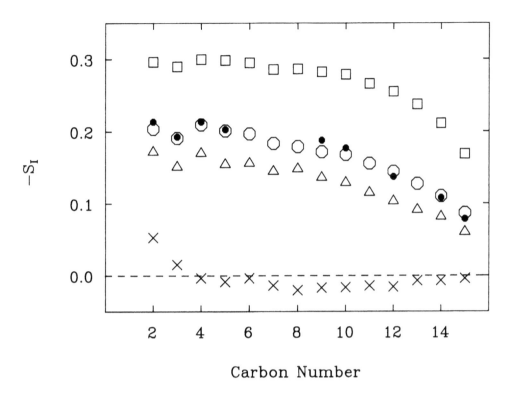

FIGURE 3. Variation of $-S_I$ as a function of carbon position calculated from dynamics simulations: $\Phi = 160$ cal/mol and $\Gamma = -4793$ cal-Å/mol (triangles); $\Phi = 180$ and $\Gamma = -9000$ (open circles); $\Phi = 180$ and $\Gamma = -9000$ (squares); $\Phi = 0$ and $\Gamma = 0$ (crosses); experimental[66] $-S_{CD}$ interpolated from 323 and 330 (filled circles). (From Pastor, R. W., Venable, R. M., and Karplus, M., in preparation. With permission.)

out at 324 K, rather than at 323 K, to facilitate comparison with the T_1 data; the field parameters were set to $\Phi = 160.14$ and $\Gamma = -4793$ to account for the change in temperature.) The simulation underestimates the magnitude of S_I for all carbons. This is the effect of torsional oscillation which is not included in the rotational isomeric model and can be compensated for by slight increases in field parameters: as shown in Figure 3, the order parameters from a 44 million step simulation with $\Phi = 180$ and $\Gamma = -9000$ converged to values close to experiment. The values for the torsion angles for the first of 90 segments of this trajectory are shown in Figure 4. (Recall that Φ_1 is the dihedral angle closest to the head group.) The chain soon departs from its initial all-*trans* configuration, with the tail dihedrals clearly more active than those near the head group. As discussed further in Section IV, over 30,000 transitions took place during the course of the entire trajectory.

The effects of the field were tested further in a 30 million step trajectory with $\Phi = \Gamma = 0$. The internal order parameters were close to zero (see Figure 3), indicating almost isotropic motion; however, a detailed analysis[22] showed dynamics very similar to that found at $\Phi = 180$ and $\Gamma = -9000$. This observation justified the use of correlation functions calculated from field values $\Phi = 180$ and $\Gamma = -9000$ to model the internal dynamics that would take place at even higher fields.

Finally, let us access the number of configurations required for accurate sampling. Even if all 30,000 transitions found in a simulation resulted in new configurations, this still represents a relatively small fraction of the over 400,000 possible rotational isomeric states. Nevertheless, the internal order parameters were reasonably converged.[22] The averages were precise for two reasons. First, many of the allowed configurations are energetically unfavorable. It was shown in Reference 22 (by averaging over the rotational isomeric states)

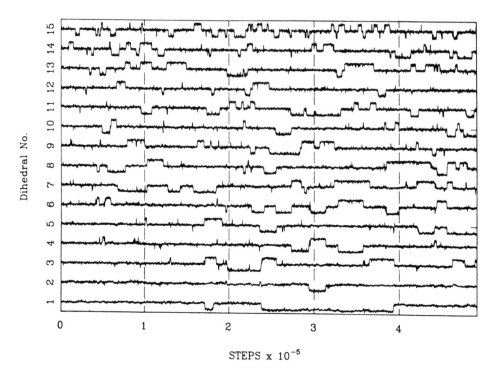

FIGURE 4.   Dihedral angle history for first segment of the mean field simulation with $\Phi = 180$ cal/mol and $\Gamma = -9000$ cal-Å/mol. The chain starts in the all-*trans* state. (From Pastor, R. W., Venable, R. M., and Karplus, M., *J. Chem. Phys.*, 89, 1112, 1988. With permission.)

that 100,000 configurations comprised 94% of the Boltzmann weight; in other words, the remaining 300,000 states only contribute 6% to the equilibrium averages. Secondly, the order parameters for both hydrogens were calculated separately and then averaged, eliminating the need to sample both mirror image configurations. Thus, many of the important states (or their mirror images) were sampled relatively early on in the simulations, as they are energetically easily accessible. Conversely, much longer trajectories would be required to sample the remaining states, highlighting the difficulties inherent in simulations of the bilayer.

C. FITS TO NMR RELAXATION DATA
1. General Formalism

An important feature of dynamics simulations is that correlation functions calculated from the trajectory can be used to evaluate dynamical experimental quantities. Arising frequently is the second-order Legendre polynomial correlation function, $<P_2(\hat{\mu}(t)\cdot\hat{\mu}(0))>$, where $\hat{\mu}$ is a unit vector in a fixed coordinate frame; it is conveniently calculated with fast Fourier transform methods[79,80] from the spherical harmonics $Y_2^m(t)$ using the x,y, and z projections of the vector as follows:

$$<P_2(\hat{\mu}(t)\cdot\hat{\mu}(0))> = (4\pi/5) \sum_{m=-2}^{2} C_2^m(t) \qquad (29)$$

where

$$C_2^m(t) = < Y_2^{m*}(t)\ Y_2^m(0) > \qquad (30)$$

and

$$C_2^{\pm 2}(t) = (45/96\pi) < (x^2(t)-y^2(t))(x^2(0)-y^2(0)) + 4x(t)y(t)x(0)y(0) > \quad (31a)$$

$$C_2^{\pm 1}(t) = (45/24\pi) < x(t)z(t)x(0)z(0) + y(t)z(t)y(0)z(0) > \quad (31b)$$

$$C_2^{0}(t) = (5/16\pi) < (3z^2(t)-1)(3z^2(0)-1) > \quad (31c)$$

The ^{13}C T_1 relaxation time for CH$_2$ group in a spherical vesicle is then given by[81,82]

$$1/NT_1 = (\hbar \gamma_C \gamma_H / r^3)^2 (1/10) \left[J(\omega_C - \omega_H) + 3J(\omega_C) + 6J(\omega_C + \omega_H) \right] \quad (32)$$

where N is the number of hydrogens bonded to the carbon, γ_C, γ_H and ω_C, ω_H are the gyromagnetic ratios and Larmor frequencies of the ^{13}C and ^{1}H nuclei, respectively, $\hbar$ is Planck's constant divided by 2π, and r is the effective CH bond distance. $J(\omega)$ is the spectral density of a correlation function involving the rotational correlation time of the vesicle, r_v, and independent lipid motions within the vesicle frame:

$$J(\omega) = \int_0^\infty C(t) \cos(\omega t) \, dt \quad (33)$$

and

$$C(t) = \exp(-t/\tau_v) < P_2(\hat{\mu}(t)\cdot\hat{\mu}(0)) > \quad (34)$$

Before proceeding to the actual calculation of T_1 for the bilayer, it is useful to consider the spectral densities associated with a single exponential decay:

$$J(\omega) = \int_0^\infty e^{-t/\tau} \cos(\omega t) \, dt = \frac{\tau}{1+(\tau\omega)^2} \quad (35)$$

Figure 5a shows the behavior of Equation 35 over the Larmor frequencies of interest (15 to 126 MHz carbon) for three values of r. $J(\omega)$ quickly decays to zero for $r = 10^{-6}$s. The radius of a single bilayer vesicle is between 125 and 150 Å,[10] so that r_v is on the order of a microsecond;[34,38] hence vesicle rotation can usually be ignored when considering T_1's.

The spectral density is constant but nonzero when $r = 10^{-10}$s; this is the motional narrowing regime: $(r\omega)^2 \ll 1$. Thus, fast motions will contribute to the magnitude, but not the frequency dependence of T_1.

Lastly, when $r = 2 \times 10^{-9}$s, $(r\omega) \approx 1$, and $J(\omega)$ shows considerable variation as the frequency changes. An interesting feature of the vesicle data is that $1/T_1$ is linearly related to $\omega_C^{-1/2}$ over the frequency range 15 to 126 MHz, indicating the possibility of collective motions.[2,3,71] Recall from Equation 32 that T_1 results from a combination of spectral densities; Figure 5b shows that for $r \approx 2$ ns, the sum $(J\omega_C - \omega_H) + 3J(\omega_C) + 6J(\omega_C + \omega_H)$ is quite linear when plotted against $\omega_C^{-1/2}$. Hence, the fact that a slow diffusive motion could fit the data discussed below is not unreasonable.[5]

2. Calculation of T_1 from Simulations

$<P_2(\hat{\mu}(t)\cdot\hat{\mu}(0))>$ describes the phospholipid dynamics within the frame of the vesicle and thus includes a wide range of possible motions. As noted earlier, these may consist of internal reorientation, axial rotation, wobble, and even collective modes. A multinanosecond-to microsecond-long simulation of many lipid chains would ideally capture all of these motions, and the calculation of an observable such as T_1 would proceed directly from the correlation function specified in Equation 29. Alternatively, if the correlation functions describe only the internal motions (as in simulations described here), it is possible to analytically include the effects of additional motions by considering an appropriate rotating frame. This approach has its advantages, as simple models can be eliminated and more complex ones can be developed as required by the experimental data.

Four models for the T_1 relaxation in vesicles were considered in our original study.[23] Spherical harmonic correlation functions calculated from the ($\Phi = 180$, $\Gamma = -9000$) simulation, denoted $\hat{C}_2^m(t)$, were used in each case to describe the internal motions. The models are outlined below, in order of increasing complexity.

Model 1 included only internal motions, and thus

$$\langle P_2(\hat{\mu}(t)\cdot\hat{\mu}(0))\rangle = (4\pi/5) \sum_{m=-2}^{2} \hat{C}_2^m(t) \tag{36}$$

Recall from the discussion of Brownian dynamics algorithms (Section II.C.2) that the time constants from the calculated correlation functions may be scaled to arbitrary collision frequency, γ. Hence, model 1 has one adjustable parameter which is related to the effective viscosity in the bilayer interior.

Model 2 consisted of internal motions with superimposed axial rotation of the entire phospholipid. The relevant correlation function is[83]

$$\langle P_2(\hat{\mu}(t)\cdot\hat{\mu}(0))\rangle = (4\pi/5) \sum_{m=-2}^{2} \exp(-m^2 D_{\parallel} t)\, \hat{C}_2^m(t) \tag{37}$$

where $D_{\parallel}$ is the axial diffusion coefficient which may be varied along with γ to fit the data. Equation 37 is approximate in that it is assumed that axial and internal rotations are not uncoupled.

Model 3 included internal motions, axial rotation, and long axis reorientation (with diffusion constant $D_{\perp}$). Then,[83]

$$\langle P_2(\hat{\mu}(t)\cdot\hat{\mu}(0))\rangle = (4\pi/5) \sum_{mn=-2}^{2} g_{mn}(t)\exp(-m^2 t(D_{\parallel}-D_{\perp}))\, \hat{C}_2^m(t) \tag{38}$$

where g_{nm} contains S_w, the order parameter associated with wobble; hence, there are a total of four adjustable parameters in model 3. The complete expression for g_{nm} is complicated and is given in Reference 23. (Note that S_w is denoted S_T, for tilt order parameter.) Model 4 was an extension of model 3, in that each of the five carbon types fitted could take on a different value of S_w, resulting in eight parameters.

As detailed in Reference 23 no range of collision frequencies or axial diffusion coefficients in models 1 and 2 provided adequate fits to the T_1 data; Figures 6a and 6b show the best fits obtained with these models. (The failure of model 2 is related to an interesting artifact in the rotational isomeric model. This is discussed in Section IV.D). The best fit parameters for model 3 ($D_{\parallel} = 2.5 \times 10^{10}$ s^{-1}, $D_{\perp} = 2.0 \times 10^{8}$ s^{-1}, $S_w = 0.54$ and $\gamma = 52$ ps^{-1}) produce results that compare very well with experiment (Figure 6c). The quantitative agreement with experiment was improved using model 4 (Figure 6d). This is to be expected, as the number of parameters increased from four to eight. However, their range was similar ($D_{\parallel} = 1.3 \times 10^{10}$ s^{-1}, $D_{\perp} = 1.3 \times 10^{8}$ s^{-1}, $\gamma = 47$ ps^{-1}, and $0.53 < (S_w)_j < 0.67$), so the fundamental description of the director fluctuations remains the same in models 3 and 4.

Naturally, these parameters can be varied somewhat; for example, S_w can be increased to 0.7 without significantly changing the good agreement with experiment. Furthermore, the correspondence between collision frequency and the bilayer viscosity as expressed in Equation 9 should be regarded as only approximate; an effective viscosity of 1 to 2 cP is a

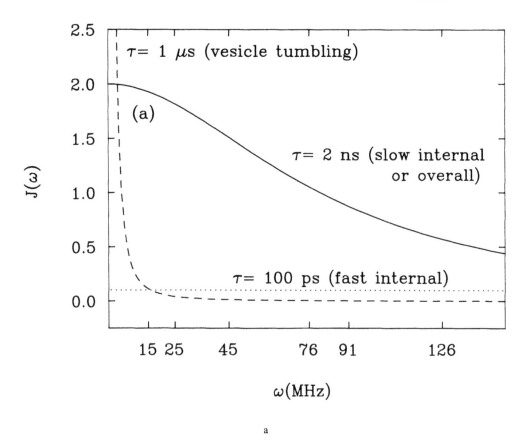

a

FIGURE 5. Spectral densities for a correlation function consisting a single exponential decay. (a) Variation over the Larmor frequency, 15 to 150 MHz (carbon), for different values of the decay constant; (b) dependence of $J(\omega_C - \omega_H) + 3J(\omega_C) + 6J(\omega_C + \omega_H)$ vs. $\omega_C^{-1/2}$ for several relaxation times on the order of a nanosecond.

reasonable estimate. Finally, we did not find it necessary to include collective modes to fit the vesicle data, although it is possible that these motions would be important in larger systems such as multilayers.

D. BUILDING IN CHAIN TILT

The fits to relaxation data discussed in the preceding subsection indicated that the assumption that internal motions alone contribute to S_{CD} is incorrect and that S_I should be increased in magnitude by a factor of $1/S_W$. This can readily be accomplished by increasing the Marcelja field parameters;[22] Figure 7 shows the required adjustment within the rotational isomeric approximation. As with the low field study, an increase in the field parameters over and above those derived from the parametrization on a lattice were required in the simulation to produce the comparable values of S_I. Figure 3 shows internal order parameters resulting from a 30 million step simulation with $\Phi = 360$ and $\Gamma = -9000$.[84] As required, the calculated internal order parameters uniformly overestimate the magnitude of experimental order parameters; the best fit to the experimental data was provided $S_W = 0.59$.

The effect of wobble can be approximated by the cone model, where we assume that the lipid is free to rotate within a cone oriented along the bilayer normal with semiangle θ_0 as sketched in Figure 1b. The relationship of θ_0 and S_W is[85]

$$S_W = (1/2) \cos\theta_0 (1 + \cos\theta_0) \qquad (39)$$

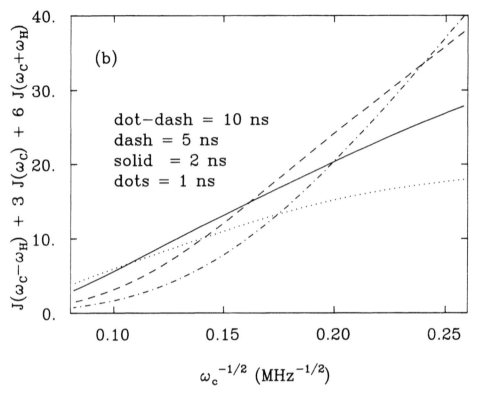

FIGURE 5B.

For example, if $S_w = 0.59$, $\theta_0 = 45.9°$.

The model of the bilayer interior is now specified. A continuous Marcelja potential modulates the populations of rotational isomers which rapidly interconvert. The lipid axially rotates and undergoes a wobbling motion on a longer time scale; at any point in time, the long axis may be found between $\pm\theta_0$.

IV. SELECTED RESULTS

A. OVERVIEW

The model presented in the preceding section was based on fits to the T_1 data using correlation functions calculated from the internal motions and two required additional modes of reorientation; axial rotation and noncollective long axis fluctuations (or wobble). Had the simulation results (i.e., the correlation functions) by themselves produced high-quality fits to the dynamic data, we would have inferred that the overall motions were too slow or too small to contribute significantly to the T_1 relaxation. In this sense, the simulation puts approximate ranges for axial ($D_\parallel$) and perpendicular ($D_\perp$) diffusion coefficients and implies that the wobble order parameter (S_w) is less than one. However, the numerical values for these parameters and for the collision frequency (γ) were derived from the fits and thus were not direct results of the simulation. Even the Marcelja field parameters Φ and Γ ultimately became entwined with the relaxation data, in that the internal order parameter (S_I) was related to S_w and S_{CD} (Equation 25).

Here we discuss simulation results that are somewhat removed from the fits. Some, such as the relative isomerization rates along the chain and degree of internal axial averaging, are almost independent of the field strength and other fitted parameters. Others, such as the

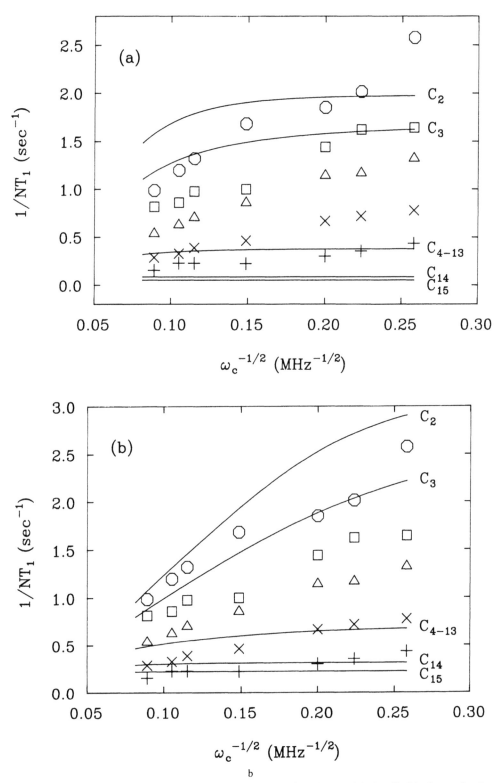

FIGURE 6. $1/NT_1$ vs. $\omega_c^{-1/2}$ calculated for a best fit for each of the four models described in the text for the range of 15 to 126 MHz. (a) Model 1, internal motions alone (Equation 36); (b) Model 2, internal motions and uncoupled axial diffusion (Equation 37); (c) Model 3, internal motions, uncoupled axial diffusion and wobble (Equation 38); (d) Model 4, internal motions, uncoupled axial diffusion and wobble (Equation 38); with a carbon-dependent wobble order parameter; experimental points:[3] C_2; □ C_3; △ $C_{4\ to\ 13}$; x C_{14}; + C_{15}. (From Pastor, R. W., Venable, R. M., Karplus, M., and Szabo, A., *J. Chem. Phys.*, 89, 1128, 1988. With permission).

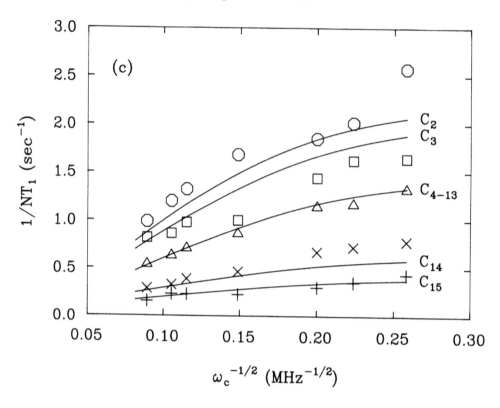

FIGURE 5C.

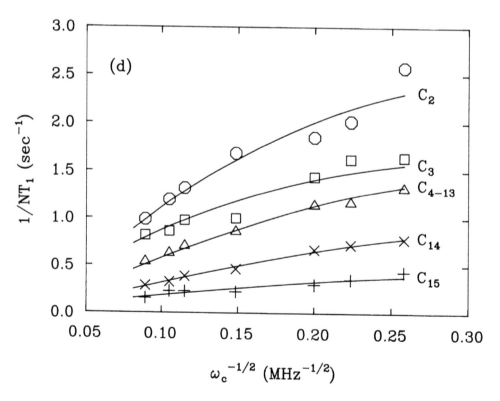

FIGURE 5D.

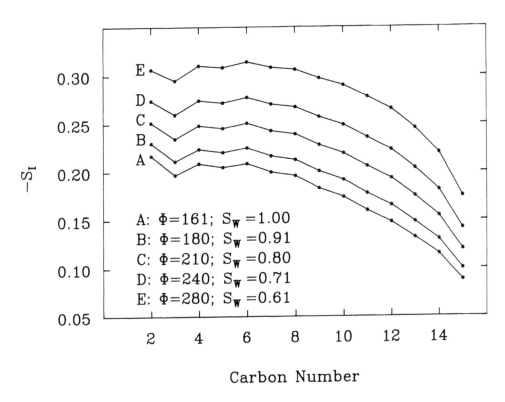

FIGURE 7. Variation of $-S_I$, the order parameter arising from internal motions, with Φ, the Marcelja mean field (in cal/mol). S_W, the tilt order parameter, is chosen for each value of Φ such that the product $(S_W)(S_I)$ most closely agrees closest with curve A, which, in turn, mostly agrees with the experimentally determined order parameter at 323 K (see Figure 3). $\Gamma = -4900$ cal-Å/mol in curve A and $\Gamma = -5000$ cal-Å/mol for curves B to E. (After Pastor, R. W., Venable, R. M., and Karplus, M., *J. Chem. Phys.*, 89, 1112, 1988. With permission.)

chain distributions, show a moderate field dependence; however, their qualitative differences from certain non-Marcelja models are important.

B. CHAIN DISTRIBUTIONS

As stated earlier, the trajectories resulted in many thousands of configurations which interconvert rapidly. Thus, average dimensions of the chain are particularly important quantities. Figure 8 shows densities for the chain carbons (excluding the anchor atoms) calculated from the trajectory consistent with $S_W = 0.59$ (i.e., $S_I \approx S_{CD}/0.59$). The distribution is relatively cylindrical, as can be seen in both the longitudinal (xz and yz) and axial (xy) projections. (The bands of higher density visible in Figure 8 result from the lattice defined by the anchor atoms and the rotational states; if the anchor atoms had been free to move, much of this detail would be lost.) The average radius of the cylinder is 3.1 Å over the range -15 Å $< z < 0$ Å.[84]

The trajectory at high field is consistent with experimental determinations chain lengths projected along the bilayer normal which are related to the bilayer thickness. Neutron diffraction measurements on deuterated DPPC at 343 K (15 degrees above the phase transition) have shown that the average distance between the C_4 and C_{12} carbons measured along the normal 6.6 Å.[86] (The present simulations were carried out at 324 K, which is 10 degrees above the phase transitions for undeuterated DPPC.) A comparison, however, first requires an estimate of the shortening of the chain projection due to the wobble; ℓ_{eff}, the projection of the chain consistent with an order parameter S_W, can be calculated using the cone model to be

$$\ell_{eff}/<z> = (1/4)(1 + (1+8S_W)^{1/2}) \tag{40}$$

where $<z>$ is the average projection without tilt.[22] For C_4 to C_{12}, $<z>$ equaled 8.09 Å in the ($\Phi = 360$, $\Gamma = -9000$) simulation; hence, for $S_W = 0.59$ $\ell_{eff} = 6.86$ Å which agrees with experiment. The C_1 to C_{16} projection after the correction for wobble was 12.5 Å.

C. COMPARISON WITH THE CRANKSHAFT MODEL

In the crankshaft model,[78,87] the only allowed conformations in the lipid chain are kinks (dihedral angle sequences $g_\pm$, t, $g_\mp$). Dihedral transitions thus only occur in pairs to form or destroy kinks. The model is intuitively appealing, as a kink causes only a slight distortion of the all-*trans* configuration, and would presumably pack well in a bilayer. The effective cylinder formed by a chain with only kinks is smaller in radius and more dense than the cylinder described in the preceding subsection. The predicted deuterium order parameters from the crankshaft model are not unreasonable: S_1 is relatively constant at -0.3 along the chain; these values could be reduced in magnitude to -0.2 by either wobble[88] or collective motion.[12] The drop-off in $-S_{CD}$ for the chain carbons close to the center of the bilayer is not explained by the crankshaft model, but one assumes that agreement with experiment might be obtained by permitting a few isolated *gauche* bonds near the chain tails.

Chains with only kinks comprise a small subset ($\sim$1800) of the over 400,000 different rotational isomeric configurations allowed in the present model. While these configurations tend to be low energy (and hence favored), an analysis[22] of the ($\Phi = 180$, $\Gamma = -9000$) trajectory showed that chain contained only kinks 5% of the time; in other words, 95% of the trajectory contained isolated *gauche* bonds and were therefore in violation of the crankshaft model. On the other hand, kinks frequently formed in the chain. Configurations with kinks and no restriction on other *gauche* bonds comprised 42% of the ($\Phi = 180$, $\Gamma = -9000$) trajectory and 34% of the ($\Phi = \Gamma = 0$) trajectory.

An insightful aspect of the crankshaft model involves the concertedness of the dihedral transitions. The crankshaft motion consists of simultaneous opposite rotations of next nearest dihedral angles as, for example, in the transition: $\ldots ttt \ldots \rightarrow \ldots g_+ tg_- \ldots$ This pathway minimizes the net motion of the chain, whereas an isolated transition might involve a large displacement of the chain. Again, just as the present model includes kinks, it includes crankshaft motions. However, as is easily seen in Figure 4, not all transitions were concerted and not all concerted transitions were of the crankshaft variety. Similar behavior was found for the ($\Phi = \Gamma = 0$) trajectory,[22] and in fact had been observed in simulations of pure alkanes by Helfand and co-workers.[18,19] Therefore, the crankshaft model, while containing elements of both structure and dynamics found in the model presented here, is also qualitatively more restrictive.

D. ERRORS ARISING FROM THE ROTATIONAL ISOMERIC APPROXIMATION

The rotational isomer (RI) model remains popular in studies of alkanes, in that it allows good statistical sampling even for a relatively large chain. If the chain is small, a complete enumeration is possible: for the 18 carbon model discussed here, the 436,755 states can be readily generated and evaluated on a minicomputer.

In limiting the degrees of freedom of each dihedral to three states, the effects of liberation in the torsional minima are lost. This was seen in Section III.B.3 when, using field parameters optimized with the RI approximation, the magnitude of the internal order parameters was systematically underestimated in the dynamics simulation. The error, however, was more quantitative than qualitative, and it is sensible to argue that the discrete Marcelja model was quite useful. This subsection considers a class of structural averages for which the RI

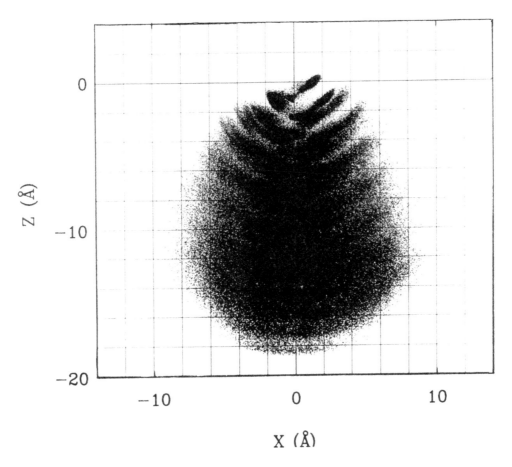

FIGURE 8. Density distributions calculated from the trajectory $\Phi = 360$ cal/mol and $\Gamma = -9000$ cal-Å/mol. The X-Z and Y-Z projections correspond to side views of the lipid in the bilayer; the X-Y projection is a view down the bilayer normal. (From Pastor, R. W., Venable, R. M., and Karplus, M., in preparation. With permission.)

approximation yields misleading results. (Here we will use the designation discrete Marcelja model to specify that states were enumerated using the RI approximation; continuous Marcelja model implies the use of a continuous torsional potentials, as in the simulations.)

The spherical harmonic correlation functions discussed in Section III were used to calculate dynamic properties; however, their plateau or long-time values contain structural information and are given by the following averages:

$$C_2^{\pm 2}(\infty) = |\langle Y_2^{\pm 2}\rangle|^2 = (45/96\pi)\left[\langle(x^2-y^2)\rangle^2 + 4\langle xy\rangle^2\right] \quad (41a)$$

$$C_2^{\pm 1}(\infty) = |\langle Y_2^{\pm 1}\rangle|^2 = (45/24\pi)\left[\langle xz\rangle^2 + \langle yz\rangle^2\right] \quad (41b)$$

$$C_2^0(\infty) = |\langle Y_2^0\rangle|^2 = (5/16\pi)\langle(3z^2 - 1)\rangle^2 \quad (41c)$$

Returning to the notation specifying that the correlation function contains only contributions from internal motion, note that the internal order parameter is related to the plateau value:

$$\hat{C}_2^0(\infty) = (5\pi/4)\,S_I^2 \quad (42)$$

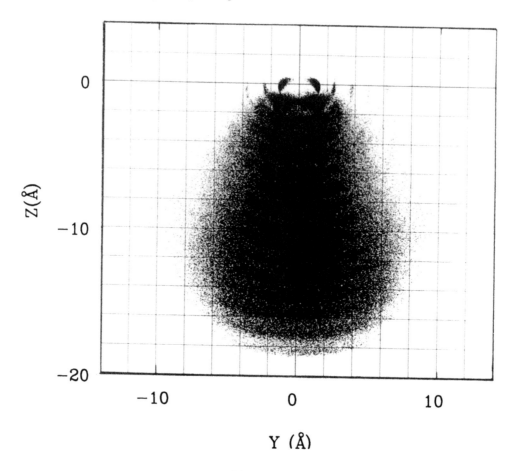

FIGURE 8B.

Thus, $\hat{C}_2^0(\infty)$ is qualitatively similar in both the continuous and discrete Marcelja model.

Table 2 shows the projections for carbons 2, 9, and 15 for two cases: the discrete model with $\Phi = 161$ and $\Gamma = -4900$ and the simulation with $\Phi = 160.14$ and $\Gamma = -4793$. For both the continuous and discrete models, $< xy >$ and $< yz >$ are either zero or close to zero, and consequently, so is $\hat{C}_2^1(\infty)$. $\hat{C}_2^2(\infty)$, however, is evaluated from the difference of $< x^2 >$ and $< y^2 >$. Compared with the discrete calculation, $< x^2 >$ is raised and $< y^2 >$ is lowered in the simulation, and, therefore, $\hat{C}_2^2(\infty)$ is significantly smaller.

The difference between the continuous and discrete models leads to different interpretations concerning the frequency dependence of axial rotation. To illustrate this argument, we write the (unnormalized) correlation function for internal motions, $\hat{C}_2^m(t)$, as a single exponential and a plateau value:

$$\hat{C}_2^m(t) = \exp(-t/\tau_m) + \hat{C}_2^m(\infty) \tag{43}$$

and look at the spectral densities that result for the three NMR models discussed in the previous section. In model 1 (internal motions only), the plateau values enter into the spectral density as a zero frequency component (i.e., the Fourier transform of a constant is a delta function). Thus, from Equation 32, the T_1 is related only to the decay of the internal correlation functions and not to their long-time values. The best fit to the relaxation data implies that the internal motions decayed rapidly and hence no frequency dependence arose from the model (Figure 6a).

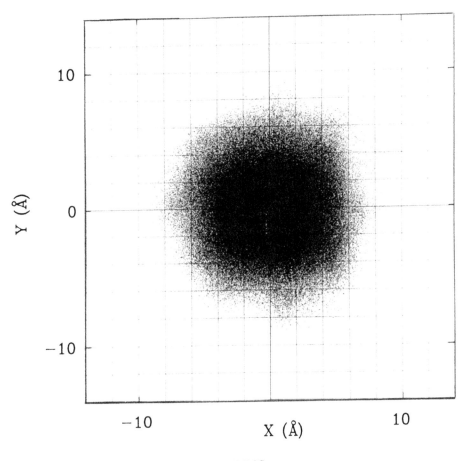

FIGURE 8C.

Model 2 included axial rotation with a diffusion constant $D_{\parallel}$, and from Equation 37 terms of the form $\hat{C}_2^1(t)\ \exp(-D_{\parallel}t)$ and $\hat{C}_2^2(t)\ \exp(-4D_{\parallel}t)$ enter into the spectral density; $\hat{C}_2^0(\infty)$ makes no contribution to $J(\omega)$ when $\omega \neq 0$. As we have just shown, an analysis using the discrete Marcelja model indicates that although $\hat{C}_2^1(\infty)$ is negligible, $\hat{C}_2^2(\infty)$ is not. On the basis is was argued that axial rotation potentially predicts the frequency dependence.[5] However, $\hat{C}_2^2(\infty)$ calculated from the simulation is nearly zero, and, as a result, model 2 could not fit the data.

Model 3 (Equation 38), by virtue of the terms $g_{0n}(t)\ \hat{C}_2^0(\infty)$, provides a coefficient, a reasonable amplitude for the slow motion, and therefore yielded agreement with experiment.

Thus, a significant amount of axial averaging is provided by internal motions, above the averaging provided by overall axial rotation or the lipid. This effect is hidden in the discrete Marcelja model. It is for this reason that wobble, rather than axial rotation, appears to be responsible for the dramatically different frequency dependence observed for the lipid chains in the bilayer and neat alkanes.

V. SUMMARY

The model presented in this Chapter supports a highly fluid-like description of the bilayer in the liquid crystal state. The physical boundary traced out by a chain is quite large (Figure 8), although porous to the other chains: density considerations stipulate that a single chain cannot individually occupy such a large cross-sectional area. The internal dynamics are very

TABLE 2
A Comparison of the Average C-H Projections for Carbons 2, 9, and 15 of DPPC Calculated from the Marcelja Model

Car	$\langle x^2 \rangle$	$\langle y^2 \rangle$	$\langle z^2 \rangle$	$\langle xy \rangle$	$\langle xz \rangle$	$\langle yz \rangle$
			Discrete ($\Phi = 161$, $\Gamma = -4900$)			
2	0.3333; 0.3333	0.4780; 0.4780	0.1886; 0.1886	-0.1024; 0.1024	-0.0273; -0.0273	0.0000; 0.0000
9	0.3333; 0.3333	0.4556; 0.4556	0.2111; 0.2111	-0.0934; 0.0934	0.0011; 0.0011	0.0000; 0.0000
15	0.3333; 0.3333	0.3920; 0.3920	0.2746; 0.2746	-0.0386; 0.0386	0.0164; 0.0164	0.0000; 0.0000
			Continuous ($\Phi = 160.14$, $\Gamma = -4793$)			
2	0.3478; 0.3468	0.4442; 0.4243	0.2080; 0.2290	0.0311; -0.0482	-0.0610; -0.0427	0.0131; -0.0063
9	0.3726; 0.3627	0.3926; 0.3871	0.2348; 0.2502	0.0188; -0.0252	0.0053; 0.0063	-0.0048; 0.0091
15	0.3548; 0.3494	0.3512; 0.3585	0.2940; 0.2921	0.0019; -0.0026	0.0056; 0.0079	0.0018; 0.0039

Note: Both hydrogens are included. The discrete results are from a systematic enumeration of states using the rotational isomeric approximation and Boltzmann weighting at T = 323 K; the continuous results are from Brownian dynamics simulations at T = 324 K.

much like a neat alkane in both the types and time scales of torsional reorientation. The model is consistent with equilibrium and dynamic properties of the DPPC bilayer as measured by deuterium line shapes and ^{13}C T$_1$ relaxation, respectively, and the average chain length obtained from neutron diffraction. As discussed in Reference 23, the parameters of the model ($D_\parallel = 2.5 \times 10^{10}$ s^{-1}, $D_\perp = 2.0 \times 10^8$ s^{-1}, $S_W = 0.54$, and $\gamma = 52$ ps^{-1}) are all physically reasonable.

What qualifications are in order? The model is based on Brownian dynamics simulations of a single chain in a mean field and fits to experiment. This approach clearly has drawbacks. Stochastic simulations even of neat liquids involve an added level of approximation when compared to full molecular dynamics simulations; the mean field describes the average interaction between chains in the bilayer and may neglect important correlations; and at least four adjustable parameters were needed to fit the T$_1$ (e.g., in model 3). Therefore, it is important to close this chapter with a statement of which results can be used with confidence and where further testing is required.

Several generally useful results that are not especially dependent on our exact procedures include:

1. That it is critical to include an analysis of dynamic data when developing an equilibrium model of the bilayer — Equilibrium properties such as the deuterium order parameters and the bilayer thickness are sensitive to both internal and overall motions the precise combination of internal order and tilt is difficult to determine from equilibrium measurements alone.

2. That the Marcelja model must be parametrized with a higher value of the mean field than is required if wobble is absent — This will change the Boltzmann weights of the individual configurations and hence their relative populations at a given temperature. When only internal degrees of freedom are included in a parametrization, an ''upper limit'' of the degree of internal disorder is provided for the model.

3. That effects of torsional flexibility, a basic property of alkane chains, should be considered — The high value of the anisotropic average $\hat{C}_2^2(\infty)$ (Section V.D) is an artifact of the rotational isomeric approximation and can be misleading. Small rotations of dihedral angles (which are often accompanied by compensating rotations of neighboring dihedrals) can reduce large van der Waals' repulsions arising from steric overlap between chains without substantially changing the conformation.

The following, more tentative, aspects of the model should be stressed:

1. It was not proven that collective motions are absent; it was shown that a particular set of T$_1$ data determined for vesicles[3] could be fit with a noncollective model. Analysis of a much wider range of data is required before more definitive conclusions can be reached.

2. Because internal reorientation was found to be in the motional narrowing limit, its dynamic details were not discernible using the NMR relaxation data. Given that wobble provides a significant contribution to the relaxation in our model, it is possible that alternative models of internal relaxation could have also fit the T$_1$ data.

3. It was assumed that overall and internal motions were uncoupled. The severity of this approximation is not yet clear; it might be tested, for example, by simulation of a complete lipid in a suitably parametrized mean field.

4. Finally, and perhaps most importantly for the reader interested in structure rather than dynamics, the assumption that a bilayer can be modeled by a mean field requires further investigation. This can probably most effectively be accomplished by molecular dynamics simulations of an ensemble of chains with an initial distribution derived

from the present model. (Several molecular dynamics simulations of bilayers have been carried out,[67,89,90] however, with different starting conditions.)

In conclusion, it is hoped that the methods and the model presented in this Chapter will provide useful tools for understanding the biological membrane.

ACKNOWLEDGMENTS

The membrane simulations and analysis reported here could not have been carried out without the help of my collaborators, Martin Karplus, Attila Szabo, and Richard Venable, and without the generous computational support provided to us by the Food and Drug Administration and the National Institutes of Health (NIH). During the initial stages of the work, I was supported by an NIH graduate training grant. I am also grateful to Frederick Carson, William Egan, and Dusanka Janezic for helpful comments on the manuscript.

REFERENCES

1. **Brown, M. F.,** Theory of spin-lattice relaxation in lipid bilayers and biological membranes. ^{2}H and ^{14}N quadrupolar relaxation, *J. Chem. Phys.,* 77, 1576, 1982.
2. **Brown, M. F.,** Theory of spin-lattice relaxation in lipid bilayers and biological membranes. Dipolar relaxation, *J. Chem. Phys.,* 80, 2808, 1984.
3. **Brown, M. F., Ribeiro, A. A., and Williams, G. D.,** New view of lipid bilayer dynamics from ^{2}H and ^{13}C relaxation time measurements, *Proc. Natl. Acad. Sci. U.S.A.,* 80, 4325, 1983.
4. **Brooks, B. R.,** Applications of molecular dynamics for structural analysis of proteins and peptides, in *Supercomputer Research in Chemistry and Chemical Engineering,* Jensen, K. F. and Truhlar, D. G., Eds., ACS Symp. Ser. 353, American Chemical Society, Washington, D.C., 1987, 123.
5. **Szabo, A.,** NMR Relaxation and the dynamics of proteins and membranes, *Ann. N.Y. Acad. Sci.,* 482, 44, 1986.
6. **Levine, Y. K., Partington, P., and Roberts, G. C. K.,** Calculation of dipolar nuclear magnetic relaxation times in molecules with multiple internal rotations. 1. Isotropic overall motion of the molecule, *Mol. Phys.,* 25, 497, 1973.
7. **London, R. E. and Avitabile, J.,** Calculation of ^{13}C relaxation times and nuclear Overhauser enhancements in a hydrocarbon chain undergoing gauche-trans isomerism, *J. Am. Chem. Soc.,* 99, 7765, 1977.
8. **Wittebort, R. J. and Szabo, A.,** Theory of NMR relaxation in macromolecules: restricted diffusion and jump models for multiple internal rotations in amino acid side-chains, *J. Chem. Phys.,* 69, 1722, 1978.
9. **Gent, M. P. N. and Prestegard, J. H.,** Nuclear magnetic relaxation and molecular motion in phospholipid bilayer membranes, *J. Magn. Reson.,* 25, 243, 1977.
10. **Bocian, D. F. and Chan, S. I.,** NMR studies of membrane structure and dynamics, *Annu. Rev. Phys. Chem.,* 29, 307, 1978.
11. **Pace, R. J. and Chan, S. I.,** Molecular motions in lipid bilayers. I. Statistical mechanic model of acyl chain motion, *J. Chem. Phys.,* 76, 4217, 1982.
12. **Pace, R. J. and Chan, S. I.,** Molecular motions in lipid bilayers. II. Magnetic resonance of multilamellar and vesicle systems, *J. Chem. Phys.,* 76, 4228, 1982.
13. **Levy, R. M., Karplus, M., and McCammon, J. A.,** Diffusive dynamics of model alkanes, *Chem. Phys. Lett.,* 65, 4, 1979.
14. **Levy, R. M., Karplus, M., and Wolynes, P. G.,** NMR relaxation parameters in molecules with internal motion: exact Langevin trajectory results compared with simplified relaxation models, *J. Am. Chem. Soc.,* 103, 5998, 1981.
15. **Rosenberg, R. O., Berne, B. J., and Chandler, D.,** Isomerization dynamics in liquids by molecular dynamics, *Chem. Phys. Lett.,* 75, 162, 1980.
16. **Montomery, J. A., Holmgren, S. L., and Chandler, D.,** Stochastic molecular dynamics study of trans-gauche isomerization processes in simple chain molecules, *J. Chem. Phys.,* 73, 3688, 1980.
17. **Knauss, D. C. and Evans, G. T.,** Liquid state torsional dynamics of butane: the Kramers rate and the torsion angle correlation times, *J. Chem. Phys.,* 73, 3423, 1980.

18. **Skolnick, J. and Helfand, E.,** Kinetics of conformational transitions in chain molecules, *J. Chem. Phys.,* 72, 5489, 1980.
19. **Helfand, E.,** Dynamics of conformational transitions of polymers, *Science,* 226, 647, 1984.
20. **van Gunsteren, W. F., Berendsen, H. J. C., and Rullmann, J. A. C.,** Stochastic dynamics for molecules with constraints: Brownian dynamics of *n*-alkanes, *Mol. Phys.,* 44, 69, 1981.
21. **Pastor, R. W. and Karplus, M.,** Inertial effects in butane stochastic dynamics, *J. Chem. Phys.,* 91, 211, 1989.
22. **Pastor, R. W., Venable, R. M., and Karplus, M.,** Brownian dynamics simulation of a lipid chain in a membrane bilayer, *J. Chem. Phys.,* 89, 1112, 1988.
23. **Pastor, R. W., Venable, R. M., Karplus, M., and Szabo, A.,** A simulation based model of NMR T_1 relaxation in lipid bilayer vesicles, *J. Chem. Phys.,* 89, 1128, 1988.
24. **Marcelja, S.,** Chain ordering in liquid crystals. II. Structure of bilayer membranes, *Biochem. Biophys. Acta,* 367, 165, 1974.
25. **Chandrasekhar, S.,** Stochastic problems in physics and astronomy, *Rev. Mod. Phys.,* 15, 1, 1943.
26. **Zwanzig, R.,** Langevin theory of polymer dynamics in solution, *Annu. Rev. Phys. Chem.,* 15, 325, 1969.
27. **Allen, M. P. and Tildesley, D. J.,** *Computer Simulation of Liquids,* Clarendon Press, Oxford, 1987.
28. **Kubo, R.,** The fluctuation-dissipation theorem, *Rep. Prog. Phys.,* 29, 255, 1966.
29. **Gordon, R. G.,** On the rotational diffusion of molecules, *J. Chem. Phys.,* 44, 1830, 1966.
30. **Skinner, J. L. and Wolynes, P. G.,** General kinetic models of activated processes in condensed phases, *J. Chem. Phys.,* 72, 4913, 1980.
31. **Bull, T. E. and Egan, W.,** Extended diffusion of rigid asymmetric molecules, *J. Chem. Phys.,* 81, 3181, 1984.
32. **Einstein, A.,** *Investigations on the Theory of Brownian Movement,* Dover, New York, 1956.
33. **Yamakawa, H.,** *Modern Theory of Polymer Solutions,* Harper & Row, New York, 1971.
34. **Canter, C. R. and Schimmel, P. R.,** *Biophysical Chemistry,* Part II, W. H. Freeman, San Francisco, 1980.
35. **Teller, D. C., Swanson, E., and de Haen, C.,** The translational friction coefficient of proteins, *Methods Enzymol.,* 61, 103, 1979.
36. **Venable, R. M. and Pastor, R. W.,** Frictional models for stochastic simulations of proteins, *Biopolymers,* 27, 1001, 1988.
37. **Hu, C. and Zwanzig, R.,** Rotational friction coefficients for spheroids with the slipping boundary condition, *J. Chem. Phys.,* 60, 4354, 1974.
38. **Berne, B. J. and Pecora, R.,** *Dynamic Light Scattering,* John Wiley & Sons, New York, 1976.
39. **Murdy, J. S. and Cotts, R. M.,** Self-diffusion in liquids: H_2O, D_2O, and Na, *J. Chem. Phys.,* 53, 4724, 1970.
40. **Garcia de la Torre, J. and Bloomfield, V. A.,** Hydrodynamic properties of complex, rigid, biological macromolecules: theory and applications, *Q. Rev. Biophys.,* 14, 81, 1981.
41. **Kirkwood, J. G. and Riseman, J.,** The intrinsic viscosities and diffusion constants of flexible macromolecules in solution, *J. Chem. Phys.,* 16, 565, 1948.
42. **Paul, E. and Mazo, R. M.,** Calculations of the diffusion coefficients on *n*-alkanes, *J. Chem. Phys.,* 48, 1405, 1968.
43. **Zimm, B. H.,** Chain molecule hydrodynamics by the Monte-Carlo method and the validity of the Kirkwood-Riseman approximation, *Macromolecules,* 13, 592, 1980.
44. **Garcia de la Torre, J., Jimenez, A., and Freire, J. J.,** Intrinsic viscosities and translational diffusion coefficients of *n*-alkanes, *Macromolecules,* 15, 148, 1982.
45. **Wang, S.-Q., Douglas, J. F., and Freed, K. F.,** Corrections to preaveraging approximation within the Kirkwood-Riseman model for flexible polymers: calculations to second order in ϵ with both hydrodynamic interaction and excluded volume interactions, *J. Chem. Phys.,* 85, 3674, 1986.
46. **Pastor, R. W. and Karplus, M.,** The parameterization of the friction constant for stochastic simulations of polymers, *J. Phys. Chem.,* 92, 2636, 1988.
47. **Ermak, D. L. and McCammon, J. A.,** Brownian dynamics with hydrodynamic interactions, *J. Chem. Phys.,* 69, 1352, 1978.
48. **Pear, M. R. and McCammon, J. A.,** Hydrodynamic interaction effects on local motions of chain molecules, *J. Chem. Phys.,* 74, 6922, 1981.
49. **Ladanyi, B. M. and Hynes, J. T.,** Hydrodynamic interaction effects on isomerization rates in chain molecules, *J. Chem. Phys.,* 77, 4739, 1982.
50. **Verlet, L.,** Computer "experiments" on classical fluids. I. Thermodynamical properties of Lennard-Jones molecules, *Phys. Rev.,* 159, 98, 1967.
51. **van Gunsteren, W. F. and Berendsen, H. J. C.,** Algorithms for Brownian dynamics, *Mol. Phys.,* 45, 637, 1982 and references therein.
52. **Brunger, A., Brooks, C. B., and Karplus, M.,** Stochastic boundary conditions for molecular dynamics simulations of ST2 water, *Chem. Phys. Lett.,* 105, 495, 1984.

53. **Pastor, R. W., Brooks, B. R., and Szabo, A.,** An analysis of the accuracy of Langevin and molecular dynamics algorithms, *Mol. Phys.,* 65, 1409, 1988.
54. **van Gunsteren, W. F. and Berendsen, H. J. C.,** Practical algorithms for dynamics simulations, in *Proc. Enrico Fermi School on Molecular-Dynamics Simulation of Statistical-Mechanical Systems,* Ciccotti, G. and Hoover, W. G., Eds., North-Holland, Amsterdam, 1986, 43.
55. **Ryckaert, J. P. and Bellemans, A.,** Molecular dynamics of liquid *n*-butane near its boiling point, *Chem. Phys. Lett.,* 30, 123, 1975.
56. **Ediden, M.,** Rotational and translational diffusion in membranes, *Annu. Rev. Biophys. Bioeng.,* 3, 179, 1974.
57. **Lakowicz, J. R.,** Fluorescence spectroscopic investigations of the dynamics properties of biological membranes, in *Spectroscopy in Biochemistry,* Vol. 1, Bull, J. E., Ed., CRC Press, Boca Raton, FL, 1981, 195.
58. **Ermak, D. and Buckholtz, H.,** Numerical integration of the Lanvevin equation: Monte Carlo simulation, *J. Comput. Phys.,* 35, 169, 1980.
59. **Allen, M. P.,** Algorithms for Brownian dynamics, *Mol. Phys.,* 47, 599, 1982.
60. **Kramers, H. A.,** Brownian motion in a field of force and the diffusion model of chemical kinetics, *Physica (The Hague),* 7, 284, 1940.
61. **Eyring, H.,** The activated complex in chemical reactions, *J. Chem. Phys.,* 3, 107, 1935.
62. **Evans, G. T.,** An analysis of the density dependence of the butane isomerization rate, *J. Chem. Phys.,* 78, 4963, 1983.
63. **Hynes, J. T.,** The theory of chemical reactions in solution, in *Theory of Chemical Reaction Dynamics,* Vol. 4, Baer, M., Ed., CRC Press, Boca Raton, FL, 1985, chap. 4 and references therein.
64. **Pollack, G. L. and Enyeart, J. J.,** Atomic test of the Stokes-Einstein law. II. Diffusion of Xe, *Phys. Rev. A,* 31, 980, 1985.
65. **Seelig, J.,** Deuterium magnetic resonance, theory and application to lipid membranes, *Q. Rev. Biophys.,* 10, 353, 1977.
66. **Seelig, A. and Seelig, J.,** The dynamic structure of fatty acyl chains in a phospholipid bilayer measured by deuterium magnetic resonance, *Biochemistry,* 13, 4839, 1974.
67. **van der Ploeg, P. and Berendsen, H. J. C.,** Molecular dynamics of a bilayer membrane, *Mol. Phys.,* 49, 233, 1983.
68. **Ryckaert, J. P., Ciccotti, G., and Berendsen, H. J. C.,** Numerical integration of the Cartesian equations of motion of a system with constraints: molecular dynamics of *n*-alkanes, *J. Comput. Phys.,* 23, 327, 1977.
69. **Pastor, R. W.,** Topics in Stochastic Dynamics of Polymers, Ph.D. thesis, Harvard University, Cambridge, 1984.
70. **Schlindler, H. and Seelig, J.,** Deuterium order parameters in relation to thermodynamic properties of a phospholipid bilayer. A statistical mechanical interpretation, *Biochemistry,* 14, 2283, 1975.
71. **deGennes, P. G.,** *The Physics and Chemistry of Liquid Crystals,* Clarendon Press, Oxford, 1974.
72. **Nagle, J. F.,** Theory of the main lipid bilayer phase transition, *Annu. Rev. Phys. Chem.,* 31, 157, 1980.
73. **Dill, K. A. and Flory, P. J.,** Interphases of chain molecules, *Proc. Natl. Acad. Sci. U.S.A.,* 77, 3115, 1980.
74. **Gruen, D. W. R.,** A statistical mechanical model of the lipid bilayer above its phase transition temperature, *Biochem. Biophys. Acta,* 95, 161, 1980.
75. **Meraldi, J.-P. and Schlitter, J.,** A statistical mechanical treatment of fatty acyl chain order in phospholipid bilayers and correlation with experimental data. A. Theory, *Biochem. Biophys. Acta,* 645, 183, 1981.
76. **Meraldi, J.-P. and Schlitter, J.,** A statistical mechanical treatment of fatty acyl chain order in phospholipid bilayers and correlation with experimental data. B. Dipalmitoyl-3-*sn*-phosphatidylcholine, *Biochem. Biophys. Acta,* 645, 192, 1981.
77. **Ben-Shaul, A. and Gelbert, W. M.,** Theory of chain packing in amphiphilic aggregates, *Annu. Rev. Phys. Chem.,* 36, 179, 1985.
78. **Cevc, G. and Marsh, D.,** *Phospholipid Bilayers,* John Wiley & Sons, New York, 1987.
79. **Bloomfield, P.,** *Fourier Analysis on Time Series: An Introduction,* John Wiley & Sons, New York, 1976.
80. **Agarwal, R. C. and Cooley, J. W.,** Fourier transform and convolution subroutines on the IBM 3090 vector facility, *IBM J. Res. Dev.,* 30, 145, 1986.
81. **Lipari, G. and Szabo, A.,** Model-free approach to the interpretation of nuclear magnetic resonance relaxation in macromolecules. I. Theory and range of validity, *J. Am. Chem. Soc.,* 104, 4546, 1982.
82. **Lipari, G. and Szabo, A.,** Model-free approach to the interpretation of nuclear magnetic resonance relaxation in macromolecules. II. Analysis of experimental results, *J. Am. Chem. Soc.,* 104, 4559, 1982.
83. **Szabo, A.,** Theory of fluorescence depolarization in macromolecules and membranes, *J. Chem. Phys.,* 81, 150, 1984.
84. **Pastor, R. W., Venable, R. M., and Karplus, M.,** A model for the lipid bilayer, in preparation.
85. **Lipari, G. and Szabo, A.,** Effect of librational motion on fluorescence depolarization and nuclear magnetic resonance relaxation in macromolecules and membranes, *Biophys. J.,* 30, 489, 1980.

86. **Zaccai, G., Buldt, G., Seelig, A., and Seelig, J.,** Neutron diffraction studies on phosphatidylcholine model membranes, *J. Mol. Biol.,* 134, 693, 1979.
87. **Trauble, H.,** The movement of molecules across lipid membranes: a molecular theory, *J. Membrane Biol.,* 4, 193, 1971.
88. **Peterson, N. O. and Chan, S. I.,** More on the motional state of lipid bilayer membranes: interpretation of order parameters from nuclear magnetic resonance experiments, *Biochemistry,* 16, 2657, 1977.
89. **Egberts, B.,** Molecular Dynamics Simulation of Multibilayer Membranes, Ph.D. thesis, Rijksuniversiteit Groningen, Groningen, 1988.
90. **Egberts, B. and Berendsen, H. J. C.,** Molecular dynamics simulation of a smectic liquid crystal with atomic detail, *J. Chem. Phys.,* 89, 3718, 1988.

Chapter 1.A.6

TAMMO: THEORETICAL ANALYSIS OF MEMBRANE MOLECULAR ORGANIZATION

Robert Brasseur

TABLE OF CONTENTS

I. INTRODUCTION

Phospholipids and proteins constitute the major components of biological membranes. They are known to occur in various proportions, ranging from approximately 25% lipid in mitochondrial inner membranes to 80% lipid in myelin. They retain, however, common structural features and presumably play the same functional role in all membranes. The consideration of biological membranes at the molecular level requires a detailed knowledge of the preferred conformations of phospholipids and the mode of insertion of amphiphilic membrane components (drugs, proteins) into the lipid matrix. Phospholipids dispersed in water often spontaneously form bilayer membranes, although other nonlamellar phases are also found, depending on composition and temperature.[1,2] X-ray diffraction,[3] (Chapters 1.B.1 and 1.B.2), neutron diffraction combined with the use of deuterated material,[4] and infrared (IR) spectroscopy[5] (Chapter 1.B.3) have provided information about the position and orientation of the molecules in lipid bilayers. This molecular approach is a prerequisite to the understanding of the organization and function of biological membranes.

This chapter describes the conformational analysis as a valuable approach to gain insight into the structure of membrane components. These theoretical predictions will be compared with the experimental data whenever available for the particular system.

Due to limitations of theoretical methods and to consideration of computing time, previous investigators have mostly limited their analysis to distinct regions of the isolated molecule (polar head group, acyl chain). More recently, such calculations were extended to whole molecules. Some of the attempts aimed at giving a molecular description of the assembly model of phospholipids in monolayers or bilayers will be described here. Examples will also be given to illustrate the relationship between the mode of insertion of a drug, a peptide, or a membrane component into the lipid matrix and the modifications of its pharmacological or biological functions. In order to facilitate a comparison between results, the atom numbering and the notation for the torsional angles proposed by Sundaralingam[6] will be used for phospholipids.

The large number of theoretical models for a lipid bilayer reflects the complexity of the physical state of the membrane. Since an exact solution to this problem is not yet available at the theoretical level, two types of approximate solutions were considered. One approach consists in assuming a simplified physical state that can be solved either exactly or by controlled approximations. This approach is both the most rigorous and meaningful. Such quantum-mechanical methods have been mostly applied to the calculation of the structure of either a single lipid molecule or of some of its structural components (hydrophilic moiety, acyl chain). In another semiempirical approach, the general model is solved by means of approximations that may, however, lose physical relevance. This approach was elaborated to yield a molecular description of the lipid structure in organized systems (bilayer, micelle, inverted micelle). The selection of this type of model is aimed at mimicking the experimental data, but should not be considered as a permanent alternative to other theoretical approaches. As will be shown further, the results of our theoretical analysis can accurately fit the experimental data and therefore enable the understanding of the basic principles underlying these experiments.

II. ENERGY FIELDS

The total conformational energy, considered as the sum of the contributions resulting from van der Waals' interactions, the torsional potential, the electrostatic interactions, and the transfer energy, is calculated for a large number of conformational orientations and modes of assembly.

A. THE LONDON-VAN DER WAALS' ENERGY OF INTERACTION BETWEEN ALL PAIRS OF NONMUTUALLY BONDED ATOMS

Buckingham's pairwise atom-atom interaction functions have been used:

$$E^{vdw} = \Sigma(A_{ij}\exp(-B_{ij}r_{ij}) - C_{ij}r_{ij}^{-6}) \tag{1}$$

were $ij = 1, 2, \ldots$ are nonbonded atoms, r_{ij} are their mutual distances, and A_{ij}, B_{ij}, and C_{ij} are coefficients assigned to atom pairs. The values of these coefficients have been reported by Liquori and co-workers.[7,8] Like other quantum mechanical results, these values emerge in part as the solution of the Schrödinger equation and in part as heuristic variables. They have been successfully applied to the conformational analysis of molecular crystals, proteins, polypeptides, and lipids. In order to compensate for the decrease of the function E^{vdw} at small r_{ij}, we have imposed an arbitrary cut-off value of:

$$E^{vdw} = 418.4 \text{ kJ/mol at } r_{ij} < 0.1 \text{ nm}$$

B. THE GENERALIZED KEESOM-VAN DER WAALS INTERACTION OR ELECTROSTATIC INTERACTION BETWEEN ATOMIC POINT CHARGES

At distances comparable to the molecular size, it becomes less accurate to deal with point dipoles rather than with atomic point-charge distributions. The coulombic interaction energies corresponding to such distributions include all higher-order terms (quadrupoles, octopoles, . . .) which are usually neglected. Formally, the energy can be written as follows:

$$E^{cb} \sum_{ij} 139.2 \left(\Sigma \frac{e_i e_j}{r_{ij}\epsilon_{ij}} \right) \tag{2}$$

where e_i and e_j are expressed in electron charge units and r_{ij} is in angstroms. ϵ_{ij} is the dielectric constant. Table 1[9,10] summarizes the values of the dielectric constant (ϵ) in model membranes determined both from experimental measurements and by theoretical estimation. To simulate the membrane interface, we assumed a dielectric constant equal to 3 above the interface, while a plane was drawn at the atom most deeply immersed in the aqueous phase, with a dielectric constant of 30. Between these two planes, the dielectric constant was assumed to increase linearly along the z-axis perpendicular to the interface.[16] The values of atomic point charge are similar to those used for polypeptides.[17]

C. THE POTENTIAL ENERGY OF ROTATION OF TORSIONAL ANGLES

The rotation around the C–C or C–O bonds was calculated according to the equation:

$$E^{Tor} \sum_{ij} \frac{U_{ij}}{2} (1 + \cos\Omega_{ij}) \tag{3}$$

where U_{ij} corresponds to the energy barrier in the eclipsed conformation during the rotation of the angle and Ω_{ij} is the torsional angle. U_{ij} is equal to 11.7 kJ/mol for the C–C bond and 7.5 kJ/mol for the C–O bond.

D. THE TRANSFER ENERGY OF EACH PART OF THE MOLECULE

The values of the transfer energies used (E^{Tr}_i) are similar to those determined experimentally by several authors (Table 2), as summarized elsewhere.[18] The E^{Tr} of a given conformation is the sum of all transfer energy changes associated with the transfer of a chemical group from the hydrophobic to the hydrophilic phase.

TABLE 1
Micropolarity Data (ϵ) on Model Membranes Determined Experimentally and by Theoretical Estimation

Model membrane	Site of determination	Method	ϵ	Ref.
Single-layer vesicles (PC)	Vesicle wall	Dielectric dispersion	10—30	11
Lipid layers	Polar head, near bulk water	Theoretical estimation	40	12
Single-layer vesicles (PC) of radius	Vesicle wall of 3.5 nm (35 Å)	Dielectric Dispersion		13
15.0 nm (150 Å)			13.9	
14.0 nm (140 Å)			15.1	
12.5 nm (125 Å)			17.3	
Multilayers (PC)	Lipid water interface	Theoretical estimation	19	14
Multilayer (PC)	Polar head interface probably near bulk water	Florescence polarity probe: ANS	32	15
Multilayer (PC)	Polar head interface near hydro-carbon core	Florescence polarity probe: NN'-DOC	25	15
Single-layered (PC, TOC)	Hydrogen belt-hydrocarbon core interface	Chemical reaction probe: DPPH-TOC	24.6	10

Note: Abbreviations: ANS, 1-anilino-8-naphtalenesulfonic acid; DPPH, 1,1-diphenyl-2-picryl-hydrazyl; ϵ, dielectric constant; N,N'-DOC, N,N'-di(octadecyl)oxacarbocyanine; PC, phosphatidylcholine; and TOC, α-tocopherol.

TABLE 2
Transfer Energy (in KJ/mol) from a Hydrophilic Phase into a Hydrophobic Domain

$-$C$-$OH	-3.482
$-$C$-$O$-$	-17.807
$>$C$=$O	-10.759
$>$C$<$	3.566
Per 1° of unsaturation	6.283

$$E^{Tr} = \sum_{\mathscr{L}} \delta E^{Tr}_k \qquad (4)$$

where δE^{Tr}_k is the transfer energy of the chemical group k from a hydrophilic into a hydrophobic domain.

III. STRATEGY

The method currently used for the study of polypeptides was modified to take into account the changes in the dielectric constant and energy of transfer when the molecule moves from one environment (hydrophilic phase) to an other (hydrophobic phase) at the simulated lipid-water interface. The method implies a three-step procedure (Figure 1):

1. Calculation of the conformation and orientation of the isolated molecule at the lipid water interface
2. Calculation of the conformation of the molecules inserted in a lipid monolayer
3. Calculation of the conformation of two interacting monolayers aimed as an approximation to mimic the behavior of a bilayer

TAMMO : Theoretical Analysis of Membrane Molecular Organization.

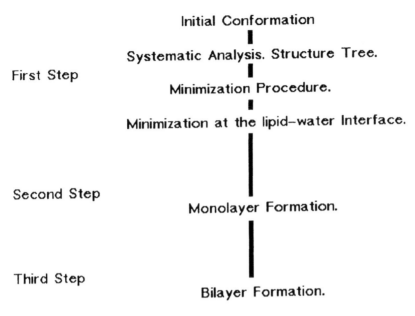

FIGURE 1. Schematic representation of the theoretical analysis of model membrane organization (TAMMO).

The main hypothesis for these types of calculations is that the total energy of a bilayer is equal to the sum of three terms:

$$E^{tol} = E^{isol.\,mol.} + E^{int.\,monolayer} + E^{int.\,bilayer} \tag{5}$$

where $E^{isol.\,mol.}$ is the energy of the isolated molecule at the lipid water interface. This term is in turn equal to the sum of four terms (Equations 1 to 4):

$$E^{isol.\,mol.} = E^{VdW} + E^{cb} + E^{tor} + E^{tr} \tag{6}$$

where $E^{int.\,monolayer}$ is the interaction energy between amphiphilic molecules within a monolayer and is equal to the sum of three terms (Equations 1, 2, and 4):

$$E^{int.\,monolayer} = E^{VdW} + E^{cb} + E^{tr} \tag{7}$$

$E^{int.\,bilayer}$ represents the energy of interaction between two monolayers of amphiphilic molecules within a bilayer. It consists of the sum of three terms (Equations 1, 2, and 4):

$$E^{int.\,bilayer} = E^{VdW} + E^{cb} + E^{tr} \tag{8}$$

IV. ISOLATED MOLECULE

The values used for the angles and bond lengths are those commonly used in conformational analysis.[17] We adopted a molecular structure in the all-*trans* conformation as initial configuration. Each molecule has n rotational angles, so that if systematic 60° changes were applied, 6^n conformations would be generated. To avoid such a large number of conformations, another procedure was selected, namely, the conformation energy was calculated for a large number of conformations in a systematic structure tree analysis, where six consecutive changes of 60° each were imposed to the n torsional angles, yielding 6^n conformers in each branch of the structure tree. The conformational energy was calculated for each of these conformers and the most probable configurations were taken as those yielding the lowest energy by the following equation:

$$P_i = \frac{e^{-E_i/kT}}{\sum_j e^{-E_j/kT}}$$ (9)

with T = 298 K and Ei and Ej corresponding to the internal energy of the ith conformer and the energies of all generated conformers, respectively. The effect of the entropy was considered as negligible at this state and, hence, the selection of the conformers was based on their energy rather than on the free energy. A structure tree includes the most probable of all configurations (a selection based upon the Boltzmann statistical weight of all configurations) together with their probability of existence as obtained after successive systematic analysis. At each step, the conformations whose probability of existence was less than 5% were discarded. After systematic analysis, the sheets of the tree were submitted to a simplex minimization procedure in order to further reduce their total energy[19] with a precision of 10° on each conformational angle. The systematic analysis and the first minimization procedure were carried out in a medium of intermediate dielectric constant representative of the membrane/water interface. The total conformational energy is calculated as the sum of three terms: the London-van der Waals' energy (E^{vdw}); the electrostatic interaction (E^{cb}); and the potential energy of rotation of torsional angles (E^{tor}).

V. ORIENTATION AT THE LIPID-WATER INTERFACE

A second minimization procedure was performed taking into account the interface properties. At this step, the total conformational energy is calculated as the sum of four terms: the London-van der Waals' energy (E^{vdw}); the electrostatic interaction (E^{cb}); the potential energy of rotation of torsional angles (E^{tor}); and the transfer energy (E^{tr}) of each part of the molecule from the hydrophilic to the hydrophobic phase. At each step, the molecule is oriented with the line joining the hydrophilic and hydrophobic centers perpendicular to the interface[16] (Figure 2). The hydrophilic center ($\vec{C}_{phi}$) is defined by the following Equation:

$$\vec{c}_{phi} = \frac{\sum E_{tr_i}^{phi} \vec{r}_i}{\sum E_{tr_i}^{phi}}$$ (10)

in which $\vec{r}_i$ are the coordinates of the ith atom. The hydrophobic center located in the hydrocarbon domain ($\vec{C}_{pho}^2$) is defined by the same equation, except that the negative transfer energies are taken into account. The interface lipid/water position ($\vec{I}$) is defined by the Equation:

$$\frac{\sum E_{tr}^{pho}}{|\vec{I} - \vec{C}_{pho}|} = \frac{\sum E_{tr}^{phi}}{|\vec{I} - \vec{C}_{phi}|}$$ (11)

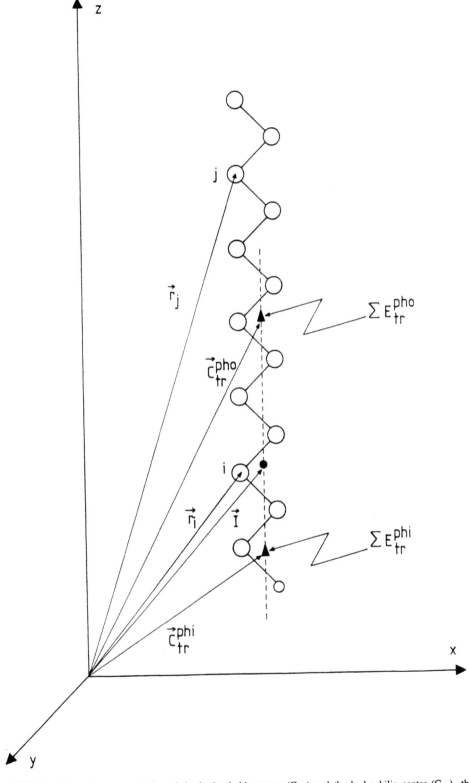

FIGURE 2. Schematic representation of the hydrophobic center (C_{pho}) and the hydrophilic center (C_{phi}), the interface position (I).

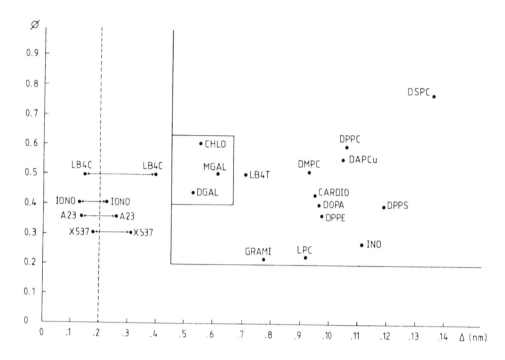

FIGURE 3. Hydrophobic-hydrophilic balance φ as a function of the distance Δ between the hydrophobic and hydrophilic centers (see text); DMPC, dimyristoylphosphatidyl; DPPC, dipalmitoylphosphatidylcholine; DSPC, distearoylphosphatidylcholine; DAPCu, diacylphosphatidylcholine unsaturated; CARDIO, cardiolipin; DOPA, dioleoylphosphatidic acid; DPPE, dipalmitoylphosphatidylethanolamine; DPPS, dipalmitoylphosphatidylserine; LPC, palmitoyllysophosphatidylcholine; GRAMI, gramicidin A; CHLO, chlorophyll a; MGAL, monogalactosyldiacylglycerol; DGAL, digalactosyldiacylglycerol; LB4T, leukotriene B4 *trans*; LB4C, leukotriene B4 *cis*; IONO, ionomycine; A23, A23187; X537, X537A or lasalocide; INO, dipalmitoylphosphatidylinositol.

VI. THE HYDROPHOBIC-HYDROPHILIC BALANCE AND THE DISTANCE BETWEEN THE HYDROPHOBIC AND HYDROPHILIC CENTERS

The hydrophobic-hydrophilic balance φ is defined by the Equation:

$$\phi = \log(\Sigma\ E_{tr}^{pho}/\Sigma\ E_{tr}^{phi}) \tag{12}$$

where Σ_{tr}^{phi} is the hydrophilic transfer energy of atom j and Σ_{tr}^{pho} is the hydrophobic transfer energy of atom i. The value of the transfer energies used for each atom or group of atoms is similar to those determined by others (see Table 2).[19] The distance Δ between the hydrophobic and the hydrophilic centers is defined by:

$$\Delta = |\vec{C}_{pho} - \vec{C}_{phi}| \tag{13}$$

The two parameters φ and Δ were calculated for several amphiphilic compounds whose mode of organization (phospholipids) or mode of insertion into a lipid bilayer (ionophores) was known. Several domains can be defined (Figure 3):

1.   φ > 0.2 and Δ > 0.43 nm. This domain is specific for molecules capable of assembling in organized structures. For these amphiphilic molecules, characterized by a large distance between the hydrophobic and hydrophilic centers, the only way to avoid the aqueous environment is to form micellar aggregates as shown experimentally (inverted

micelles for monogalactosyldiacylglycerol, micelles for lysopalmitoyl-phosphatidylcholine, and bilayers for dipalmitoylphosphatidylcholine, Figure 3, and dimyristoyl- and distearoylphosphatidylcholine). It is noteworthy that the components of the thylakoid membranes (monogalactosyldiacylglycerol, digalactosyldiacylgly-cerol, and chlorophyll a) are located in the $0.40 < \phi < 0.64$ and $0.43 < \Delta < 0.65$ nm domain. Phospholipid constituents of the bilayer membranes, such as saturated or unsaturated phosphatidylcholines, phosphatidylethanolamine, cardiolipin, phosphati-dylinositol, and phosphatidylserine, are assembled in the $\phi > 0.2$ and $\Delta > 0.43$ nm domain. The location of gramicidin A next to lysophosphatidylcholine in the ϕ-A map might look surprising. It was recently demonstrated, however, that gramicidin A, mixed with lysophosphatidylcholine in a 1:4 molar ratio, could form a bilayer (Chapter 1.A.8). This result suggests that for similar ϕ- and Δ-values, maximal interactions between amphiphilic molecules can be expected, even when the structures of the two molecules differ significantly. Such a hypothesis would account for the presence of molecules as different as chlorophyll a, monogalactosyldiacylglycerol, and digalac-tosyldiacylglycerol, a native thylakoid membrane. On the contrary, amphiphilic mol-ecules with different ϕ- and Δ-values such as dimyristoylphosphatidylcholine and distearoylphosphatidylcholine will form bilayers, but will segregate into two separate phases inside a liposomal structure. A different behavior should be expected for di-myristoylphosphatidylcholine and dipalmitoylphosphatidylcholine with similar ϕ- and Δ-values. This hypothesis is fully supported by the experimental data showing that these two lipids are randomly distributed inside a liposome.

2. $\phi > 0.2$ and $0.20 <= \Delta < 0.43$ nm. This second domain is characteristic of molecules which do not assemble in organized structures. In this case, the ϕ- and Δ-values will determine their respective domains: either in the lipid phase, at the lipid-water interface, or in the aqueous phase. This applies to several ionophores, among which the compound A23187 is able to transport Ca^{2+} ions across lipid bilayers. We recently demonstrated (Chapter 2.2) that this process implies the existence of two isomers: an interfacial structure which enables the ion binding and release at the lipid-water interface and a hydrophobic structure which transports Ca^{2+} ions across the hydrophobic region of the bilayer. The isomerization process is mediated by the degree of penetration of the ionophore into either the aqueous or the hydrophobic phase. In our analysis method, the degree of penetration is simulated by a variation of the dielectric constant at the interface. For all ionophores studied, we could define two regions characterizing the interfacial ($\phi > 0.2$ and $\Delta > 0.20$ nm) and hydrophobic ($\phi > 0.2$ and $\Delta < 0.20$ nm) conformations as illustrated in Figure 3 for the X537A ionophore. It is interesting to note that the energy required for the structural isomerization is quite low (less than 4.18 kJ/mol) and the ionophore-lipid interaction remains weak. It has been observed that the *trans*-isomer of leukotriene B4 is unable to transfer Ca^{2+} ions. This molecule is located inside the lipid domain as a result of the significant increase of the distance between hydrophobic and hydrophilic centers compared to the leukotriene B4 *cis*-isomer which acts as a Ca^{2+} carrier (Chapter 2.1). Its enhanced amphiphilic character, together with a high energy of interaction with lipids, abolishes its carrier properties which require a high mobility within the bilayer.

3. Our conformational analysis method enables the prediction of the mode of organization of amphiphilic structures. Two parameters are required in order to define the location of an amphiphilic compound either at the lipid-water interface, in the aqueous phase, or in the lipid phase. This method of calculation provides a unique opportunity to investigate how minor structural modifications of a membrane compound can affect its location in the lipid membrane. It should be stressed that the domains defined in Figure 3 were obtained from the comparison with a limited number of amphiphilic molecules rather than drawn on a theoretical basis. Therefore, the borderlines between

different domains are only indicators of regions corresponding to a possible model of organization for amphiphilic molecules.

VII. MONOLAYER FORMATION

Two methods were developed for monolayer formation.

A. SEQUENTIAL METHOD[20]

1. The position of lipid B is modified along the x-axis (Figure 4a) in steps of 0.05 nm (0.05 nm). (The phosphate atom was used to define the distance separating two molecules.) At each separation distance, lipid B is rotated by an angle of 30° around its own axis z and around lipid A (Figure 4b). Among the 14,400 possible orientations, only the structure corresponding to the minimal energy is considered.
2. The position of lipid A is kept constant and lipid B is allowed to move along the z-axis perpendicular to the lipid water interface (Figure 4c). Here again, only the structure with the minimal energy is considered.
3. The orientation of lipid B around the z-axis compared to lipid A can be modified (Figure 4c). This procedure enables to ultimately define the most probable packing of the two lipid molecules. The intermolecular energy of interaction was calculated as the sum of the London-van der Waals' energy of interaction (E^{vdw}), the electrostatic interaction (E^{cb}), and the transfer energy of atoms or groups of atoms from a hydrophobic phase to a hydrophilic phase (E^{tr}). The extension of these calculations to a system with three molecules implies a similar approach. The packing of the first two molecules is maintained and the orientation of the third molecule around them is studied systematically. The assembly procedure is completed when the central molecule interacts with a defined number of surrounding molecules.

B. HYPERMATRIX METHOD[21]

The procedure used to surround one molecule A with other B molecules is a modification of the method used to surround one drug with lipid molecules (sequential method) and can be described as follows (Figure 5). After orienting of molecule A at the air/water interface, its position and orientation were fixed. A second molecule B was oriented at the interface and it was allowed to move along the x-axis in steps of 0.05 nm. For each position, the second molecule was rotated in steps of 30° around its long axis z' and around the first molecule: 1 is the number of positions along the x-axis, m is the number of rotations of the second molecule around the first one, and n is the number of rotations of the molecule itself. For each set of values, 1, m, and n, the intermolecular energy of interaction was calculated as the sum of the London-van der Waals' energy of interactions (E^{vdw}), the electrostatic interaction (E^{cb}), and the transfer energy of atoms or groups of atoms from a hydrophobic to a hydrophilic phase (E^{tr}). Then, the second molecule was allowed to move in steps of 0.05 nm along the z'-axis perpendicular to the interface and the position of the z'-axis was varied in steps of 5° with respect to the z-axis, such that the lowest interaction energy state could be obtained for each set of values, 1, m, and n. The energy values together with the coordinates associated to each set of 1, m, and n were stored in a hypermatrix and classified according to decreasing values of the interaction energy. The position of the third molecule C is defined as the first energetically favorable orientation stored in the hypermatrix, but taking into account the sterical and energetic constraints imposed by the presence of the second molecule. Thus, orientations are disregarded in which overlap of atomic coordinates of two molecules occurs and in which the interaction energy between the two molecules was positive. In order to minimize further the conformational energy, the position of the second and third molecule is then alternatively modified in steps according to the energy

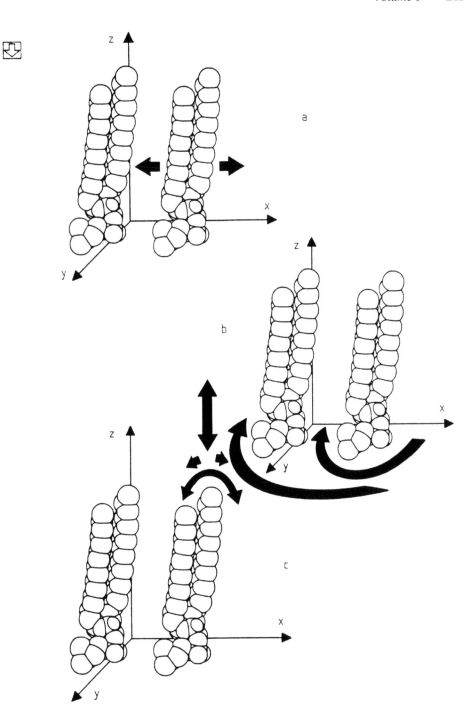

FIGURE 4.   Schematic representation of the packing procedure of lipid molecules assembled in monolayer by the sequential method.

classification of the hypermatrix. For the fourth molecule, the same process is repeated, but now the positions of the three surrounding molecules are modified alternatively in order to find the lowest energy state. In this calculation, the interaction energy between all monomers in the aggregate is considered and minimalized until the lowest energy state of the entire aggregate is reached. We limited this approach to the number of molecules sufficient to surround one central molecule. The mean molecular area occupied by the hydrophobic and

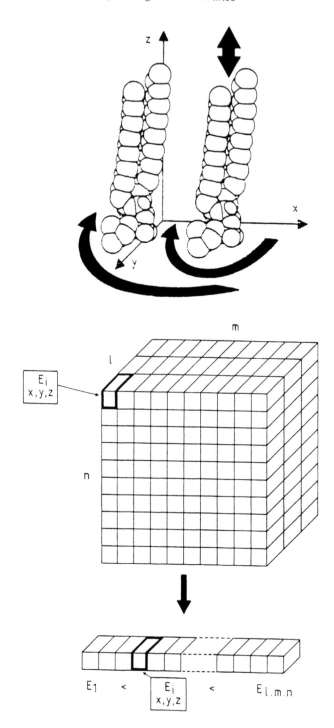

FIGURE 5.   Schematic representation of the packing procedure of lipid molecules assembled in monolayer by the hypermatrix method.

hydrophilic moieties was estimated by projection on the x-y plane using a grid of squares, each with a 0.1 mm side.

VIII. BILAYER FORMATION

1. The position of monolayer B is modified along the z-axis. Again, each separating distance is equal to 0.1 nm (1 Å) (Figure 6b). A rotation angle of 30° is imposed on monolayer B around the z-axis (Figure 6a). Monolayer A is fixed.
2. The orientation of monolayer B around the z-axis can be modified (Figures 6d and c). The position of monolayer A is fixed.

Figure 7 summarizes the conformational analysis steps for dipalmitoylphosphatidylcholine (DPPC). First, a systematic analysis was performed in which the torsional angles relative to the polar head groups ($\alpha6$, $\alpha5$, $\alpha4$, $\alpha3$, $\alpha2$, $\alpha1$, $\Theta1$) were varied by increments of 60°. In the second step, the angles $\beta1$, $\beta2$, $\beta3$, $\beta4$, $\tau1$, $\tau2$, $\tau3$, $\tau4$, $\Theta3$ relative to the hydrocarbon domain were varied with increments of 60°. The combination of the two procedures yields six final structures for the entire DPPC molecule. The energy minimum associated to each of these structures was calculated using the simplex minimization procedure. An assembly procedure finally yields the molecular structure of the monolayer and the bilayer.

In each case, only the bilayer structure with the minimal energy is retained. For dipalmitoylphosphatidylcholine,[16] the most probable conformation is characterized by the close proximity of the phosphate residue associated with the hydrophilic moiety of one lipid and the choline residue associated with the adjacent lipid. The electrostatic interaction between the two residues stabilizes the lipid structure. Based upon the knowledge of the lipid structure within a monolayer, the organization of the lipid bilayer could be extrapolated theoretically and compared with the available experimental data. The data obtained from neutron diffraction experiments, combined with the use of selectively deuterated lipids.[4] This approach was applied to bilayer membranes consisting of dipalmitoylphosphatidylcholine deuterated at 12 different positions in the hydrocarbon chain and the polar head group. The experimental and theoretical distances between the center of the bilayer and each deuterated atom were in excellent agreement (Table 3). The isolated molecules were assembled as described in the sequential method. This theoretical approach was performed without introducing any parameter associated with the crystal structure. This method had also been successfully applied to the prediction of other modes of organization of lipid aggregates such as micelles or hexagonal H_{II} types of configuration.[21,22]

IX. COMPUTER SYSTEM

All calculations were performed using as hardware an IBM-compatible personal computer (PC) and a 8087, 80287, or a 80387 or 8046 processor and using as software the PC-TAMMO + (Theoretical Analysis of Molecular Membrane Organization) and the PC-MSA + (molecular structure analysis) procedures. Graphs were drawn with the PC-MGM + (Molecular Graphics Manipulation) program.

X. CONCLUSION

A comparison with the experimental data is a prerequisite to the demonstration of the validity of the predictive methods. Such a comparison could be carried out in a few cases and supported the theoretical approach. Further refinements are, moreover, required to solve some of the limiting factors of the conformational analysis procedure described above, especially its failure to take into account the conformational changes that might result from

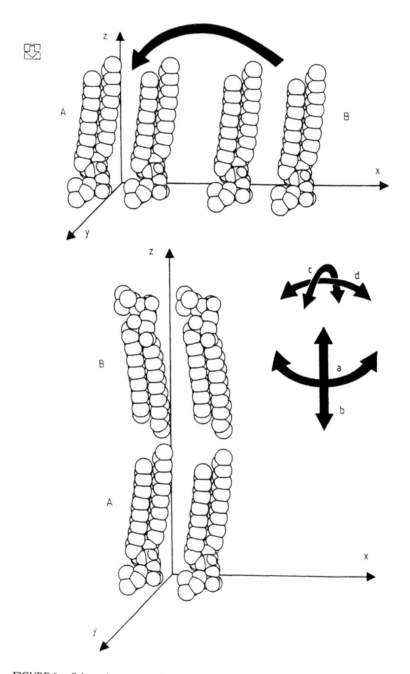

FIGURE 6.   Schematic representation of the packing procedure of lipid molecules assembled in bilayer.

molecular interactions. Moreover, extensive efforts are required to extend this theoretical analysis to the description of the mode of insertion of proteins into a lipid matrix. Such a type of conformational analysis, applied to the different types of helices present in lipid-associating proteins, should enable the computation of the parameters accounting for the different properties of such helices. According to our primary results, the orientation of the line joining the hydrophobic and hydrophilic centers of the helix seems to determine its orientation at the lipid/water interface. This parameter should usefully contribute to the

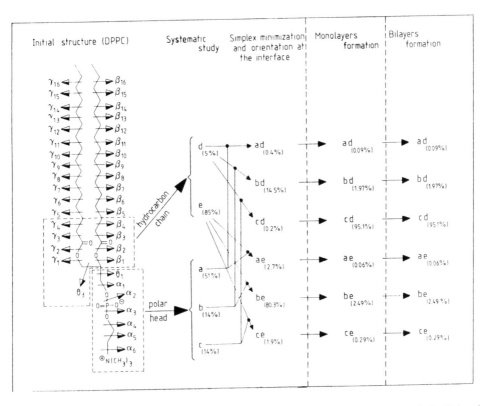

FIGURE 7. Schematic representation of dipalmitoylphosphatidylcholine (DPPC) structure analysis. Values in percent indicate the percent of probability of structures in each step of analysis.

TABLE 3
Summary of the Mean Carbon Positions of Dipalmitoylphosphatidylcholine in the Bilayer

Methyl	Neutron diffraction[4]	TAMMO
	Distance from the center of the bilayer (nm)	
C	2.51 ± 0.06	2.52
C	2.48 ± 0.07	2.5
C	2.45 ± 0.07	2.4
GC-C	2.31 ± 0.10	2.22
C2(2)	2.00 ± 0.10	2.02
C2(1)	1.81 ± 0.10	1.73
C-4	1.62 ± 0.06	1.56
C-5	1.50 ± 0.06	1.47
C-9	1.01 ± 0.10	1.00
C-14	0.41 ± 0.06	0.47
C-15	0.29 ± 0.06	0.35

Note: TAMMO, theoretical analysis of membrane molecular organization.

differentiation between an amphiphilic helix, orientated parallel to the interface, and a transmembrane helix, orientated perpendicularly.[23]

The representation of these segments at the molecular level and the visualization of their orientation in a phospholipid environment contribute to the understanding of their mode of insertion into a lipid bilayer. This computer modeling approach should usefully complement the statistical analysis carried out on these helices, based on their hydrophobicity and hydrophobic moment.

We reported recently (Chapter 3.6) that a peptide can take an oblique orientation compared to the lipid water-interface.[24,25] The unusual orientation of the N-terminal peptide of the fusion protein of the paramyxovirus prevents a parallel orientation of the phospholipid acyl chains and consequently perturbs the lipid organization. Since the existence of such an amphipathic asymmetrical peptide is related to a polymorphism of the viral protein, this might represent the initial events in the virus/cell fusion. In Chapters of Volumes I and II, we moreover demonstrate that this type of conformational analysis enables a molecular description of the mode of assembly of amphiphilic membrane components, such as phospholipids, together with the prediction of the mode of insertion of amphiphilic molecules, such as drugs and peptides, into a lipid matrix.

REFERENCES

1. **Luzzati, V.,** in *Biological Membranes*, Vol. 1, Chapman, D., Ed., Academic Press, London, 1968, 71.
2. **Cullis, P. R. and de Kruijff, B.,** *Biochim. Biophys. Acta*, 559, 399, 1979.
3. **Hauser, H., Pascher, L., Pearson, R. H., and Sundell, S.,** Preferred conformation and molecular packing of phosphatidylethanolamine and phosphatidylcholine, *Biochim. Biophys. Acta*, 650, 21, 1981.
4. **Buldt, G., Gally, H. U., Seelig, A., Seelig, J., and Zaccai, G.,** Neutron diffraction studies on selectively deuterated phospholipid bilayers, *Nature (London)*, 271, 182, 1978.
5. **Goormaghtigh, E., Brasseur, R., Huart, P., and Ruysschaert, J.-M.,** Study of the adriamycin-cardiolipin complex using ATR-IR spectroscopy, *Biochemistry*, 26, 1789, 1987.
6. **Sundaralingam, M.,** Molecular structures and conformations of the phospholipids and sphingomyelins, *Ann. N.Y. Acad. Sci.*, 195, 324, 1972.
7. **Liquori, A. M., Giglio, E., and Mazzarella, L.,** van der Waals interactions and the packing of molecular crystal. II. Adamantane, *Nuovo Cimento B*, 55, 57, 1968.
8. **Giglio, E., Liquori, A. M., and Mazzarella, L.,** van der Waals' interactions and the packing of molecular crystals. IV. Orthorhombic sulfur, *Nuovo Cimento*, 56, 57, 1968.
9. **Fragata, M. and Bellemare, F.,** Model of singlet oxygen scavenging by α-tocopherol in biomembrane, *Chem. Phys. Lipids*, 27, 93, 1980.
10. **Bellemare, F. and Fragata, M.,** Polarity studies on the head group of single-layered phosphatidylcholine-α-tocopherol, *J. Colloid Interface Sci.*, 77, 243, 1980.
11. **Schawn, H. P., Takashima, S., Miyamoto, U. K., and Stoeckenius, H. P.,** Electrical properties of phospholipid vesicles, *Biophys. J.*, 10, 1102, 1970.
12. **Gillespie, C. J.,** Ion sorption and the potential profile near a model lecithin membrane, *Biochim. Biophys. Acta*, 203, 47, 1970.
13. **Redwood, W. R., Takashima, S., Schwan, H. P., and Thompson, T. E.,** Dielectric studies on homogeneous phosphatidylcholine vesicles, *Biochim. Biophys. Acta*, 255, 557, 1972.
14. **Colbow, K. and Jones, B. L.,** in *Biological Membranes*, Colbow, K., Ed., Simon Fraser University, Burnaby, British Columbia, 1975,
15. **Colbow, K. and Chong, C. S.,** in *Biological Membranes*, Colbow, K., Ed., Simon Fraser University, Burnaby, British Columbia, 1975,
16. **Brasseur, R. and Ruysschaert, J. M.,** Conformation and mode of organization of amphiphilic membrane components: a conformational analysis, *Biochem. J.*, 238, 1, 1986.
17. **Hopfinger, A. J.,** in *Conformational Properties of Macromolecules*, Academic Press, New York, 1973,
18. **Tanford, C.,** in *The Hydrophobic Effect: Formation of Micelles and Biological Membranes*, John Wiley & Sons, New York, 1973,
19. **Nelder, J. A. and Mead, R.,** A simplex method for function minimization, *Comput. J.*, 7, 308, 1965.

20. **Brasseur, R., Goormaghtigh, E., and Ruysschaert, J.-M.,** Theoretical conformational analysis of phospholipids bilayers, *Biochem. Biophys. Res. Commun.,* 103, 301, 1981.
21. **Brasseur, R., Killian, J. A., de Kruijjff, B., and Ruysschaert, J.-M.,** Conformational analysis of gramicidin-gramicidin interaction at the air-water interface suggests that gramicidin aggregates into tube-like structures similar as found in the gramicidin-induced hexagonal H_{II} phase, *Biochim. Biophys. Acta,* 903, 11, 1987.
22. **Brasseur, R., de Kruijff, B., and Ruysschaert, J.-M.,** Mode of organization of lipid aggregates: a conformational analysis, *Biosci. Rep.,* 4, 259, 1984.
23. **Brasseur, R., de Loof, H., Ruysschaert, J. M., and Rosseneu, M.,** Conformational analysis of lipid-associating proteins in a lipid environment, *Biochim. Biophys. Acta,* 943, 95, 1988.
24. **Brasseur, R., Lorge, P., Goormaghtigh, E., Ruysschaert, J.-M., Espion, D., and Burny, A.,** Mode of insertion into lipid matrix of the paramyxovirus F1 N-terminus, first step in host cell-virus fusion, *Virus Genes,* 1, 325, 1988.
25. **Brasseur, R., Cornet, B., Burny, A., Vandenbranden, M., and Ruysschaert, J. M.,** Mode of insertion into lipid membrane of the N-terminus HIV gp 41 peptide segment, *AIDS Res. Hum. Retrovirus,* 4, 83, 1988.

Chapter 1.A.7

MOLECULAR CONFORMATIONS OF PHORBOL ESTERS IN A SIMULATED LIPID/WATER INTERFACE

Michel Deleers, Jean-Marie Ruysschaert, and Robert Brasseur

TABLE OF CONTENTS

I. INTRODUCTION

Certain phorbol esters, such as 12-*O*-tetradecanoylphorbol 13-acetate (TPA) and phorbol 12,13-didecanoate (PDD), are potent tumor-promoting agents, while other phorbol esters are biologically inactive.[1-3] Phorbol 12,13-dibutyrate (PDB) is a weak cocarcinogenic agent, and 4-α-phorbol 12,13-didecanoate (4-α-PDD), the isomer of PDD, is biologically inactive. These phorbol esters also exert early effects on different cell types.[1,3] For instance, tumor-promoting phorbol esters stimulate insulin release, whereas nontumor-promoting phorbol esters fail to do so.[4-6] The biological response to phorbol esters is thought to be solely due to their binding to membrane receptors.[7-10] The determination of several functional parameters in isolated pancreatic islets exposed to biologically active phorbol esters led some to postulate that these agents affect Ca^{2+} fluxes in islet cells, possibly by facilitating Ca^{2+} transport mediated by native ionophores.[5,11,12] In order to explore such a hypothesis further, we investigated the interaction of phorbol ester with artificial lipid monolayers or bilayers,[13-17] a study that was initiated earlier.[18-19]

Under suitable experimental conditions, the relative biological potency of disting phorbol esters parallels their capacity to interact with phospholipids[5,6,13,14] and to interfere with ionophore-mediated calcium transport in model membranes.[6,13,15,16] Moreover, several aspects of a specific binding of phorbol esters can be mimicked in artificial membranes formed solely of phospholipids.[16,17] Thus, phorbol esters could be first located in the lipid domain of cell membranes and cause a primary disorder in the physicochemical properties of such a domain.[18-20] Indeed, there is a sequence of inhibition of the binding of [20-^{3}H(N)]-phorbol-12,13-dibutyrate to liposomes solely formed of egg yolk phosphatidylcholine.

The latter finding raises the idea that the biological potency of phorbol esters may be somehow related to the modalities of their insertion between and interaction with membrane lipids. Since the latter modalities may themselves depend on the structural configuration and orientation of the phorbol ester molecules, we have analyzed the conformation of phorbol esters at a simulated membrane/water interface. We have then investigated the configuration and assembly of both tumor-promoting and biologically inactive agents at a simulated lipid-water interface. We have also applied the same procedure to visualize the insertion of distinct phorbol esters within a phospholipid monolayer.

On the other hand, it is well known that tumor-promoting phorbol esters like diacylglycerols strongly bind to protein kinase C/phospholipid complex and also activate this enzyme.[10,21,22] Both structurally unrelated classes of activators, phorbol esters and diacylglycerols, were shown to compete for the same binding site on the kinase.[23] Specific structural features appear to be required. We therefore finally analyzed the conformation of potent diacylglycerols and phorbol esters when inserted into phospholipids and looked for structural analogies.

II. METHODS

The method used for the conformational analysis of each of the four phorbol esters (TPA, PDD, 4-α-PDD, and PDB) is based on a strategy described elsewhere in a preceeding chapter. In this method, the total conformational energy is empirically calculated as the sum of the contributions resulting from the van der Waals' interaction, the torsional potential, and the electrostatic interaction. The equations and parameters used for such a purpose were described extensively. The electrostatic interaction was calculated for a dielectric constant of 16. In a first systematic study, the 5 to 8 first torsional angles of the hydrocarbon chains underwent successive increments of 60° each, yielding 6^5 to 6^8 different conformations derived from an all-*trans* conformer, taken arbitrarily as the initial configuration. The conformations derived from the first systematic study and yielding a low internal energy, i.e.,

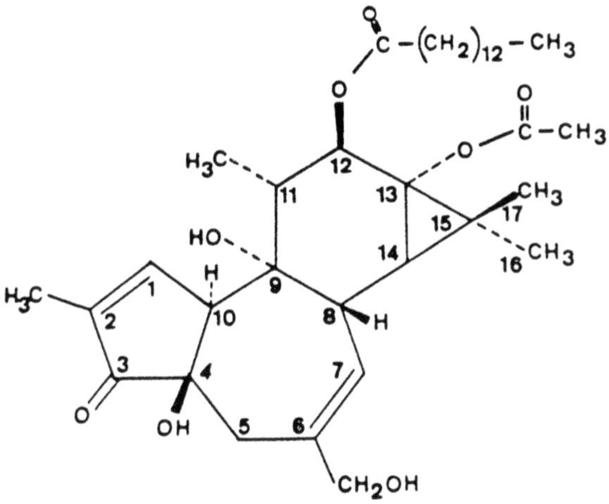

FIGURE 1. Chemical formula and configuration of the phorbol backbone with myristoyl and acetyl chains on C_{12} and C_{13}. This figure also indicates the numbering of the four-ring system of phorbol.

those with a statistical weight of at least 5%, were then submitted to a second analysis, using simplex minimization procedure.

In the last step of the procedure, the assembly of molecules in the monolayer was computed as follows. The position of a molecule B relative to a reference molecule A was assessed by stepwise and successive changes of the five following parameters: the distance between the hydrophilic centers of A and B, the rotation of molecule B around its own z-axis, the gravitation of molecule B around molecule A, the up-and-down migration of molecule B along the z-axis perpendicular to the lipid-water interface, and the oscillation of molecule B around its z-axis.

In each case, the interaction between molecules A and B was calculated from the van der Waals and electrostatic energies. The configuration of the A and B pair yielding the lowest energy was then used as reference to assess the position of a third molecule C. The same procedure was then repeated up to a total of five molecules, at which point the mean molecular area was found to reach a fairly stable value. When the configuration of the cluster of five molecules had been established, the mean molecular area was calculated from both the area occupied by each molecule and the intermolecular area, which were estimated after projection on the x-y plane and using a grid of squares, each with a 0.1-nm side.

III. RESULTS

A. ISOLATED PHORBOL ESTERS

In our conformational analysis of TPA, PDD, or PDB, the phorbol backbone was designed, in the light of previous study, with 4-OH *cis*, 8-H *cis*, 9-OH *trans*, 10-H *trans*, 11-CH$_3$ *trans*, 12-OH *cis*, and 13-OH *trans* (Figure 1). Due to the presence of a three-carbon cycle (C_{13}–C_{14}–C_{15}), the six carbon cycle (C_8–C_9–C_{11}–C_{12}–C_{13}–C_{14}) was set in the boat form with the bonds C_9–C_{11} and C_{13}–C_{14} parallel to each other. Because of the double bond between C_6 and C_7, the bonds from C_5 to C_8 were kept coplanar. The five-carbon cycle (C_1–C_2–C_3–C_4–C_{10}) was also planar.

In the phorbol backbone of 4-α-PDD as distinct from the other phorbol esters, 4–OH is *trans*. This single difference affected markedly the conformational organization of the phorbol backbone. Indeed, both the orientation of the five-carbon planar cycle and the conformation of the seven-carbon ring depended strongly on the position of OH on C_4.[24]

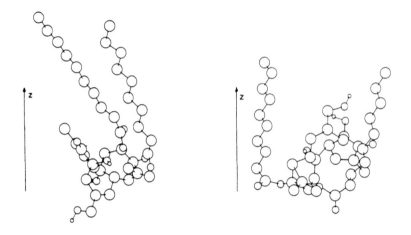

FIGURE 2.   Comparison between the most probable configurations of PDD and 4-α-PDD after energy minimization procedure and reorientation of the molecule at the simulated interface. The molecule is shown in a frontal view, with z-axis pointing toward the hydrophobic domain.

TABLE 1
Most Probable Conformers of Four Phorbol Esters After the Energy Minimization Procedures

Agent	PMA		PDD	4-α-PDD		PDB	
Probability (%)	60	20	99	74	8	56	10
Distance between hydrophilic and hydrophobic centers (nm)							
	0.325	0.458	0.525	0.257	0.480	0.130	0.126
Molecular area (nm²/molecule)							
	0.64	0.59	0.69	1.15	0.60	0.72	0.52
Number of surrounding lipids							
	7	—	8	9	—	6	—

Figure 2 illustrates the two most probable conformers for PDD and 4-α-PDD, respectively, selected from a first systematic study on 1,679,616 conformers in each case and obtained after application of a simplex minimization procedure and reorientation of the molecule at the simulated lipid-water interface. The two phorbol esters are shown in frontal view, being drawn in a plane perpendicular to the simulated interface. All other conformers for 4-α-PDD presented a probability of existence below 8%. The most striking difference between the most probable conformers for PDD and 4-α-PDD, respectively, consisted in the position of the two decanoyl chains which were close and parallel to each other in the PDD molecule, but not close in the 4-α-PDD molecule.

A comparable systematic procedure was applied to the three first torsional angles of the myristoyl chain and the two first torsional angles of the acetyl chain in the TPA molecule and on the three first torsional angles of both butyryl chains in the PDB molecule, yielding, respectively, 6^5 (TPA) and 6^6 (PDB) conformers. The most probable conformers derived from the analysis of the isolated molecule of each phorbol ester were taken as those yielding the lowest internal energy, such a selection being based on a statistical weight (Boltzmann) of all configurations. The most probable conformers with a probability of existence of 60 and 20%, respectively, were selected for study in the monolayer model.

B. PHORBOL ESTERS MONOLAYERS

The principle results of the assembly in the monolayers are shown in Table 1. It is clear

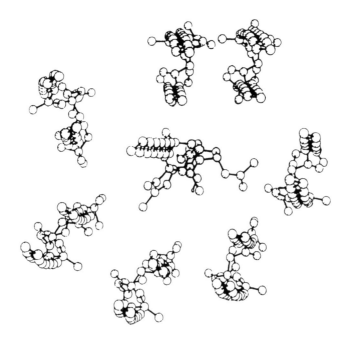

FIGURE 3. Projection on the interfacial plane of a mixed monolayer of PMA and DPPC at a simulated membrane-water interface.

that the molecular area of PDD, as well as those of PMA conformers, were strikingly lower than that of the most probable conformer of 4-α-PDD (see Table 1). These data coincide with experimental measurements performed at an air-water interface, indicating that at low surface pressures (<10 dyn/cm), the molecular area of 4-α-PDD exceeds that of PMA or PDD.[13,14,18]

At higher surface pressures (e.g., 15 to 20 dyn/cm), however, these three phorbol esters display closely similar molecular areas. Therefore, the low theoretical area here found for the less probable conformer of 4-α-PDD suggests that an increase in surface pressure may lead to a change in configuration, the energy of compression compensating for the increase in conformational energy.[25]

C. MIXED PHORBOL ESTERS—PHOSPHOLIPID MEMBRANES

In the third step of this study, conformational analysis has been extended to visualize the insertion of distinct phorbol esters within a dipalmitoylphosphatidylcholine (DPPC) monolayer. The position of a first molecule of DPPC relative to a molecule of phorbol esters was then assessed by systematic changes of the five parameters: distance between hydrophilic centers, rotation of the lipid molecule about its z-axis, gravitation of DPPC about the phorbol ester, up-and-down migration of the lipid molecule, and oscillation about the z-axis.

The procedure is repeated until the phorbol ester molecule was completely surrounded by phospholipids. The results obtained with PMA are illustrated in Figure 3 which represents a projection in the interface plane of the mixed monolayer. Table 1 provides further data obtained with either PMA, PDB, PDM (phorbol-12,13-dimyristate), or 4-α-PDM. Figure 4 represents a comparison of results obtained with PDD and 4-α-PDD. The minor difference between the total area of the monolayer assembly and that expected from the summation of individual areas suggests limited attractive interaction, in good agreement with experimental data collected in mixed monolayers spread at an air-water interface.

It should be noted that, at each step of the computation procedure, the initial molecule of phorbol ester or the assembly formed by one molecule of phorbol ester and one or more

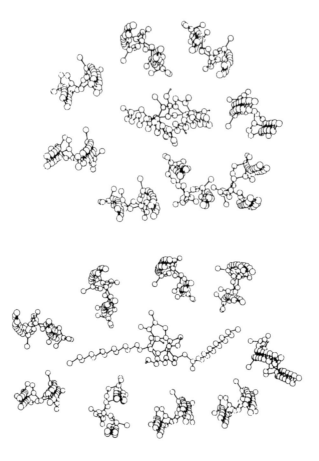

FIGURE 4. (a) Projection on the interfacial plane of a mixed monolayer of PDD and DPPC at a simulated membrane-water interface (top); (b) projection on the interfacial plane of a mixed monolayer of 4-α-PDD and DPPC at a simulated membrane-water interface (bottom).

molecule(s) of DPPC was given the opportunity to interact with either a second molecule of phorbol ester or a further DPPC molecule. In all cases, however, the interaction with DPPC was eventually selected because of a lower energy. This clearly indicates a low probability of existence for monolayers comprising close-to-equal numbers of DPPC and phorbol ester molecules.[26]

D. ANALOGIES WITH PROTEIN KINASE C ACTIVATORS

In the last study of this chapter, the minimum-energy configuration of diacyl 1,2- and 1,3-glycerols, distearin and diolein, was first examined as isolated molecules. Diacylglycerol molecules have 35 rotational angles which give rise to 10^{27} conformers when submitted to systematic 60° changes. The analysis was actually performed on the 9 first angles and yields 1,679,616 conformers per molecule. Then we have determined the most probable association between the diacylglycerols and the DPPC molecules, the conformation of which was previously predicted and experimentally confirmed by neutron diffraction analysis. Two parameters describing this association, namely, molecular area and interaction energy were calculated.

It appears that the active diacyl glycerol form occupies the largest molecular area and interacts less tightly with the phospholipid neighborhood.[27] Here we focus on the orientation of the CH$_2$-OH group at C3 of 1,2-diacylglycerol. The angles formed by C2–C3 (a) and C3–OH (b) bonds with the plane of the lipid/water interface obviously show that the orientation of CH$_2$-OH group strongly depends on the nature of the acyl chain since the saturation of the *cis*-double bond markedly changes the orientation of C2–C3 and C3–OH bonds and disfavors the potency. The CH-OH group at C2 yields inactive compounds irrespective of the nature of the chain. The molecular structure of phorbol didecanoate (PDD) and 4-phorbol didecanoate (4-α-PDD) as well as the angles formed by the C6–C20 (a) and C20–OH (b) bonds with the lipid/water interface reveals a striking similarity between the orientation of the CH$_2$-OH group at C20 of potent phorbol didecanoate (a = 55˙, b = −15˙) and that of the same group at C3 of potent diolein (a = 50˙, b = 20˙). The importance of the primary alcohol group at C20 for biological activity of phorbol esters has already been emphasized since esterification or etherification of this position gives rise to inactive compounds.

IV. DISCUSSION AND CONCLUSIONS

The present work aims at characterizing the most probable conformation of phorbol esters at a simulated membrane/water interface. The four phorbol esters under study were selected on the basis of their vastly different biological potencies. Our conformational analysis emphasizes the existence of differences in the configuration of distinct phorbol esters at the simulated membrane-water interface. Although PDD and 4-α-PDD only differ from one another by the position of the hydroxyl group on C$_4$, their configuration at the interface was strikingly dissimilar. Such a dissimilarity may help in understanding differences in the biological potency, if one assumes that the insertion of these esters in a lipid bilayer is relevant to the expression of their tumor-promoting action and other biological properties. For instance, the biological inactivity of 4-α-PDD could be explained, at least in part, by hindrance to its insertion into the lipid bilayer. It is indeed obvious from the configurations illustrated here that the lesser amphiphilic character and the greater distance between the two decanoyl chains of 4-α-PDD, as distinct from PDD, both represent unfavorable attributes for insertion in a lipid bilayer.

In our study, TPA, which is biologically somewhat more potent than PDD, appeared less amphiphilic than PDD, this difference being attributable to the presence of only one long acyl chain in TPA. However, the presence of this single chain orientated toward the lipophilic domain may facilitate the insertion of TPA along the acyl chains of endogenous phospholipids. In the same perspective, the more globular conformation of PDB could account for the much lower biological potency of this phorbol ester relative to that of TPA.

The data presented here also reinforce the view that the interaction of phorbol esters with phospholipids may play an important role in the expression of their biological potency. The present work also indicates that the conformational analysis of mixed monolayers formed of distinct amphiphilic molecules may provide useful information to predict the insertion of drugs in the phospholipid domain of biological membranes. Finally, we also show that the orientation of the CH$_2$-OH group at C3 of 1,2-diolein is remarkably similar to that of the same group at C20 of phorbol didecanoate and is crucial for potency in activating the enzyme via the proposed mechanism of binding to receptors.[28,29]

The present results support the possibility that the hydrophobic domain of diacylglycerols (acyl chains at C1 and C2) and phorbol esters (acyl chain at C12) is required for[17] interactions with adjacent lipid microenvironment and that, in addition, highly specific electrophilic interactions involving the CH$_2$-OH group (at C3 of diacylglycerols and C20 of phorbol esters) are essential for binding to the protein moiety of the protein kinase C/phospholipid complex and subsequent enzyme activation.[28] However, the apparent affinity of 1,2-diolein for activating the kinase is two to three orders of magnitude less than that of potent phorbol esters,[21] suggesting that additional interactions occurred in the vicinity of the CH$_2$-OH group in C20 which may confer to the molecule a higher stereospecificity.

It is certainly of interest to note here that the elucidation of the precise conformation of potent phorbol esters and diacylglycerols when inserted into phospholipids should contribute to design drugs which may be used in preventing the effects of tumor promoters as well as in controlling protein kinase C-mediated processes, such as platelet aggregation, phosphatidyl inositol turnover, neurite development, protein release, and Ca movements.[28-38] It is always tempting to propose, as a working hypothesis, that phorbol esters provoke an early (binding to phospholipid, modification of microviscosity, alterations of some Ca movements, . . .) and a late (specific binding to protein kinase-C, phosphatidyl inositol turnover, secondary Ca movements, general biological response, etc.) phase.

REFERENCES

1. **Boutwell, R. K.,** The function and mechanism of promoters of carcinogenesis, *CRC Crit. Rev. Toxicol.,* 2, 207, 1974.
2. **Blumberg, P. M.,** In vitro studies on the mode of action of the phorbol esters, potent tumor promoters. I, *CRC Crit. Rev. Toxicol.,* 8, 153, 1980.
3. **Blumberg, P. M.,** In vitro studies on the mode of action of the phorbol esters, potent tumor promoters. II, *CRC Crit. Rev. Toxicol.,* 9, 199, 1981.
4. **Virji, M. A. G., Steffes, M. W., and Estensen, R. D.,** Phorbol myristate acetate: effect of a tumor promoter on insulin release from isolated rat islets of Langerhans, *Endocrinology,* 102, 706, 1978.
5. **Malaisse, W. J., Sener, A., Herchuelz, A., Carpinelli, A. R., Polczek, P., Winand, J., and Castagna, M.,** Insulinotropic effect of the tumor promoter 12-O-tetratdecanoyl-13-acetate in rat pancreatic islets, *Cancer Res.,* 40, 3827, 1980.
6. **Deleers, M., Castagna, M., and Malaisse, W. J.,** Phorbol esters exert parallel effects on tumor promotion, insulin release and calcium ionophoresis, *Cancer Lett.,* 14, 109, 1981.
7. **Driedger, P. E. and Blumberg, P. M.,** Specific binding of phorbol esters tumor promoters, *Proc. Natl. Acad. Sci. U.S.A.,* 77, 567, 1980.
8. **Horowitz, A. D., Greenbaum, E., Nicolaides, M., Woodward, K., and Weinstein, I. B.,** Inhibition of phorbol ester receptor binding by a factor from human serum, *Mol. Cell. Biol.,* 2, 545, 1982.
9. **Solanki, V. and Slaga, T. J.,** Specific binding of phorbol ester tumor promoters to intact primary epidermal cells from Sencar mice, *Proc. Natl. Acad. Sci. U.S.A.,* 78, 2549, 1981.
10. **Ashendel, C. L., Statler, J. M., and Boutwell, R. K.,** Identification of a calcium- and phospholipid dependent phorbol ester binding activity in the soluble fraction of mouse tissues, *Biochem. Biophys. Res. Commun.,* 111, 340, 1983.
11. **Malaisse, W. M., Lebrun, P., Herchuelz, A., and Malaisse-Lagae, F.,** Synergistic effect of a tumor promoting phorbol ester and a hypoglycemic sulfonylurea upon insulin release, *Endocrinology,* 113, 1870, 1983.
12. **Castagna, M., Deleers, M., and Malaisse, W. J.,** *Carcinogenesis, a Comprehensive Survey,* Raven Press, New York, 1982, 555.
13. **Deleers, M., Defrise-Quertain, F., Ruysschaert, J. M., and Malaisse, W. J.,** Interactions of phorbol esters with lipid bilayers: thermotropic changes in fluorescence polarization, phase transition and calcium ionophoresis, *Res. Commun. Chem. Pathol. Pharmacol.,* 34, 423, 1981.
14. **Deleers, M., Ruysschaert, J. M., and Malaisse, W. J.,** Interaction between phorbol esters and phospholipid in a monolayer model membrane, *Chem. Biol. Interact.,* 42, 271, 1982.
15. **Deleers, M. and Malaisse, W. J.,** Influence of phorbol esters on ionophore-mediated calcium exchange diffusion in liposomes, *Chem. Phys. Lipids,* 31, 1, 1982.
16. **Malaisse, W. J. and Deleers, M.,** Insertion of phorbol esters with lipid monolayers or bilayers, *Colloids Surface,* 10, 257, 1984.
17. **Deleers, M. and Malaisse, W. J.,** Binding of tumor-promoting and biologically inactive phorbol esters to artificial membranes, *Cancer Lett.,* 17, 135, 1982.
18. **Jacobson, K., Wenner, C. E., Kemp, G., and Papahadjopoulos, D.,** Surface properties of phorbol esters and their interaction with lipid monolayers and bilayers, *Cancer Res.,* 35, 2991, 1975.
19. **Castagna, M., Rochette-Egly, C., Rosenfeld, C., and Mishal, Z.,** Altered lipid microviscosity in lymphoblastoid cells treated with 12-O-tetradecanoyl phorbol-13-acetate, a tumor promoter, *FEBS Lett.,* 100, 62, 1979.

20. **Tran, P. L., Ter-Minassian-Saraga, L., Madelmont, G., and Castagna, M.,** Tumor promoters 12-*O*-tetradecanoyl phorbol-13-acetate alters state, fluidity and hydration of 1,2 diacyl-sn-glycero 3-phosphocholine bilayers, *Biochim. Biophys. Acta,* 727, 31, 1983.
21. **Castagna, M., Takai, Y., Kaibuchi, K., Sano, K., Kikkawa, N., and Nishizuka, Y.,** Direct activation of calcium-activated phospholipid dependent protein kinase by tumor promoting phorbol esters, *J. Biol. Chem.,* 257, 7847, 1982.
22. **Ashendel, C. L.,** The phorbol ester receptor: a phospholipid-regulated protein kinase, *Biochim. Biophys. Acta,* 822, 219, 1985.
23. **Sharkey, N. A., Leach, K. L., and Blumberg, P. M.,** Competitive inhibition by diacylglycerol of specific phorbol ester binding, *Proc. Natl. Acad. Sci. U.S.A.,* 81, 607, 1984.
24. **Deleers, M., Brasseur, R., Ruysschaert, J. M., and Malaisse, W. J.,** Conformational analysis of phorbol esters at a simulated membrane-water interface, *Biophys. Chem.,* 17, 313, 1983.
25. **Brasseur, R., Deleers, M., Ruysschaert, J. M., and Malaisse, W. J.,** Conformational analysis of phorbol esters monolayers, *Biochem. Int.,* 5, 659, 1982.
26. **Brasseur, R., Deleers, M., Ruysschaert, J. M., and Malaisse, W. J.,** Conformational analysis of mixed monolayers of phorbol esters and phospholipid, *Biochem. Int.,* 7, 71, 1983.
27. **Brasseur, R., Cabiaux, V., Huart, P., Castagna, M., Baztar, S., and Ruysschaert, J. M.,** Structural analogies between protein kinase C activators, *Biochem. Biophys. Res. Commun.,* 127, 969, 1985.
28. **Blumberg, P. M., Jaken, S., Konig, B., Sharkey, N. A., Leach, K. L., Jeng, A. Y., and Yeh, E.,** Mechanism of action of the phorbol ester tumor promoters: specific receptors for lipophilic ligands, *Biochem. Pharmacol.,* 33, 933, 1984.
29. **Leeb-Lundberg, L. M. F., Cotechia, S., Lomasmey, J. M., Debernardis, J. R., Lefkowitz, R. J., and Caron, M. G.,** Phorbol esters promote α_1-adrenergic receptor phosphorylation and receptor uncoupling from inositol phospholipid metabolism, *Proc. Natl. Acad. Sci. U.S.A.,* 82, 5651, 1985.
30. **Daniel, L. W.,** Phosphatidyl inositol turnover in Madin-Darby cells: comparison of stimulation by A23187 and 12-*O*-tetradecanoyl-phorbol-13 acetate, in *Inositol and Phosphoinositides: Metabolism and Regulation,* Humana Press, N.J., 1985, 537.
31. **Mobley, A. and Tai, T.-H.,** Synergistic stimulation of thromboxane biosynthesis by calcium ionophore and phorbol ester or thrombin in human platelets, *Biochem. Biophys. Res. Commun.,* 130, 717, 1985.
32. **Schimmel, S. D. and Hallam, T. J.,** Rapid alterations in Ca^{2+} content and fluxes in phorbol 12-myristate-13-acetate treated myoblasts, *Biochem. Biophys. Res. Commun.,* 92, 624, 1980.
33. **Zurgil, N. and Zisapel, N.,** Phorbol esters and calcium act synergistically to enhance neurotransmitter release by brain neurons in culture, *FEBS Lett.,* 185, 257, 1985.
34. **Baraban, J. M., Gould, R. J., Peroutka, S. J., and Snyder, S. H.,** Phorbol ester effects on neurotransmission: interaction with neurotransmitters and calcium in smooth muscle, *Proc. Natl. Acad. Sci. U.S.A.,* 82, 604, 1985.
35. **Albert, P. R. and Tashjian, A. H.,** Dual actions of phorbol esters on cytosolic free Ca^{2+} concentrations and reconstitution with ionomycin of acute thryrotropin-releasing hormone responses, *J. Biol. Chem.,* 260, 8746, 1985.
36. **Hsu, L.,** Neurite-promoting effects of 12-*O*-tetradecanoyl-phorbol-13-acetate on chick embryo neurons, *Neurosci. Lett.,* 62, 283, 1985.
37. **Valone, F. H. and Johnson, B.,** Modulation of platelet-activating-factor-induced calcium influx and intracellular calcium release in platelets by phorbol esters, *Biochem. J.,* 247, 669, 1987.
38. **Reinders, J. H., Vervoorn, R. C., Verweij, C. L., van Mourik, J. A., and de Groot, P. G.,** Perturbation of cultured human vascular endothelial cells by phorbol ester or thrombin alters the cellular von Willebrand factor distribution, *J. Cell. Physiol.,* 133, 79, 1987.

Chapter 1.A.8

DEFORMATION OF THE LIPID/WATER INTERFACE MEDIATED BY PHOSPHOLIPIDS OR PEPTIDES

Jean-Marie Ruysschaert and Robert Brasseur

TABLE OF CONTENTS

I. INTRODUCTION

Phospholipids are essential constituents of biological membranes. Their amphipathic structure is responsible for their tendency to aggregate in aqueous media in organized structures. This organization depends on the type of lipid and the experimental conditions. In excess aqueous buffer, at physiological conditions of temperature and ionic strength, isolated membrane phospholipids will adopt either a bilayer (dipalmitoylphosphatidylcholine), micellar (lysophosphatidylcholine), or hexagonal H_{II} (phosphatidylethanolamines, protonated dioleoylphosphatidic acid) type of configuration.[1] In particular, the abundant occurrence of the H_{II} type of lipids together with the notion of a new lipid structure, the interbilayer lipidic particle,[2] and the involvement of nonbilayer lipid structures in some membrane functions has greatly renewed the interest in lipid polymorphism to explain the phase preferences of lipids. A shape-structure model[2] has been proposed which relates the dynamical shape of the molecule (including head group hydration and intra- and intermolecular interactions) to the structure of the aggregate. In this model, cylindrical molecules prefer bilayers, with cone- and inverted cone-shaped molecules preferring H_{II} and micellar organizations, respectively[1] (Figure 1).

We present here evidence that the mode of organization of lipids can be predicted from a conformational analysis of the lipid structure. This approach has already been used to assess the mode of association of dipalmitoylphosphatidylcholine (DPPC) in bilayers.[3] We bring here evidence that from conformational analysis of palmitoyl lysophosphatidylcholine (LPC), protonated dioleoylphosphatidic acid (DOPA), and gramicidin, aggregate states can be calculated which are fully compatible with the phase preferences of these lipids.

II. CONFORMATIONAL ANALYSIS OF PHOSPHOLIPIDS

We started by calculating the conformation of the isolated molecule at the air-water interface. The torsional angles of the glycerol, Θ_3, the torsional angles in the τ-segment (τ_1, τ_2, τ_3, τ_4), and the torsional angles in the β-segment (β_1, β_2, β_3, β_4) except for lysophosphatidylcholine were given successive increments of 60°, yielding 6^9 conformers for DPPC and DOPA and 6^5 conformers for LPC (Figure 2). Only structures with a statistical weight of at least 1% were retained.

Secondly, the torsional angles of the bonds located in the polar head group (Θ_1, α_1, α_2, α_3, α_4, α_5, α_6) for DPPC and LPC and Θ_1, α_1, α_2 for DOPA were given successive increments of 60°, yielding 6^7 conformers for DPPC and DOPA and 6^3 for LPC. Again, only structures with at least 1% of statistical weight were retained. As described elsewhere[3] for DPPC, combination of the three most probable structures obtained for the polar head group and the two most probable structures for the hydrophobic chain gives six structural possibilities. Application of the simplex minimization procedure and orientation at the interface for each structure made it possible to define one structure of minimal energy. This structure was assembled in monolayers using the sequential method (see Chapter 1.A.6) and only a structure with 95% probability was retained. The calculated structures were in excellent agreement with neutron diffraction data of hydrated DPPC.[3] The important point is that the hydrophobic part and hydrophilic part after projection on the membrane were equal in size, 0.58 nm², allowing a tight packing in a bilayer type of structure (Figure 3). Application of the same procedure to the LPC molecule resulted in the most probable conformer. This type of structure does not assemble into a bilayer, but instead forms an aggregate which adopts the classical micelle (see Figure 3) organization as has been demonstrated experimentally by Tanford.[4] The molecular reason for this mode of aggregation is associated with the large difference between the area of the hydrophobic (0.2 nm²) and the hydrophilic (0.59 nm²) moiety. To the best of our knowledge, this is the first computational approach describing the mode of organization of lysophosphatidylcholine in micelles. It should be realized that

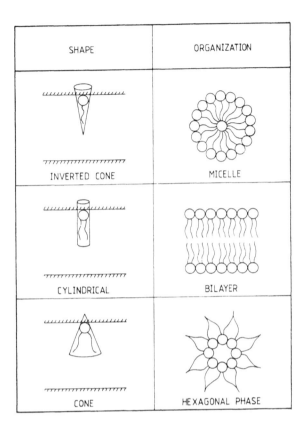

SHAPE	ORGANIZATION
INVERTED CONE	MICELLE
CYLINDRICAL	BILAYER
CONE	HEXAGONAL PHASE

FIGURE 1. Shape-structure model. Relationship between the dynamical shape of lipids and their state of organization in excess water. For the hexagonal phase, a cross section through one tube in which which this phase is composed is shown.

palmitoylisophosphatidylcholine undergoes a gel state lamellar-micellar transition at approximately 3°C.[5,6] This transition is accompanied by chain melting. Since our calculations are carried out for molecules at 25°C, an all-*trans* chain appears to be the most probable conformation. It can be argued that, for instance, chain interactions in the aggregate would not show up in our analysis and that this interaction could cause the formation of *cis*-conformers. However, in a recent conformational study on 1-palmitoyl-2-oleoylphosphatidylcholine, *cis*-conformers were found in the palmitoyl acyl chains; this demonstrates that indeed, chain-chain interactions contribute to the conformational state of the acyl chain and show up in our calculations.

The conformer of DOPA obtained after minimization, orientation at the air-water interface, and assembly in monolayer is represented in Figure 3 with the corresponding torsional angles given in Table 1. The calculations demonstrate that the double bond of the oleic acyl chain greatly increases the volume of the hydrophobic segment (0.90 nm²) as compared to the calculated head group area (0.59 nm²). After assembly, the structure of the aggregate resembles part of an inverted micelle in which the head groups point inward. This result is fully compatible with the observations of the hexagonal H_{II} phase and inverted micellar structures in DOPA-containing model membranes.[7]

III. CONFORMATIONAL ANALYSIS OF GRAMICIDIN

Gramicidin A is a linear pentadecapeptide which in a dimer conformation forms ion-selective channels in membranes.[8-10] The mode of insertion of gramicidin in a lipid bilayer

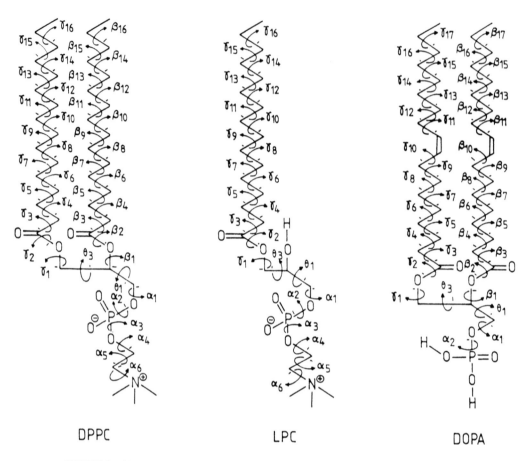

FIGURE 2. Notation of the different chains and torsional angles in DPPC, DOPA, and LPC.

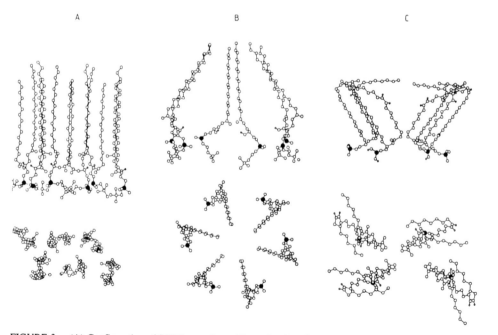

FIGURE 3. (A) Configuration of DPPC monolayer (Six molecules of the most probable conformer of DPPC are shown in a frontal view, upper, and from above, lower); (B) configuration of LPC monolayer, same presentation as in (A); (C) configuration of DOPA monolayer, same presentation as in (A).

TABLE 1
Conformers of Lipids After Minimization and Orientation to the Lipid-Water Interface

Torsion Angles	DPPC	DOPA	LPC
α_6	10	—	12
α_5	59	—	179
α_4	117	—	177
α_3	59	—	185
α_2	62	238	77
α_1	210	146	263
Θ_1	70	190	157
Θ_3	210	300	174
β_1	105	179	—
β_2	131	176	—
β_3	240	60	—
β_4	89	60	—
β_5	177	186	—
τ_1	134	178	181
τ_2	140	180	178
τ_3	200	179	230
τ_4	180	180	309
τ_5	185	174	179
τ_{10}	180	160	180
τ_{11}	180	263	180
τ_{12}	180	157	181

Note: The table indicates the values of all torsion angles. A torsional angle around a given j bond is taken as positive when the distal (j + 1) bond rotates clockwise relative to the proximal (j − 1) bond. All other torsional angles obtained for β-segment and τ-segment are 180° ± 5°. The precision of the minimization is equal to 10°.

has been extensively studied and four classes of models have been proposed: the aminoterminal to aminoterminal $\beta^{6.3}$ helical dimer,[11,12] the carboxy terminal to carboxy terminal helical dimer,[13] and parallel[14,15] and antiparallel[15] double helices. The N-N-terminal $\beta^{6.3}$ helical dimer was originally proposed by Urry et al.[11] as the channel conformation and is presently largely accepted on the basis of ^{13}C-NMR,[11,12,16] infrared (IR),[17] and circular dichroism[18] studies.

Gramicidin A was oriented in the left-handed β-helical structure at the air/water interface using the data published by Venkatachalam and Urry.[19] From the hydrophobic transfer energy (Σ_j E$^-$tr$_j$ = 959.7 KJ/mol) and the hydrophilic transfer energy (Σ_j Etr$_j$ = 594.4 KJ/mol) associated to the entire molecule, we calculated the position of the hydrophobic and hydrophilic centers. The most probable orientation of the isolated gramicidin A at the air/water interface, which was calculated to run through tryptophan 9, is that with the hydrophobic center located in the hydrophilic medium, i.e., with the C-terminal tryptophans 13 and 15 bearing part pointing toward the hydrophobic medium (Figure 4). Figure 5 gives a representation of the gramicidin A structure in real volume, showing the cone-shaped structure of the molecule. The calculated areas of the hydrophobic and hydrophilic moiety responsible for this cone-shaped structure were equal to 1.37 and 0.47 nm^2 per molecule. This compares favorably with the value of 1.30 and 1.45 nm^2 per molecule reported as limiting values at the air/water interface.[20,21] The calculated energy required to orient gramicidin A with the tryptophans directed toward the hydrophilic medium was calculated to be 133.8 KJ/mol which is of the order of magnitude of the energy required to reorient lipids with the acyl

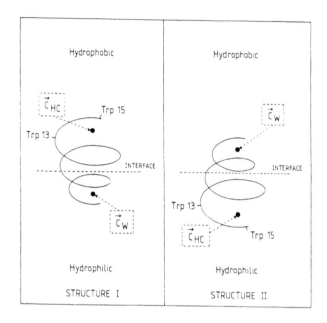

FIGURE 4.   Schematic representation of the two possible orientations of gramicidin at the lipid water interface.

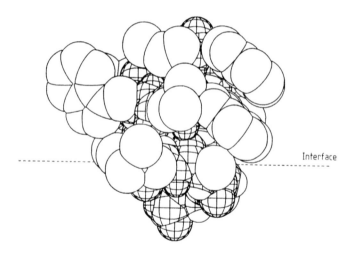

FIGURE 5.   Space-filling drawing of gramicidin A showing the cone-shaped dynamical structure of the molecule. The plane delineates the hydrophobic (above) and the hydrophilic (below) medium. Gramicidin A is a pentadecapeptide with the following chemical structure: $HCO-_LVal_1-_DGly_2-_LAla_3-_DLeu_4-_LAla_5-_DVal_6-$ $_LVal_7-_DVal_8-_LTrp_9-_DLeu_{10}-_LTrp_{11}-_DLeu_{12}-_LTrp_{13}-_DLeu_{14}-_Ltrp_{15}-NHCH2CH2OH$.

chains pointing into the aqueous phase. We assumed that gramicidin A could adopt two orientations.

The present calculations clearly suggest a preferred orientation of the gramicidin molecule in the $\beta^{6.3}$ helical structure with its C-terminal end directed toward the hydrophobic medium, in good agreement with the data on the effect of gramicidin on lipid polymorphism,[22-25] but in contradiction with other studies.[11,12,16-18] The reason for this discrepancy is unknown, but might be related to the ability of the gramicidin molecule to adopt a variety of different structures, depending on the environmental conditions. However, it should be noted that the conformational analysis methods we have used are still crude and, for instance, do not take into account a possible change in structure due to gramicidin-gramicidin interaction.

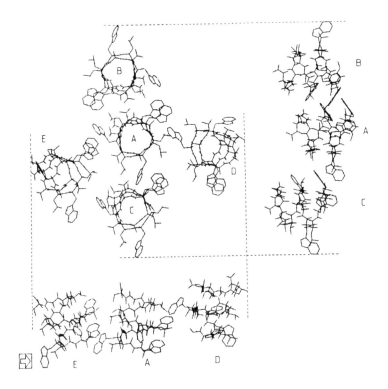

FIGURE 6.   Top and front view of four gramicidin molecules (B, C, D, and E) which surround one gramicidin molecule (A). In the front view, for sake of clarity, only three molecules are shown.

Gramicidin A is a potent modulator of membrane lipid structure. In aqueous mixtures with lysophosphatidylcholine, a bilayer is formed, despite the preferred micellar organization of the pure lipid.[22,23,26,27] Furthermore, it is the best-known example of a hydrophobic peptide which can induce bilayer → hexagonal$_{II}$ phase transitions in model membranes composed of a variety of different phospholipids with acyl chain length in excess of 16 carbon atoms[28] and even in the membrane of the human erythrocyte.[40] From DSC,[29] NMR,[30,31] X-ray diffraction, and sucrose density centrifugation experiments, it could be concluded that this pentadecapeptide has a tendency to aggregate in the bilayer and that this aggregation is a prerequisite for H$_{II}$ phase formation. Interestingly also for channel formation, it appears that lateral aggregation of the peptide might be involved.[32,33] In the case of 18:1$_c$/18:1$_c$ PC, a lipid which has been studied most thoroughly,[30,31,34] the H$_{II}$ phase is very rich in gramicidin (gramicidin/PC > 1:7 molar). The structural parameters of this phase seem to be mainly determined by the peptide itself[28] which because of its pronounced cone shape, due to the location of the four bulky tryptophan residues all at the C terminus of the peptide, seems to be ideally suited to fit in the tubes of which the H$_{II}$ phase is formed. This shape of the peptide also is supposed to be the main determinant for bilayer formation with the oppositely shaped lysophosphatidylcholine.[27]

In order to get a better theoretical understanding of the importance of gramicidin aggregation for hexagonal H$_{II}$ phase formation, we report in this study the results of computations on the energetics of gramicidin-gramicidin interactions at the air/water interface. The most probable structure of the gramicidin aggregate was obtained using methods similar to those previously used to obtain insight in the conformation and interfacial location of pure lipids[35] and lysophosphatidylcholine-gramicidin aggregates.[27]

After assemblage of four gramicidin molecules around one fixed gramicidin molecule at the air/water interface, a lowest-energy organization is obtained which is as a top view depicted in the left-hand corner of Figure 6. The channel present within the molecules is

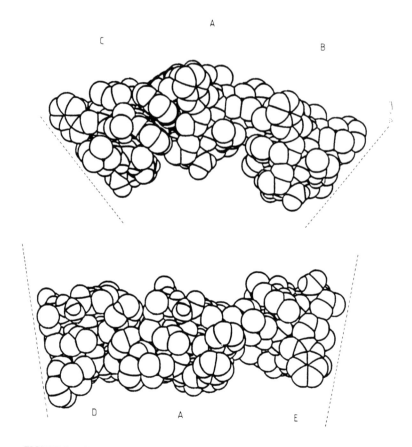

FIGURE 7.   Space-filling drawings of side views of the BAC and EAD assemblage.

clearly visible. Due to the cone shape of gramicidin which is, for instance, apparent in the side view of molecule A, two kinds of assemblage occur in the pentameric aggregate. One results in a linear association, such as is found in the direction of the molecules E, A, and D (Figure 7a), and one results in a curved association, such as is found in the direction of the molecules B, A, and C (Figure 7b). The mean energy of interaction between gramicidin molecules is higher along the BAC axis (mean interaction energy between monomers, −41.8 KJ/mol) than along the DAE axis (mean interaction energy between monomers, −25.1 KJ/mol). When these numbers are compared to the calculated interaction energy between two $18:1_c/18:1_c$ molecules (−28.4 KJ/mol) and between one gramicidin and one $18:1_c/18:1_c$ PC molecule (−27.2 KJ/mol), then it can be concluded that the curved self-association of gramicidin is the preferred organization even in a $18:1_c/18:1_c$ PC monolayer.

Interactions between tryptophans, but also aliphatic amino acid side chains, are responsible for the stronger interaction along the BAC axis. For instance, the energy of interaction between A and B is higher than the energy of interaction between A and D. This difference is the result of the close proximity of Trp_9 and Trp_{15} of molecule A and Trp_{13} of molecule B and of Trp_{13} associated with molecule A and Trp_9 and Trp_{15} associated with molecule B (Figure 8). In the arrangement of molecules A and B, there is also a strong possible interaction between the leucine side chains. Such a possibility does not exist in the AD association. Furthermore, in this case, the Trp-Trp interaction is limited to Trp_{11} (of D) and Trp_9 and Trp_{15} (of A). The calculations further revealed the exact distances between the tryptophan residues which are compared in Figure 9.

The two modes of organization calculated to be present in a pentameric lateral aggregate of gramicidin at the air/water interface provide new insight in the ability of gramicidin to

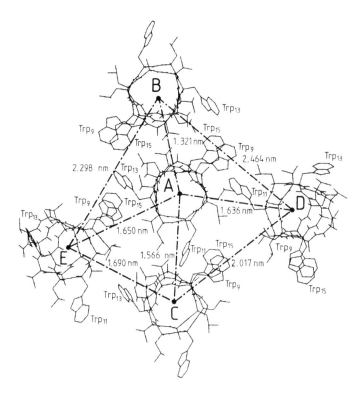

FIGURE 8. Top view of the pentametric assemblage with location of tryptophans and distances between gramicidin molecules within the aggregate. The labeling of each gramicidin is the same as used in Figure 6.

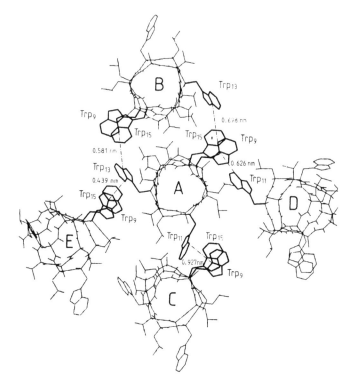

FIGURE 9. Distance between atomic centers of tryptophan in the pentameric gramicidin aggregate. The labeling of each gramicidin is the same as used in Figure 5.

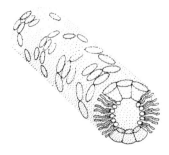

FIGURE 10.   Schematic representation of one tube of the gramicidin-induced H_{II} phase in 18:1$_c$/18:1$_c$ PC.

TABLE 2
Tube Diameter of H_{II} Phases Induced by Gramicidin in Different (Model) Membrane Systems

	Tube diameter (Å)	Ref.
18:1$_c$/18:1$_c$ PE	74 (40—60°C)	29
18:1$_c$/18:1$_c$ PC	71 (20°C)	31
	70 (70°C)	31
18:1$_c$/18:1$_c$ PG	72 (25°C)	37
18:1$_c$/18:1$_c$ PS	70 (25°C)	37
Cardiolipin (beef heart)	72 (25°C)	37
22:1$_c$/22:1$_c$ PC		
PC/gramicidin = 5 M	86	25
PC/gramicidin = 2.5 M	72	25
Total lipid extract		
Human erythrocytes	69 (37°C)	—[a]
Human erythrocytes ghosts	64 (37°C)	—[a]

Note: The tube diameter is calculated as two times the second-order (1/√3) reflection in small-angle diffraction patterns of the samples.

[a]   Tournois, H., unpublished data.

induce the H_{II} phase in membrane systems. The curved association would be ideally suited to fit into a cylindrical structure such as those found in the gramicidin-induced H_{II} phase. The linear assemblage would then parallel the axis of the cylinder. Extrapolation of the association of the gramicidin molecules B, A, and C (Figure 10) toward a circular arrangement requires 12 gramicidin molecules. From this arrangement and the length of the gramicidin monomer in the $\beta^{6.3}$ helical conformation, it can be estimated that the outer diameter of such circular arrangement is 7 nm. This value is very close to the tube diameters reported for a number of gramicidin-induced H_{II} phases which are summarized in Table 1. The relative insensitivity of the diameter of the gramicidin-containing tubes with respect to the nature of the membrane lipid constituents, together with the remarkably temperature insensitivity of the tube diameter (see Table 2) and acyl chain order,[31] as opposed to the strong temperature-dependent tube diameter and acyl chain order in the hexagonal H_{II} phases formed by phosphatidylethanolamine,[29,31] supports the view[30] that gramicidin in a laterally aggregated manner forms the structural backbone of the H_{II} phase.

Because phospholipids can rapidly diffuse around the tubes present in the gramicidin-induced H_{II} phase (as inferred from ^{31}P and ^2H-NMR data[30,31]) and acyl chains dynamics are decreased by the gramicidin-18:1$_c$/18:1$_c$ PC interaction in this phase,[31] we have to propose that the tubes of the H_{II} phase are composed of both cylindrical aggregates of gramicidin and phospholipids. A schematic representation of the peptide and lipid organization in a tube is shown in Figure 10. The calculated importance of intermolecular Trp-Trp interactions for stabilization of the structure of the cylindrical gramicidin aggregate supports recent experimental observations that N-formylation of these residues completely blocks H_{II} phase formation[36] and that replacement of Trp$_9$ and Trp$_{11}$ by a phenylalanine residue results in a large decrease in extent of H_{II} phase formation.[34] Both types of modification are expected to cause considerable changes in possibilities for aromatic-aromatic interactions. The importance of intramolecular Trp-Trp interactions for the structure of the gramicidin monomer is indicated by the close proximity of Trp$_9$ and Trp$_{15}$ in the $\beta^{6.3}$ helical configuration.[38]

IV. CONCLUSION

The present results demonstrate the feasibility of the prediction of the aggregate structure by molecular conformation analysis. Inverted micellar structures were also predicted using this approach for monogalactosyldiglycerides constituting the thylakoid membrane.[39] The conformational analysis here described is applicable to any groups of amphipatic molecules. It opens the way to describe in detail the influence of proteins, peptides, and drugs on membrane structure.

REFERENCES

1. **Cullis, P. R. and de Kruijff, B.,** Lipids polymorphism and the functional roles of lipids in biological membranes, *Biochim. Biophys. Acta,* 559, 399, 1979.
2. **de Kruijff, B., Verkley, A. J., van Echteld, C. J. A., Gerritsen, W. J., Mombers, C., Noordam, P. C., and de Gier, J.,** The occurrence of lipidic particles in lipid bilayers as seen by ^{31}P NMR and freeze-fracture electron microscopy, *Biochim. Biophys. Acta,* 555, 200, 1979.
3. **Brasseur, R., Goormaghtigh, E., and Ruysschaert, J.-M.,** Theoretical conformational analysis of phospholipids bilayers, *Biochem. Biophys. Res. Commun.,* 103, 301, 1981.
4. **Tanford, C.,** in *The Hydrophobic Effect. Formation of Micelles and Biological Membranes,* John Wiley & Sons, New York, 1973,
5. **van Echteld, C. J. A., de Kruijff, B., and de Gier, J.,** Differential miscibility properties of various phosphatidylcholine/lysophosphatidylcholine mixtures, *Biochim. Biophys. Acta,* 595, 71, 1980.
6. **van Echteld, C. J. A., de Kruijff, B., Mandersloot, J. G., and de Gier, J.,** Effects of lysophosphatidylcholines on phosphatidylcholine and phosphatidylcholine/cholesterol liposome systems as revealed by ^{31}P NMR, electron microscopy and permeability studies, *Biochim. Biophys. Acta,* 649, 211, 1981.
7. **Cullis, P. R., de Kruijff, B., Hope, M. J., Verkley, A. J., Mayar, R., Farren, S. B., Tilcoch, C. P. S., Madden, T. D., and Bally, M. B.,** in *Membrane Fluidity in Biology,* Vol. 2, Aloia, R. C., Ed., Academic Press, New York, 1982,
8. **Urry, D. W.,** The gramicidin A transmembrane channel: a proposed $\pi_{(L,D)}$ helix, *Proc. Natl. Acad. Sci. U.S.A.,* 68, 672, 1971.
9. **Hladky, S. B. and Haydon, D. A.,** Ion transfer across lipid membranes in the presence of gramicidin A — studies of the unit conductance channel, *Biochim. Biophys. Acta,* 274, 294, 1972.
10. **Apell, H. J., Bamberg, E., and Alpes, H.,** Dicarboxylic acid analogs of gramicidin A: dimerization kinetics and single channel properties, *J. Membrane Biol.,* 50, 271, 1979.
11. **Urry, D. W., Trapane, T. L., and Prasad, K. U.,** Is the gramicidin A transmembrane channel single-stranded or double-stranded helix? A simple unequivocal determination, *Science,* 221, 1064, 1983.
12. **Weinstein, S., Wallace, B. A., Blout, E. R. N., Morrow, J., and Veatch, W. R.,** Conformation of gramicidin A channel in phospholipid vesicles: a ^{13}C and ^{19}F nuclear magnetic resonance study, *Proc. Natl. Acad. Sci. U.S.A.,* 76, 4230, 1979.
13. **Bradley, R. J., Urry, D. W., Okamoto, K., and Rapaka, R.,** Channel structures of gramicidin: characterization of succinyl derivatives, *Science,* 200, 435, 1978.

14. **Veatch, W. R., Fossel, E. T., and Blout, E. R.,** The conformation of gramicidin A, *Biochemistry*, 13, 5249, 1974.

15. **Arseniev, S. A., Barsukov, I. L., and Bystrov, V. F.,** NMR solution structure of gramicidin A complex with caesium cations, *FEBS Lett.*, 180, 33, 1985.

16. **Urry, D. W., Trapane, T. L., Romanowski, S., Bradley, R. J., and Prasad, K. U.,** Use of synthetic gramicidins in the determination of channel structure and mechanism, *Int. Peptide Protein Res.*, 21, 16, 1983.

17. **Naik, V. M. and Krimm, S.,** The structure of crystalline and membrane-bound gramicidin A by vibrational analysis, *Biochem. Biophys. Res. Commun.*, 125, 919, 1984.

18. **Wallace, B. A.,** Gramicidin A adopts distinctly different conformations in membrane and in organic solvents. III, *Biopolymers*, 22, 397, 1983.

19. **Venkatachalam, C. M. and Urry, D. W.,** Theoretical conformational analysis of the gramicidin A transmembrane channel. I. Helix sense and energetics of head-to-head dimerization, *J. Comp. Chem.*, 4, 461, 1983.

20. **Cornell, B. A., Sacré, M. M., Peel, W. E., and Chapman, D.,** The modulation of lipid bilayer fluidity by intrinsic polypeptides and proteins, *FEBS Lett.*, 90, 29, 1978.

21. **Kemp, G., Jacobson, K. A., and Wenner, C. E.,** Solution and interfacial properties of gramicidin pertinent to its effect on membranes, *Biochim. Biophys. Acta*, 255, 493, 1972.

22. **Killian, J. A., de Kruijff, B., van Echteld, C. J. A., Verkleij, A. J., Leunissen-Bijvelt, J., and de Gier, J.,** Mixtures of gramicidin and lysophosphatidylcholine form lamellar structures, *Biochim. Biophys. Acta*, 728, 141, 1983.

23. **Pasquali-Ronchetti, E., Spisni, A., Casali, E., Masotti, L., and Urry, D. M.,** Gramicidin A induces lysolecithin to form bilayers, *Biosci. Rep.*, 3, 127, 1983.

24. **van Echteld, C. J. A., van Stigt, R., de Kruijff, B., Leunissen-Bijvelt, J., Verkleij, A. J., and de Gier, J.,** Gramicidin promotes formation of the hexagonal H_{II} phase in aqueous dispersions of phosphatidylethanolamine and phosphatidylcholine, *Biochim. Biophys. Acta*, 648, 287, 1981.

25. **van Echteld, C. J. A., de Kruijff, B., Verkleij, A. J., Leunissen-Bijvelt, J., and de Gier, J.,** Gramicidin induces the formation of non-bilayer structures in phosphatidylcholine dispersions in a fatty acid length dependent way, *Biochim. Biophys. Acta*, 692, 126, 1982.

26. **Killian, J. A., Borle, F., de Kruijff, B., and Seelig, J.,** Comparative ^{2}H- and ^{31}P-NMR study on the properties of palmitoyllysophosphatidylcholine in bilayers with gramicidin, cholesterol and dipalmitoylphosphatidylcholine, *Biochim. Biophys. Acta*, 854, 133, 1986.

27. **Brasseur, R., Cabiaux, V., Killian, J. A., de Kruijff, B., and Ruysschaert, J.-M.,** Orientation of gramicidin A at the lysophosphatidylcholine-water interface: a semi-empirical conformational analysis, *Biochim. Biophys. Acta*, 855, 317, 1986.

28. **Killian, J. A. and de Kruijff, B.,** The influence of proteins and peptides on the phase properties of lipids, *Chem. Phys. Lipids*, 40, 259, 1986.

29. **Killian, J. A. and de Kruijff, B.,** Thermodynamic motional, and structural aspects of gramicidin-induced hexagonal H_{II} phase formation in phosphatidylethanolamine, *Biochemistry*, 24, 7881, 1985.

30. **Killian, J. A. and de Kruijff, B.,** Importance of hydratation for gramicidin-induced hexagonal H_{II} phase formation in dioleoylphosphatidylcholine model membrane, *Biochemistry*, 24, 7890, 1985.

31. **Chupin, V., Killian, J. A., and de Kruijff, B.,** ^{2}H-nuclear magnetic resonance investigations on phospholipid acyl chain order and dynamics in the gramicidin-induced hexagonal H_{II} phase, *Biophys. J.*, 51, 395, 1987.

32. **Stark, G., Strässle, M., and Takàcz, Z.,** Temperature-jump and voltage-jump experiments at planar lipid membranes support and aggregational (micellar) model of the gramicidin A ion channel, *J. Membrane Biol.*, 89, 23, 1986.

33. **Spisni, A., Pasquali-Ronchetti, I., Casali, E., Lindner, L., Cavatorta, P., Masotti, L., and Urry, D. W.,** Supramolecular organization of lysophosphatidylcholine-packaged gramicidin A, *Biochim. Biophys. Acta*, 732, 58, 1983.

34. **Killian, J. A., Burger, K. N. J., and de Kruijff, B.,** Phase separation and hexagonal H_{II} phase formation by gramicidins A, B and C in dioleoylphosphatidylcholine model membranes. A study on the role of the tryptophan residues, *Biochim. Biophys. Acta*, 897, 269, 1987.

35. **Brasseur, R. and Ruysschaert, J.-M.,** Conformation and mode of organization of amphiphilic membrane components: a conformational analysis, *Biochem. J.*, 238, 1, 1986.

36. **Killian, J. A., Timmermans, W. J., Keur, S., and de Kruijff, B.,** The tryptophans of gramicidin are essential for the lipid structure modulating effect of the peptide, *Biochim. Biophys. Acta*, 820, 154, 1985.

37. **Killian, J. A., van den Berg, C. W., Tournois, H., Keur, S., Slotboom, A. J., van Scharrenburg, G. J. M., and de Kruijff, B.,** Gramicidin-induced hexagonal H_{II} phase formation in negatively charged phospholipids and the effect of N- and C-terminal modification of gramicidin on its interaction with zwitterionic phospholipids, *Biochim. Biophys. Acta*, 857, 13, 1986.

38. **Brasseur, R., Killian, J. A., de Kruijff, B., and Ruysschaert, J. M.,** Conformational analysis of gramicidin-gramicidin interactions at the air/water interface suggest that gramicidin aggregates into tube-like structures similar as found in the gramicidin-induced hexagonal H_{II} phase, *Biochim. Biophys. Acta,* 903, 11, 1987.

39. **Brasseur, R., de Meutter, J., Goormaghtigh, E., and Ruysschaert, J. M.,** Mode of organization of galactolipids: a conformational analysis, *Biochem. Biophys. Res. Commun.,* 115, 666, 1983.

40. **Tournois, H.,** unpublished data.

Part 1B. Experimental Data

Chapter 1.B.1

X-RAY DIFFRACTION ANALYSIS OF MEMBRANE LIPIDS

Thomas J. McIntosh

TABLE OF CONTENTS

I. INTRODUCTION

The lipid bilayer is the core of biological membranes and plays essential role in the diverse functions which membranes perform. It provides a suitable environment for the many enzymes and transport proteins which are membrane bound and for the glycoproteins and glycolipids which are thought to mediate interactions of cells with their environment. Since the lipid bilayer is a highly efficient permeability barrier for ions and certain other charged molecules, it is a key element in the compartmentalization of cells and cellular organelles. Moreover, the permeability barrier to ions provided by the bilayer is necessary in many cellular functions. For instance, the impermeability of the bilayer of the inner mitochondrial membrane to hydrogen ions is essential in the synthesis of ATP, and the sequestering of calcium by the sarcoplasmic membrane is critical to the regulation of skeletal muscle contraction. Bilayers also play important roles in membrane fusion events which occur during protein secretion, endocytosis, and cell division. Membrane fusion involves the close apposition and subsequent joining of the membrane lipid bilayers.

Most membrane lipids are amphipathic — containing both a polar or hydrophilic head group and a nonpolar or hydrophobic hydrocarbon tail. There are a great number of lipids present in biological membranes, with diversity in both the head group and hydrocarbon tails of the lipid molecules. Specific membranes often have their own characteristic lipid composition.[1,2] For instance, the inner mitochondrial membrane has a distinctly different lipid composition than the endoplasmic reticulum membrane, and the plasma membrane differs in composition from most organelle membranes in that it contains glycolipids and relatively high concentrations of cholesterol.[1]

The reasons for the immense diversity in lipids found in biological membranes are only partially understood at present. Some possible roles for specific lipids include membrane stabilization,[3-5] signal transduction,[6,7] regulating the fluidity of the membrane interior,[8] and binding of ions, toxins, and lectins.[9-12] The activities of certain membrane-bound proteins, such as receptors, transporters, and enzymes, are functions of lipid head group type, hydrocarbon chain length, and degree of unsaturation of the fatty acid chains.[13-19] In addition, the roles of various classes of lipids in membrane fusion events have been the subject of intense investigation.[20-23]

Many of these functional roles for membrane lipids depend strongly on the structural details of the bilayer formed by each lipid. For example, in order for a given intrinsic protein to "fit" in the hydrocarbon core of the membrane, the thickness of the hydrocarbon chain region of the bilayer must nearly match the thickness of the hydrophobic stretch of amino acids in the protein.[24,25] As another example, the passive permeability of the membrane to ions and nonelectolytes decreases in proportion to the thickness of the bilayer hydrocarbon region. In addition, membrane surface properties depend on the lipid head group type and its orientation.[25]

In this article, X-ray diffraction structural studies are presented on specific examples of the three major classes of membrane lipids — phospholipids, sterols, and glycolipids. The two phospholipids examined, phosphatidylethanolamine (PE) and phosphatidylcholine (PC), are the two most prevalent phospholipids in many biological membranes. The structural effects of the sterol cholesterol, which accounts for as much as 40% of some plasma membranes, are studied in both PE and PC bilayers. We also determine the structure of bilayers containing the glycolipid ganglioside GM1 which is found in plasma membranes in the brain and intestine and is the receptor for cholera toxin.[10] For each of these systems, electron density maps are used to determine the bilayer hydrocarbon thickness and the modifications in fluid thickness between bilayers caused by the different head group types. These structural results are related to the functional role of each lipid in native biological membranes.

II. MATERIALS AND METHODS

The ganglioside GM1 was purified from bovine brain by the methods of Felgner et al.[26] The other purified lipids were used as obtained from commercial sources. Egg phosphatidylcholine (EPC), 1-palmitoyl-2-oleoylphosphatidylcholine (POPC), dilauroylphosphatidylethanolamine (DLPE), and bacterial phosphatidylethanolamine (BPE) were purchased from Avanti Polar Lipids, cholesterol was obtained from Sigma, and dipalmitoylphosphatidylcholine (DPPC), distearoylphosphatidylcholine (DSPC), and dilauroylphosphatidylcholine (DLPC) were obtained from both Avanti Polar Lipids and Calbiochem. The same lipids from different commercial sources gave identical diffraction patterns. Lipid purity was checked by thin-layer chromotography. A single spot was observed for each commercial sample tested (100 μg of lipid), and the GM1 was found to be greater than 90% pure.[27] Europium-labeled GM1 was prepared by codissolving equal molar ratios of europium chloride (Alfa Inorganics Inc.) and GM1 in methanol/water (33:1), followed by evaporation of the solvent. Poly(vinylpyrrolidone) (PVP) was obtained from Sigma and triply distilled water was used to make PVP-water solutions in the range of 0 to 60% w/w. These PVP solutions were used to vary the fluid spaces between adjacent bilayers in order to determine the phase angles for the X-ray reflections (see Section III, Results).

Lipid suspensions consisting of unoriented multilamellar vesicles were prepared by the following procedure. A single lipid or lipid mixture was dissolved in an appropriate organic solvent, usually ethanol or chloroform. The solvent was removed by rotary evaporation, leaving a thin lipid layer. The lipid was hydrated by adding water or water-PVP solution and allowing the suspensions to incubate several hours at temperatures above the lipid phase transition temperature. For most experiments, an excess amount (greater than 70% by weight) of water or water-PVP solution was added. In these specimens, the excess phase was visible either by direct observation or by light microscopy.

For X-ray diffraction experiments, these suspensions were sealed in quartz glass capillary tubes and mounted in a temperature-controlled specimen holder in either a pinhole collimation camera or a double-mirror camera. Diffractions patterns were recorded with a flat plate film cassette containing three or more sheets of Kodak® DEF-5 X-ray film. Specimen-to-film distance was usually 10 cm, and typical exposure times were 3 to 10 h. X-ray films were processed by standard techniques and densitometered in a radial direction from the center of the pattern with a Joyce-Loebl Model MKIIIC microdensitometer. The background curve was subtracted, and the integrated intensity, $I(h)$, for each diffraction order h was obtained by measuring the area under the diffraction peak. For these unoriented suspensions, the structure amplitude, $|T(h)|$, was set equal to $|T(h)| = [h^2 I(h)]^{1/2}$, i.e., for the unoriented specimens, a correction factor of h^2 was applied to the observed intensity data. One factor of h is due to the intersection of the reciprocal lattice of the multilayer with the Ewald sphere (the Lorentz correction).[28] The second factor of h is a geometrical correction which arises from scanning the X-ray film in a radial direction across the circular reflections with a microdensitometer slit of small fixed height.[28]

Oriented multilayer specimens were obtained by evaporation of lipid from organic solvent on a flat glass substrate. The oriented multilayers on the supporting plate were placed in a constant relative humidity chamber and oriented on a Unican oscillation camera so that the planes of the bilayers were approximately parallel to a pinhole collimator. The specimen was oscillated through an appropriate angle so that diffraction orders out to $(6 \text{ Å})^{-1}$ could be recorded.[29] The size of the pinhole collimator was selected so that the entire width of the specimen was in the X-ray beam at all angles of oscillation. The resulting diffraction patterns consisted of sharp reflections of constant height which depended on the size of the pinhole. Densitometer traces were obtained scanning from the beam stop through the center of each reflection and integrated intensities, $I(h)$, were obtained as described above. For this camera, geometry, the Lorentz-polarization factor for oscillation photographs was used,[29] so that $|T(h)| = [hI(h)]^{1/2}$. To record wide-angle reflections from the lipid hydrocarbon chains, the specimen was held stationary or oscillated through a smaller angle.[29]

For each series of experiments with a particular bilayer system, the structure amplitudes were normalized according to the method of Blaurock.[30] The electron density distribution across the bilayer on a relative electron density scale is given by

$$\rho(x) = \sum e^{i\phi(h)} |T(h)| \cos(2\pi xh/d)$$

where $\phi(h)$ is the phase angle for each order h. For these centrosymmetric bilayers, $\phi(h)$ must be 0 or 180° for each diffraction order. The phase angles were calculated, as illustrated in Section III, Results, by varying the fluid spaces between adjacent bilayers and therefore tracing out the continuous Fourier transform of each bilayer.[31,32]

III. RESULTS

A. LOW- AND WIDE-ANGLE DIFFRACTION PATTERNS

For each specimen investigated, the X-ray diffraction pattern consisted of a series of sharp low-angle reflections (in the range of 90 to 6 Å) which indexed as orders of a lamellar repeat and one or two sharp or broad wide-angle reflections (in the range of 4 to 5 Å). The fact that the low-angle reflections are sharp and index on a lamellar lattice indicates that each specimen consists of well-ordered arrays of bilayers. Profiles, which give the distribution of electron density across the multilayers, can be calculated from these low-angle reflections once the proper phase angle for each reflection is determined. The wide-angle reflections are due to the hydrocarbon chain packing in the plane of the bilayer; sharp wide-angle reflection indicates ordered chain packing, whereas broad bands indicate a more fluid organization of the chains. Thus, the low-angle X-ray data can be used to determine the width of the bilayer and the fluid separation between adjacent bilayers, and the wide-angle reflections provide direct information on the organization of the hydrocarbon core of the bilayer.

Examples of diffractions patterns from oriented and unoriented multibilayer specimens are shown in Figures 1 and 2, respectively. Figure 1 shows oriented specimens of DLPC (Figure 1A and C), 2:1 molar ratio DLPC:cholesterol (Figure 1B), DPPC (Figure 1D), and 2:1 molar ratio DPPC:cholesterol (Figure 1E) in various relative humidity atmospheres.[29] In all patterns in this figure, the multilayers are stacked so that the bilayer planes are in the horizontal direction. Thus, low-angle diffraction from the stacking of the bilayers is along the vertical axis (meridian of the X-ray film). Figure 1A and B are low-angle patterns, showing the first eight lamellar orders of diffraction from DLPC and DLPC:cholesterol multilayers. Note the sharpness and uniform lateral dimension of each diffraction order. Wide-angle patterns, taken with a shorter specimen-to-film distance, are shown in Figure 1C, D, and E. The patterns in Figure 1C and D are from lipids with ordered hydrocarbon chains (called the "gel" state), as indicated by the presence of sharp reflections at 4.2 Å (arrows). In the pattern taken at low relative humidity (Figure 1C), the wide-angle reflections are centered near the horizontal axis (equator) of the X-ray film, whereas in the pattern taken at high relative humidity (Figure 1D), the reflections are located off the equator by an angle of about 24°. For cylindrical structures, such as gel state lipid hydrocarbon chains, most of the scattered intensity will be observed in a direction perpendicular to the cylinder's axis. Thus, these patterns indicate that the orientation of the hydrocarbon chains in gel state PC bilayers is a function of the relative humidity. PC bilayers at low humidity contain little water, and the hydrocarbon chains are nearly perpendicular to the plane of the bilayer (Figure 1C). However, PC bilayers at high relative humidity absorb moisture from the atmosphere and the hydrocarbon chains of these partially hydrated bilayers (Figure 1D) are tilted relative

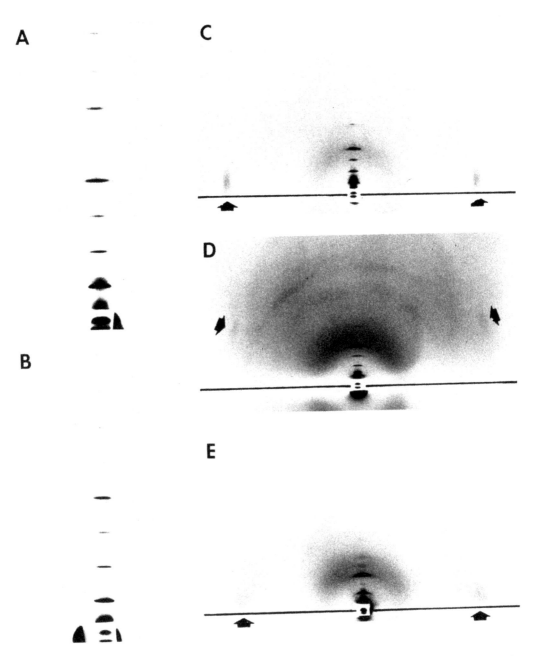

FIGURE 1.   Typical (A,B) low-angle and (C,D,E) wide-angle X-ray diffraction patterns from (A, C) DLPC; (B) 2:1 DLPC:cholesterol; (D) DPPC; and (E) 2:1 DPPC:cholesterol multilayers oriented on glass substrates. One half of each diffraction pattern is shown, and a black line has been drawn on the equator of the wide-angle patterns. Before each exposure was taken, the beam stop was removed for a few seconds so that the direct beam is seen in the middle of the equator as a black circle. The light line through this circle is due to absorption of the X-rays by the glass support. The low-angle patterns, which have been photographically enlarged, show the first eight lamellar orders of diffraction. In the wide-angle patterns, a few of these lamellar orders are visible above the beam stop, and the arrows point to the wide-angle reflections. (From McIntosh, T. J., *Biochim. Biophys. Acta*, 513, 43, 1978. With permission.)

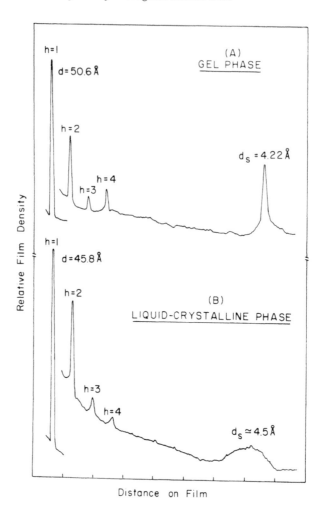

FIGURE 2.   Densitometer traces of diffraction patterns of unoriented, fully hydrated suspensions of DLPE in the gel phase (A) and the liquid-crystalline phase (B). For both phases, four orders of a lamellar repeat period d are observed. For both phases, orders two to four and the wide-angle reflections (d_s) are from traces of the first films in the cassette, whereas the first orders (h = 1) are from the third films in the pack. (From McIntosh, T. J. and Simon, S. A., *Biochemistry*, 25, 4948, 1986. With permission.)

to the planes of the bilayer.[29,33] In the diffraction pattern from DPPC:cholesterol (Figure 1E), the wide-angle reflection is considerably broader and located on the equator at a larger spacing (4.5 Å). This indicates that cholesterol removes the hydrocarbon chain tilt and makes the DPPC chains more fluid and the hydrocarbon chain region of the bilayer more disordered. Note, however, that cholesterol does not appreciably modify the orderliness of the stacking of the bilayers, as indicated by the sharpness of the low-angle reflections in Figure 1B. This type of organization, with long-range bilayer stacking order chain yet disordered hydrocarbon chain packing is often referred to as the ''liquid-crystalline'' phase.

Microdensitometer traces of patterns from fully hydrated and unoriented specimens are shown in Figure 2.[34] The traces were taken in a radial direction across the reflections which are concentric rings on the X-ray film. These patterns are from DLPE at 20°C in the gel phase (Figure 2A) and at 35°C in the liquid-crystalline phase (Figure 2B). Both patterns consist of four lamellar diffraction orders, plus one wide-angle reflection. In the case of gel phase DLPE, the wide-angle reflection is extremely sharp, indicating the ordered packing of the hydrocarbon chains. For the liquid-crystalline phase, the reflection is considerably broader.

B. ANALYSIS OF THE LAMELLAR DIFFRACTION DATA

In this Section, we present structural analysis of various types of lipid bilayers based primarily on low-angle lamellar diffraction data, such as shown in Figures 1 and 2.

1. Phosphatidylcholine

Figure 3A and B show structure amplitudes obtained from DPPC in the gel phase and EPC in the liquid-crystalline phase. These data were obtained from unoriented liposomes in water and various PVP-water solutions.[35] PVP is a neutral polymer which is too large to enter the fluid space between adjacent bilayers. It therefore competes for water with the lipid multilayers and causes water to flow from the interbilayer space to the polymer solution.[35-37] The amount of water removed from the lipid lattice depends on the concentration of the PVP-water solution. Therefore, different concentrations of polymer solution can be used to vary the fluid space between adjacent bilayers and change the lamellar repeat period, d. The circles in Figure 3A and B represent structure factors obtained at different PVP-water concentrations — 11 experiments for DPPC and 10 experiments for EPC. For DPPC, d ranged from 63.6 Å in water to 57.8 Å in 60% PVP, while for EPC, d ranged from 63.2 Å in water to 51.7 Å in 60% PVP.

Diffraction theory shows that if the structure of the bilayer remains the same during this modification of the fluid space, then the structure amplitudes obtained at different values of d should fall on a smooth curve — the absolute value of the Fourier transform of the bilayer.[31,32] In fact, for both DPPC and EPC, the structure amplitudes do fall very close to the smooth curve drawn with solid lines in Figure 3A and B. These solid lines were obtained by the use of the sampling theorem which calculates the continuous Fourier transform from any one set of lamellar diffraction structure amplitudes, provided the phase of each reflection and the structure amplitude at the origin of reciprocal space are known.[29,32] Unfortunately, neither the phases or the zero order structure amplitude are directly observable. However, they can be calculated by use of the additional sets of structure factors obtained through the PVP-water experiments.[35] In brief, the zero-order structure amplitude is obtained by analytical continuing to the origin of reciprocal space the curve traced out by the swelling experiments.[38] Then, for each possible phase combination (if there are 5 diffraction orders, there are $2^5 = 32$ possible phase assignments), the continuous transform is calculated by the use of the sampling theorem. Each of these possible transforms is then compared to the structure amplitude data from all PVP-water solutions. The correct phase combination produces a transform which most closely fits all the structure amplitude data.[32,35] The solid lines in Figure 3A and B represent the mean values of all transforms calculated using each data set (11 for DPPC and 10 for EPC) and the correct phase choice. The dashed curves show ±1 SD from the mean. None of the other phase combinations fit all the structure factors so closely or produce such small standard deviations from the mean. Transforms similar to those shown in Figure 3 have been derived for both DPPC and EPC both by similar swelling experiments[39] and also by recording diffraction patterns from dispersions of single-walled vesicles.[40,41]

The continuous transforms for DPPC (Figure 3A) and EPC (Figure 3B) are somewhat similar in shape, but have their nodes and maxima at different positions in reciprocal space. In particular, the nodes for the DPPC transform are shifted to smaller values of reciprocal space coordinate than the corresponding nodes in EPC. This indicates that the bilayer is wider for DPPC than for EPC.

Figure 4 shows electron density profiles calculated for DPPC and EPC in excess water using the phase combinations determined as described above. For each profile, the two

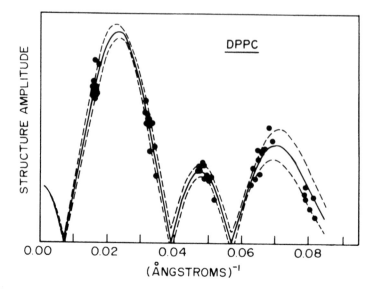

A

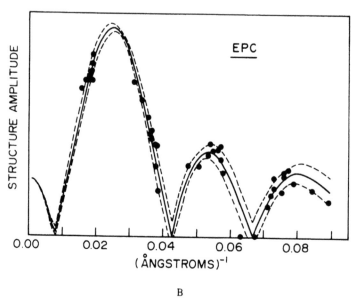

B

FIGURE 3.   Structure amplitudes for (A) DPPC and (B) EPC. The circles represent structure amplitudes for liposomes in water and water-PVP and water-dextran solutions. The solid curves are means of all transforms calculated using the different sets of structure amplitudes and the phase angles $(0,\pi,0,\pi)$ for the first four observed nodes in the transforms. The dashed curves show ± 1 SD (standard deviation) from the mean. (From McIntosh, T. J. and Simon, S. A., *Biochemistry*, 25, 4058, 1986. With permission.)

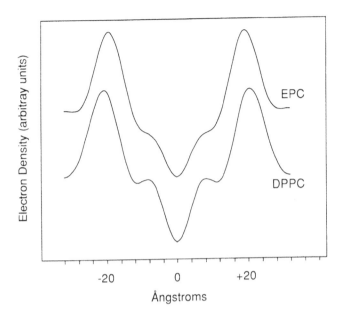

FIGURE 4.   Electron density profiles of DPPC and EPC in excess water.

highest electron density peaks correspond to the lipid polar head groups, and the trough at 0 Å is in the geometric center of the bilayer and corresponds to the localization of the terminal methyl group of the hydrocarbon chains. The medium density regions between the head group peaks and the terminal methyl trough correspond to the methylene groups, and the narrow medium density regions at the outer edges of each profile correspond to the fluid layers between adjacent bilayers. In the profile of the gel state bilayer (DPPC), the terminal methyl trough is deeper, indicating more ordered hydrocarbon chains in this phase as compared to the liquid-crystalline phase (EPC).

The distance between head group peaks across the bilayer for the experiments shown in Figure 3 is 41.9 ± 0.6 Å (mean ± SD; N = 11 experiments) for DPPC and 37.8 ± 0.8 Å (N = 10) for EPC.[35] The distance between the head group peaks across the fluid space between adjacent bilayers is a function of the concentration of the PVP-water solution, and for DPPC varies from 21.7 Å in water to 15.9 Å in 60% PVP solution and for EPC varies from 25.4 Å in water to 13.9 Å in 60% PVP solution.

2. Phosphatidylethanolamine

Figure 5 shows electron density profiles for DLPE in the gel and liquid-crystalline phases obtained from the diffraction patterns shown in Figure 2.[34] These profiles are similar to those of PC (see Figure 3) in that the high-density peaks correspond to the lipid head groups and the low-density troughs at 0 Å correspond to the localization of the lipid terminal methyl groups in the geometric center of the bilayer. For DLPE, the transition from the gel to liquid-crystalline phase causes the distance between head group peaks across the bilayer to decrease from 37.2 ± 0.3 Å (N = 3 experiments) to 33.0 ± 0.6 Å (N = 3). Notice that this decrease in distance between head group peaks is, within experimental uncertainty, equal to the decrease in lamellar repeat period between the two phases, 50.5 − 46.1 = 4.4 Å. Most of the volume change observed upon melting the hydrocarbon chains occurs in the hydrocarbon region of the bilayer.[42] Therefore, the observation that the difference in observed repeat periods and head group peak separations is the same provides strong evidence that (1) the thickness of the fluid layer between bilayers remains nearly constant upon melting and (2) the conformation of the phosphate moiety-glycerol backbone portion of the DLPE molecule is approximately the same in gel and liquid-crystalline phases.[34]

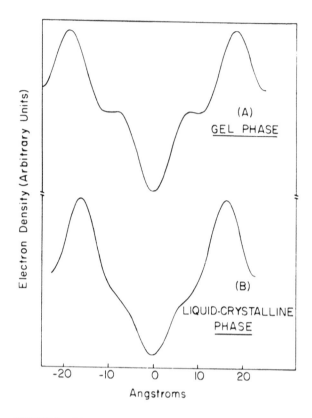

FIGURE 5.   Electron density profiles of fully hydrated DLPE in the gel and liquid-crystalline phases. (From McIntosh, T. J. and Simon, S. A., *Biochemistry*, 25, 4948, 1986. With permission.)

Although the profiles of gel and liquid-crystalline phase PCs (see Figure 4) and PEs (see Figure 5) resemble each other, there is one important difference, i.e., the width of the fluid space in fully hydrated DLPE is considerably smaller than that of either gel or liquid-crystalline phase PC. For DLPE, the distance between head group peaks across the fluid space is 13.3 and 13.1 Å in the gel and liquid-crystalline phase, respectively, compared to 21.7 and 25.4 Å for fully hydrated DPPC and EPC, respectively. These differences in fluid spaces between PC and PE bilayers may help to explain why bilayers containing PE fuse more readily than do bilayers composed of PC (see Section IV, Discussion).

The electron density profiles and wide-angle diffraction patterns, along with published dilatometry data,[42] can be used to calculate the area per lipid molecule as well as the number and distribution of water molecules in the system.[34] The area in the liquid crystalline-phase, A_l, is equal to

$$A_l = A_g + A_g(\Delta V/V_g - \Delta H/H_g)(H_g/H_l)$$

where A_g is the area per molecule in the gel phase and $\Delta H/H_g$ and $\Delta V/V_g$ are the relative changes in hydrocarbon thickness and volume of the bilayer, respectively, obtained upon going through the gel to liquid-crystalline phase transition. $\Delta H/H_g$ can be estimated[34] from the electron density profiles (see Figure 5) and $\Delta V/V_g$ has been measured by dilatometry.[42] Since the hydrocarbon chains in the gel state of saturated PEs are oriented perpendicular to the plane of the bilayer and packed in a hexagonal array,[43] A_g can be directly calculated from the wide-angle gel spacing, d_s, by $A_g = 2(2/\sqrt{3})(d_s)^2 = 41.0 \pm 0.2$ Å^2.[34] The above equation then gives $A_l = 50.6$ Å^2.[34] Now, since the area per molecule and lamellar repeat

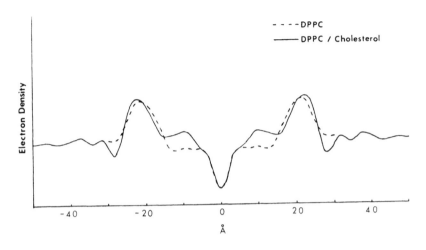

FIGURE 6. Electron density profiles of DPPC and 2:1 DPPC:cholesterol. (From McIntosh, T. J., *Biochim. Biophys. Acta,* 513, 43, 1978. With permission.)

period are known, the volume of the unit cell can be obtained for both gel and liquid-crystalline bilayers. The approximate number of water molecules associated with the lipid can be obtained by subtracting the volume of the anhydrous molecule from the unit cell dimensions of the hydrated lipid. McIntosh and Simon[34] have used this procedure to show that there are about seven and ten water molecules per DLPE molecule in the gel and liquid-crystalline phases, respectively. These values can be compared to estimates of 15 and 25 waters per lipid molecule for gel state DPPC[44] and liquid-crystalline phase EPC,[45] respectively. Thus, fully hydrated DLPE contains significantly less water than PC bilayers, as also evidenced in the electron density profiles by the narrower width of the fluid spaces between DLPE bilayers (see Figure 5) than between DPPC or EPC bilayers (see Figure 4).

The electron density profiles of DLPE in the gel and liquid-crystalline phases (see Figure 5) and the values of A_g and A_l can be used to determine the approximate distribution of these water molecules between the interbilayer fluid space and the bilayer head group region, i.e., the electron density profiles can be used to estimate the thickness of the fluid space between bilayers, and this distance multiplied by the area per molecule gives the volume of the fluid space. Dividing this fluid space volume by the volume of a water molecule (about 30 $Å^3$) gives the number of water molecules in the fluid space. This analysis shows that roughly half of the water is located in the fluid spaces between adjacent bilayers, and the remaining water molecules are intercalated into the bilayer, presumably in the head group region. That is, for fully hydrated DLPE in the liquid-crystalline phase, there are four to five water molecules per lipid molecule in the fluid space between bilayers and five to six water molecules intercalated into the bilayer head group region.[34]

3. Phospholipid/Cholesterol

Figure 6 shows electron density profiles of gel phase DPPC and 2:1 DPPC:cholesterol bilayers. These profiles were obtained from diffraction patterns from oriented specimens in relative humidity atmospheres (such as shown in Figure 1), and the resolution is somewhat higher than the profiles from the unoriented, fully hydrated specimens shown in Figures 4 and 5. The profile for DPPC:cholesterol was calculated from the continuous transform of a single bilayer obtained by varying the lamellar repeat period with different relative humidities. Therefore, in this case, the fluid space between bilayers appears to be indefinitely wide. Note that cholesterol has two major effects on the bilayer profile. First, it increases the bilayer thickness, since it decreases hydrocarbon chain tilt as indicated by wide-angle patterns

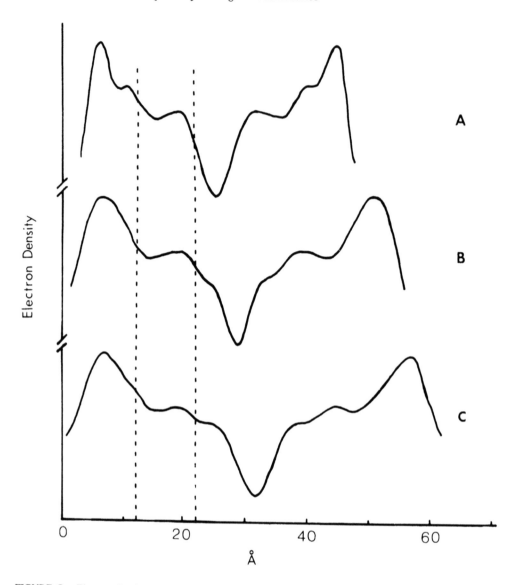

FIGURE 7. Electron density profiles of (A) 2:1 DLPC:cholesterol; (B) 2:1 DPPC:cholesterol; and (C) 2:1 DSPC:cholesterol. The dotted lines delimit regions in the profiles where the electron density has been raised due to the cholesterol sterol rings. (From McIntosh, T. J., *Biochim. Biophys. Acta,* 513, 43, 1978. With permission.)

such as those shown in Figure 1D and E. Second, it adds density to the methylene chain region of the bilayer, adjacent to the lipid head group. This is because the steroid rings of cholesterol are more electron dense than the fatty acid chains of DPPC.

Figure 7 shows electron density profiles of PC:cholesterol bilayers with PCs of different length hydrocarbon chains.[29] Figure 7A, B, and C are bilayers of DLPC:cholesterol, DPPC:cholesterol, and DSPC:cholesterol, respectively. DLPC, DPPC, and DSPC contain 12, 16, and 18 carbons per fatty acid chain, respectively. In this figure, the origin has been shifted to the edge of the unit cell of DSPC:cholesterol and the head group regions of the three profiles have been aligned in vertical register. The two dotted lines delimit the evaluations in electron density caused by the cholesterol sterol rings (see Figure 6). These elevations are adjacent to the head group region in all cases, indicating that cholesterol is localized in the same position relative to the phosphocholine group in each bilayer, independent of fatty acid chain length.[29]

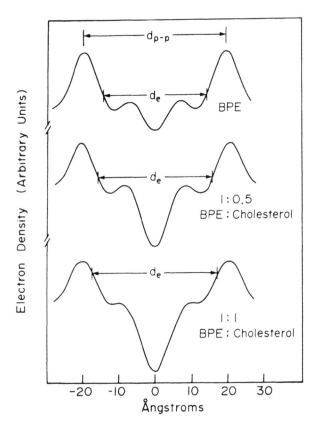

FIGURE 8. Electron density profiles of fully hydrated BPE and BPE:cholesterol liposomes. The dielectric thickness of each bilayer, d_e, was measured by specific capacitance measurements on planar bilayers of the same compositions. (From McIntosh, T. J., Simon, S. A., and Dilger, J. F., in *Water Transport in Biological Membranes*, Benga, G., Ed., CRC Press, Boca Raton, FL).

Electron density profiles of fully hydrated liquid-crystalline phosphatidylethanolamine bilayers, in the presence and absence of cholesterol, are shown in Figure 8. The lipid used in these studies is bacterial phosphatidylethanolamine (BPE), derived from *Escherichia coli* membranes. Increasing amounts of cholesterol raise the density of the hydrocarbon region next to the head group relative to the trough in the center of the bilayer. Cholesterol has only a small effect on bilayer thickness, increasing the head group separation across the bilayer by less than 1 Å. Moreover, cholesterol has little effect on the width of the fluid space between adjacent bilayers; the distance between head group peaks across the fluid space is 14.1, 13.9, and 14.1 Å for BPE, 2:1 BPE:cholesterol, and 1:1 BPE:cholesterol, respectively.

The electron density profiles of BPE and BPE:cholesterol are also useful because they can be compared to specific capacitance measurements of bilayers made from the same lipids. BPE is one of the few lipids which forms liposomes in water suitable for diffraction studies and also forms stable, "solvent-free" single planar bilayers useful for electrical capacitance studies. Specific capacitance measurements give the width of the low dielectric region of the bilayer, d_e. Measured values of d_e taken from Simon et al.[46] for BPE and BPE:cholesterol bilayers are shown superimposed on the corresponding electron density profiles in Figure 8. Notice that although the bilayer thickness, as indicated by the head group separation across the bilayer in electron density profiles, is increased by less than 1

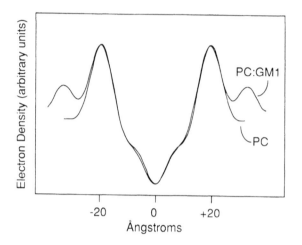

FIGURE 9.   Electron density profiles of PC and PC:GM1 bilayers.

Å by the incorporation of cholesterol, d_e is 6.0 Å greater for 1:1 BPE:cholesterol bilayers than for BPE bilayers, i.e., the effective thickness of the low dielectric region of the bilayer increases upon incorporation of cholesterol, whereas the geometric thickness of the bilayer remains nearly the same. Water has a dielectric constant of about 80 and the bilayer hydrocarbon region has a dielectric constant of about 2. Therefore, these data imply that cholesterol, whose steroid rings are localized in the hydrocarbon region of the bilayer adjacent to the lipid head group, displaces water molecules from the bilayer head group region, thereby increasing the thickness of the low dielectric region of the bilayer.

4. Phospholipid/Ganglioside GM1

Electron density profiles for POPC and POPC:GM1 bilayers are shown in Figure 9. Note that the incorporation of GM1 has little effect on the structure of the interior of the bilayer. However, GM1 does increase the total thickness of the membrane by adding a region of moderately high density outside the phospholipid head group peak. This indicates that the ganglioside sugar residues are localized in this region, extending beyond the plane of the PC head groups and into the fluid space between adjacent bilayers. The high density region caused by the ganglioside extends at least 15 Å from the center of the PC head group. To more quantitatively determine the conformation of the GM1 head group, labeling experiments with europium were performed.[48] Europium has been shown to bind to the carboxylate group of the GM1 sialic acid moiety.[49] Electron density profiles for labeled and unlabeled POPC:GM1 bilayers are shown in Figure 10, along with a difference profile which gives the distribution of the europium label. The width of the label in the difference profile is large, probably because europium binds both to the PC head group as well as to the GM1 sialic acid moiety. Model calculations give a best fit to the observed data with the GM1 carboxylate group located 10 Å from the center of the PC head group. Based on molecular models of GM1, these data indicate that the hydrated GM1 head group is extended, approximately perpendicular to the plane of the bilayer.

IV. DISCUSSION

The analysis of lamellar and wide-angle diffraction patterns provides many important details concerning the organization of specific lipid bilayers. In this section, several of these structural observations are related to the functional roles which these lipids perform in native biological membranes.

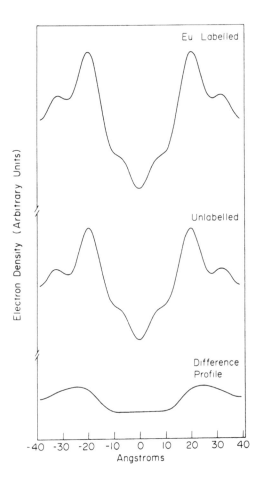

FIGURE 10. Electron density profiles of europium-labeled and unlabeled PC:GM1 bilayers. The difference profile was obtained by subtracting the unlabeled profile from the labeled profile. (From McDaniel, R. V. and McIntosh, T. J., *Biophys. J.*, 49, 94, 1986. With permission.)

One important difference observed between phosphatidylcholine and phosphatidylethanolamine bilayers is the width of the fluid space between adjacent bilayers. For both fully hydrated gel and liquid-crystalline phases, the fluid space between bilayers is significantly smaller for PE than for PC bilayers. In fact, for PE bilayers, the fluid spaces are small enough that one or two water molecules could span the space between adjacent bilayers.[34] This observation may help to explain why bilayers containing PE fuse more readily than do bilayers containing PC.[23] As noted by Duzgunes et al.,[23] the steps involved in liposome fusion are aggregation, destabilization of the bilayer structure, and finally vesicle fusion. Based on the X-ray evidence, aggregated bilayers containing large amounts of PE are significantly closer together than those containing large amounts of PC. This may mean that when bilayer destabilization occurs, e.g., as a result of different surface energies of the inner and outer monolayers of the bilayer,[50] PE-containing bilayers are close enough to fuse, whereas bilayers containing large amounts of PC are too far apart for fusion to occur.[34]

Cholesterol is an important component of many plasma membranes. Its location in the bilayer has been determined by X-ray diffraction studies,[29,51] such as those presented in this paper. The molecule lies approximately parallel to the lipid hydrocarbon chains in the bilayer. The electron dense sterol rings can be observed in electron density profiles to be localized in the hydrocarbon chain region of the bilayer, near the head group region. Cholesterol has several important effects on bilayer structure. First, it effects the "fluidity" of the bilayer interior.[8,52] When added to gel state bilayers, it fluidizes the hydrocarbon chains (see Figure 1D and E). However, when added to liquid-crystalline lipids, it condenses the bilayer, i.e., it reduces the area per molecule and increases order in the hydrocarbon chain region — especially in the initial segments of the chains near the head group. Thus, bilayers containing cholesterol have hydrocarbon chain packing which is more fluid than gel bilayers, yet more ordered than most liquid-crystalline bilayers.

Cholesterol also has an important effect on the distribution of water in bilayers. Combined X-ray diffraction and electrical capacitance analysis indicates that cholesterol removes water molecules from the head group region of PE bilayers,[46,47] i.e., by occupying space at the boundary between the head group and the hydrocarbon chain regions of the bilayer, cholesterol displaces the deepest water molecules from the head group region. This has the effect of moving the water/hydrocarbon interface, so that the low-dielectric region of the bilayer is about 6 Å wider when cholesterol is added. Since the passive permeability of the bilayer decreases in proportion to the hydrocarbon thickness, cholesterol may have a significant effect on membrane permeability. In fact, it has been observed that the addition of cholesterol decreases the passive permeability of bilayers to various nonelectrolytes, including water.[53] In addition, as previously noted,[47] the ability of cholesterol to increase the effective hydrophobic thickness of the bilayer might be important in terms of lipid-protein interactions, i.e., intrinsic membrane proteins are thought to be embedded in the bilayer so that the hydrophobic regions of the protein coincide with the hydrophobic core of the lipid bilayer. Increasing the width of the bilayer hydrophobic region may thus have an important effect on the solubility of proteins in bilayers.[47]

Gangliosides are glycolipids which are found on the outer surface of many plasma membranes, especially neurons and epithelial cells. In particular, the ganglioside GM1 is the receptor in intestinal epithelial cells for cholera toxin.[10] X-ray diffraction analysis of bilayers containing GM1 shows two important features which may be shared by other membrane receptors: (1) GM1 does not alter or perturb the structure of the bilayer and (2) the sugar moiety extends well out into the fluid space. The electron density profiles in Figure 9 clearly show that GM1 fits into PC bilayers without appreciably modifying the structure of the bilayer; the electron density profiles of PC and PC:GM1 superimpose in the region of the bilayer between the PC head group peaks. This means that GM1 can be incorporated into the bilayer in large quantities (up to 30 mol%) without changing the bilayer thickness or bilayer hydrocarbon packing, which, as discussed above, are important in determining membrane permeability and in protein-lipid interactions. The electron density maps also show that the GM1 head group extends out from the PC head group peak, i.e., the GM1 head group is oriented nearly perpendicular to the plane of the bilayer, so that the receptor portion of the molecule is extended as far as possible into the fluid space. This orientation of the head group in intestinal cells would make the binding site maximally accessible to the contents of the intestine, Moreover, as noted by McDaniel and McIntosh,[48] because the fixed charge on GM1 is located about 10 Å away from the center of the phospholipid head group, the potential at the hydrocarbon/water interface of these bilayers is smaller than that of charged phospholipid bilayers.

Thus, these bilayers of different lipid composition have distinct structural features which may be related to their roles in native biological membranes. One significant structural feature that these different lipid bilayers have in common should be noted, i.e., for each of these bilayer systems, the structure of the bilayer remains nearly constant as water is removed from the fluid space between adjacent bilayers. This is demonstrated by the observations that, as bilayers move from their equilibrium separation in excess water to within about 5 Å of each other, the X-ray structure factors fall on a smooth curve (see Figure 3A and B and also Reference 35) and the distance between head group peaks across the bilayer in electron density profiles remains nearly constant.[35] This implies that bilayers are relatively incompressible, in agreement with measured compressibility moduli,[54] and that the lipid environment for proteins remains relatively constant in structure as water between membrane surfaces is removed. However, recent structural analysis indicates that significant changes in bilayer structure and hydrocarbon chain packing do occur when enough water is removed so that apposing bilayers come into steric hindrance.[55]

ACKNOWLEDGMENTS

The author wishes to express his gratitude to Dr. Sidney Simon for many extremely useful comments, suggestions, and insights throughout the course of these studies and to Dr. Alan Magid for assistance with the PVP experiments and computer graphics and for many helpful suggestions. This work was supported in part by a grant from the National Institutes of Health (GM 27278).

REFERENCES

1. **Rouser, G., Nelson, G. J., Fleischer, S., and Simon, G.,** Lipid composition of animal cell membranes, organelles, and organs, in *Biological Membranes, Physical Fact and Function,* Chapman, D., Ed., Academic Press, London, 1968, 5.
2. **Korn, E. D.,** Current concepts of membrane structure and function, *Fed. Proc.,* 28, 6, 1969.
3. **Pascher, I.,** Molecular arrangements in sphingolipids. Conformation and hydrogen bonding of ceramide and their implications on membrane stability and permeability, *Biochim. Biophys. Acta,* 455, 433, 1976.
4. **Tilcock, C. P. S., Bally, M. B., Farren, S. B., Cullis, P. R., and Gruner, S. M.,** Cation-dependent segregation phenomena and phase behavior in model membrane systems containing phosphatidylserine: influence of cholesterol and acyl chain composition, *Biochemistry,* 23, 2696, 1984.
5. **Curatolo, W.,** Glycolipid function, *Biochim. Biophys. Acta,* 906, 137, 1987.
6. **Fain, J. N. and Berridge, M. J.,** Relationship between hormonal activation of phosphatidylinositol hydrolysis, fluid secretion and calcium flux in the blowfly salivary gland, *Biochem. J.,* 178, 45, 1979.
7. **Burgess, G. M., Godfrey, P. P., McKinney, J. S., Berridge, M. F., Irvine, R. F., and Putney, J. W.,** The second messenger linking receptor activation to internal Ca release in liver, *Nature (London),* 309, 63, 1984.
8. **Oldfield, E. and Chapman, D.,** Molecular dynamics of cerebroside-cholesterol and shingomyelin-cholesterol interactions: implications for myelin membrane structure, *FEBS Lett.,* 21, 303, 1972.
9. **Behr, J.-P. and Lehn, J.-M.,** The binding of divalent cations by purified gangliosides, *FEBS Lett.,* 31, 297, 1973.
10. **Van Heyningen, S.,** Cholera toxin: interaction of subunits with ganglioside GM1, *Science,* 183, 656, 1974.
11. **Moss, J., Osborne, J. C., Fisnman, P. H., Nakaya, S., and Robertson, D. C.,** *Escherichia coli* heat labile enterotoxin, *J. Biol. Chem.,* 256, 12,861, 1981.
12. **Curatolo, W., Yau, A. O., Small, D. M., and Sears, B.,** Lectin-induced agglutination of phospholipid/glycolipid vesicles, *Biochemistry,* 17, 5740, 1978.
13. **Baldwin, P. A. and Hubbell, W. L.,** Effects of lipid environment on the light-induced conformational changes of rhodopsin. II. Roles of lipid chain length, unsaturation, and phase state, *Biochemistry,* 24, 2633, 1985.
14. **Fong, T. M. and McNamee, M. G.,** Correlation between acetylcholine receptor function and structural properties of membranes, *Biochemistry,* 25, 830, 1986.
15. **Boheim, G., Hanke, W., and Eibl, H.,** Lipid phase transition in planar bilayer membrane and its effect on carrier- and pore-mediated ion transport, *Proc. Natl. Acad. Sci. U.S.A.,* 77, 3403, 1980.
16. **Poon, R., Richards, J. M., and Clark, W. R.,** The relationship between plasma membrane lipid composition and physical-chemical properties. II. Effect of phospholipid fatty acid modulation on plasma membrane physical properties and enzymatic activities, *Biochim. Biophys. Acta,* 649, 58, 1981.
17. **Moore, B. M., Lentz, B. R., Hoechli, M., and Meissner, G.,** Effect of lipid membrane structure on the adenosine 5-triphosphate hydrolyzing activity of the calcium-stimulated adenosinetriphosphatase of sarcoplasmic reticulum, *Biochemistry,* 20, 6810, 1981.

18. **Criado, M., Eibl, H., and Barrantes, F. J.,** Functional properties of the acetylcholine receptor incorporated in model lipid membranes. Differential effects of chain length and head group of phospholipids on receptor affinity states and recepto-mediated ion translocation, *J. Biol. Chem.,* 259, 9188, 1984.

19. **Spector, A. A. and Yorek, M. A.,** Membrane lipid composition and cellular function, *J. Lipid Res.,* 26, 1015, 1985.

20. **Papahadjopoulos, D., Vail, W. J., Jacobson, K., and Poste, G.,** Cochleate lipid cylinders: formation by fusion of unilamellar lipid vesicles, *Biochim. Biophys. Acta,* 394, 483, 1975.

21. **Bentz, J., Ellens, H., Lai, M.-Z., and Szoka, F. C.,** On the correlation between HII phase and the contact-induced destabilization of phosphatidylethanolamine-containing membranes, *Proc. Natl. Acad. Sci. U.S.A.,* 82, 5742, 1985.

22. **Verleij, A. J., Humbel, B., Studer, D., and Muller, M.,** "Lipid particle" systems as visualized by thin-section electron microscopy, *Biochim. Biophys. Acta,* 812, 591, 1985.

23. **Duzgunes, N., Straubinger, R. M., Baldwin, P. A., Friend, D. S., and Papahadjopoulos, D.,** Proton-induced fusion of oleic acid-phosphatidylethanolamine liposomes, *Biochemistry,* 24, 3091, 1985.

24. **Israelachvili, J. N.,** Refinement of the fluid-mosaic model of membrane structure, *Biochim. Biophys. Acta,* 469, 221, 1977.

25. **Israelachvili, J. N., Marcelja, S., and Horn, R. G.,** Physical principles of membrane organization, *Q. Rev. Biophys.,* 13, 121, 1980.

26. **Felgner, P. L., Friere, E., Barenholz, Y., and Thompson, T. E.,** Kinetics of transfer of gangliosides from their micelles to dipalmitoylphosphatidylcholine vesicles, *Biochemistry,* 20, 2168, 1982.

27. **McDaniel, R. V. and McIntosh, T. J.,** X-ray diffraction studies of the cholera toxin receptor, GM1, *Biophys. J.,* 49, 94, 1986.

28. **Herbette, L., Marquardt, J., Scarpa, A., and Blasie, J. K.,** A direct analysis of lamellar X-ray diffraction from oriented multilayers of fully functional sarcoplasmic reticulum, *Biophys. J.,* 20, 245, 1977.

29. **McIntosh, T. J.,** The effect of cholesterol on the structure of phosphatidylcholine bilayers, *Biochim. Biophys. Acta,* 513, 43, 1978.

30. **Blaurock, A. E.,** Structure of the nerve myelin membrane: proof of the low-resolution profile, *J. Mol. Biol.,* 56, 35, 1971.

31. **Moody, M. F.,** X-ray diffraction pattern of nerve myelin: a method for determining the phases, *Science,* 142, 1173, 1963.

32. **Worthington, C. R., King, G. I., and McIntosh, T. J.,** Direct structure determination of multilayered membrane-type systems which contain fluid layers, *Biophys. J.,* 13, 480, 1973.

33. **Tardieu, A., Luzzati, V., and Reman, F. C.,** Structure and polymorphism of the hydrocarbon chains of lipids: a study of lecithin-water phases, *J. Mol. Biol.,* 75, 711, 1973.

34. **McIntosh, T. J. and Simon, S. A.,** Area per molecule and distribution of water in fully hydrated dilauroylphosphatidylethanolamine bilayers, *Biochemistry,* 25, 4948, 1986.

35. **McIntosh, T. J. and Simon, S. A.,** Hydration force and bilayer deformation: a reevaluation, *Biochemistry,* 25, 4058, 1986.

36. **LeNeveu, D. M., Rand, R. P., Parsegian, V. A., and Gingell, D.,** Measurement and modification of forces between lecithin bilayers, *Biophys. J.,* 18, 209, 1977.

37. **Parsegian, V. A., Rand, R. P., Fuller, N. L., and Rau, D. C.,** Osmotic stress of the direct measurement of intermolecular forces, *Methods Enzymol.,* 127, 400, 1986.

38. **King, G. I. and Worthington, C. R.,** Analytic continuation as a method of phase determination, *Phys. Lett. A,* 35, 259, 1971.

39. **Torbet, J. and Wilkins, M. H. F.,** X-ray diffraction studies of lecithin bilayers, *J. Theor. Biol.,* 62, 447, 1976.

40. **Lesslauer, W., Cain, J. E., and Blasie, J. K.,** X-ray diffraction studies of lecithin bimolecular leaflets with incorporated fluorescent probes, *Proc. Natl. Acad. Sci. U.S.A.,* 69, 1499, 1972.

41. **Wilkins, M. H. F., Blaurock, A. E., and Engelman, D. M.,** Bilayer structure in membranes, *Nature (London) New Biol.,* 230, 72, 1971.

42. **Wilkinson, D. A. and Nagle, J. F.,** Dilatometry and calorimetry of saturated phosphatidylethanolamine dispersions, *Biochemistry,* 20, 187, 1981.

43. **McIntosh, T. J.,** Differences in hydrocarbon chain tilt between hydrated phosphatidylethanolamine and phosphatidylcholine bilayers: a molecular packing model, *Biophys. J.,* 29, 237, 1980.

44. **Janiak, M. J., Small, D. M., and Shipley, G. G.,** Temperature and compositional dependence of the structure of hydrated dimyristoyl lecithin, *J. Biol. Chem.,* 254, 6068, 1979.

45. **Reiss-Husson, F.,** Structure des phases liquide-cristallines de differents phospholipides, monoglycerides, sphingolipides, anhydres ou en presence d'eau, *J. Mol. Biol.,* 25, 363, 1967.

46. **Simon, S. A., McIntosh, T. J., and Latorre, R.,** The influence of cholesterol on water penetration into bilayers, *Science,* 216, 65, 1982.

47. **McIntosh, T. J., Simon, S. A., and Dilger, J. F.,** Location of the water-hydrocarbon interface in lipid bilayers, in *Water Transport in Biological Membranes,* Benga, G., Ed., CRC Press, Boca Raton, FL, in press.
48. **McDaniel, R. V. and McIntosh, T. J.,** X-ray diffraction studies of the cholera toxin receptor, GM1, *Biophys. J.,* 49, 94, 1986.
49. **Sillerud, L. O., Prestegard, J. H., Yu, R. K., Schafer, D. E., and Konigsberg, W. H.,** Assignment of the C nuclear magnetic resonance spectrum of aqueous ganglioside GM1 micelles, *Biochemistry,* 17, 2619, 1978.
50. **Hall, J. E. and Simon, S. A.,** A simple model for calcium induced exocytosis, *Biochim. Biophys. Acta,* 436, 613, 1976.
51. **Franks, N. P.,** Structural analysis of hydrated egg lecithin and cholesterol bilayers. I. X-ray diffraction, *J. Mol. Biol.,* 100, 345, 1976.
52. **Jain, M. K.,** Role of cholesterol in biomembranes and related systems, in *Current Topics in Membranes and Ion Transport,* Vol. 6, Bronner, R. and Kleinzeller, A., Eds., Academic Press, New York, 1975, 1.
53. **Cohen, B. E.,** The premeability of liposomes to nonelectrolytes. II, *J. Membrane Biol.,* 20, 235, 1975.
54. **Kwok, R. and Evans, E.,** Thermoelasticity of large lecithin bilayer vesicles, *Biophys. J.,* 35, 637, 1981.
55. **McIntosh, T. J., Magid, A. D., and Simon, S. A.,** Steric repulsion between phosphatidylcholine bilayers, *Biochemistry,* in press.

Chapter 1.B.2

PREFERRED CONFORMATION OF THE DIACYLGLYCEROL MOIETY OF PHOSPHOLIPIDS

H. Hauser, I. Pascher, and S. Sundell

TABLE OF CONTENTS

I. INTRODUCTION

Long-chain phospholipids are amphiphiles that are practically insoluble in water and have a great tendency to form regular aggregates. These are usually referred to as phases comprising structures such as bilayers (smetic phase), cylinders (hexagonal phases), and more complex three-dimensional networks (cubic phases). Phospholipids are important constituents of biological membranes; there is now unambiguous evidence that phospholipids are present as bilayer structures in these membranes. For this reason, the physicochemical properties of lipid bilayers have been the subject of extensive studies. The knowledge of the structure and dynamics of phospholipids in bilayers and biological membranes is a prerequisite for an understanding of their functional role. Information pertinent to structural (conformational) and dynamic properties of lipids in bilayers has been derived mainly from X-ray diffraction studies, in particular single-crystal analyses, and spectroscopic methods such as nuclear magnetic resonance (NMR), electron spin resonance (ESR), infrared (IR), and Raman and fluorescence spectroscopy.

This chapter is addressed to the question of whether or not the diacyl (dialkyl) glycerol group of glycerophospholipids adopts preferred conformations. To shed light on this question, existing single-crystal structures of glycerophospholipid and related relevant compounds will be summarized and discussed. The solid state structures serve as a reference and give insight into possible energy-minimum conformations of the diacylglycerol part. Next we ask the question whether the diacylglycerol group of glycerophospholipids maintains one or more preferred conformations in the liquid crystalline state which is a highly dynamic state with rapid molecular and segmental motion. The latter comprise fast oscillations and isomerizations about C–C and C–O bonds of the hydrocarbon chains and various bonds of the lipid polar group. Any preferred conformation present in the liquid crystalline state would have to be compatible with the dynamics of this state.

II. STRUCTURAL AND CONFORMATIONAL NOTATION

The atom numbering and notation for torsion angles used here are shown in Figure 1.[1,2] For reasons discussed in a previous review,[1] this atom numbering is better suited for the discussion of phospholipid and sphingolipid conformation than the stereospecific numbering widely used in biochemical work. The glycerol backbone is regarded as the central part of the glycerophospholipid molecule and its C atoms are numbered C(1), C(2), and C(3). The atom numbering is such that the polar group or α-chain (with torsion angles α) is attached to C atom C(1) of the glycerol group; the two hydrocarbon chains designated β- and γ-chain are linked through ester or ether bonds to atoms C(2) and C(3), respectively (see Figure 1). The first numeral of the atom number is 1, 2, or 3 referring to the α-, β-, or γ-chain, respectively; the second numeral is the running number of the C and O atoms of the chain. The torsion angles of the three substituent chains α, β, and γ are denoted α_n, β_n, and γ_n, respectively, with n increasing along each chain, starting from the glycerol backbone (see Figure 1). The torsion angles we will be concerned with in this paper are defined in Table 1. For describing approximate conformations of two substituents about a C–C bond, i.e., for defining torsion angle ranges, the conformational notation of Klyne and Prelog[3] is used (Table 2). Other structural parameters we shall make use of in this article are depicted in Figure 2. (For details, see Reference 1.)

Chain stacking, i.e., the parallel alignment of hydrocarbon chains, is a fundamental property of lipid aggregates (lipid phases). This is true for lipids with one hydrocarbon chain and also for lipid molecules with two and more hydrocarbon chains. With the former class of lipids, the result is intermolecular chain stacking; with the latter, both intra- and intermolecular chain stacking occur. The driving forces behind chain stacking are van der Waals' forces and hydrophobic interactions leading to a significant gain in free energy. It is this

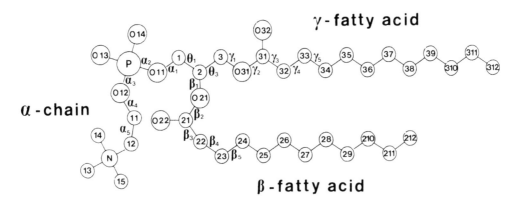

γ-fatty acid

α-chain

β-fatty acid

FIGURE 1.   Atom numbering and notation for torsion angles.[2]

TABLE 1
Notation for Torsion Angles

θ_1	O(11)–C(1)–C(2)–C(3)	β_1	C(1)–C(2)–O(21)–C(21)
θ_2	O(11)–C(1)–C(2)–O(21)	β_2	C(2)–O(21)–C(21)–C(22)
θ_3	C(1)–C(2)–C(3)–O(31)	β_3	O(21)–C(21)–C(22)–C(23)
θ_4	O(21)–C(2)–C(3)–O(31)	β_4	C(21)–C(22)–C(23)–C(24)
		β_5	C(22)–C(23)–C(24)–C(25)
α_1	C(2)–C(1)–O(11)–P	γ_1	C(2)–C(3)–O(31)–C(31)
α_2	C(1)–O(11)–P–O(12)	γ_2	C(3)–O(31)–C(31)–C(32)
α_3	O(11)–P–O(12)–C(11)	γ_3	O(31)–C(31)–C(32)–C(33)
α_4	P–O(12)–C(11)–C(12)	γ_4	C(31)–C(32)–C(33)–C(34)
α_5	O(12)–C(11)–C(12)–N	γ_5	C(32)–C(33)–C(34)–C(35)
α_6	C(11)–C(12)–N–C(13)		

Note: For atom numbering, see Figure 1.

TABLE 2
Notation for Torsion Angle Ranges According
to Klyne and Prelog[3]

Torsion angle range	Notation
$0 \pm 30°$	Synperiplanar (sp)
$+60 \pm 30°$	+ Synclinal (sc) or + gauche
$+120 \pm 30°$	+ Anticlinal (ac)
$180 \pm 30°$	Antiperiplanar (ap)
$+240 \pm 30°$ or $-120 \pm 30°$	− Anticlinal
$+300 \pm 30°$ or $-60 \pm 30°$	− Synclinal

Note: Abbreviations are in parenthesis.

gain in free energy due to van der Waals' and hydrophobic forces that is also responsible for the insolubility of lipids in H_2O and their great tendency to aggregate in this solvent.

Since the two fatty acyl chains of diacylglycerophospholipids are bound to the C(2) and C(3) atoms of the glycerol group, chain stacking of diacylglycerophospholipids is expected to result in a preferred conformation about the C(2) – C(3) glycerol bond. The conformation about this bond is defined by torsion angles θ_3 = C(1)–C(2)–C(3)–O(31) or θ_4 = O(21)–C(2)–C(3)–O(31) (see Table 1). The three possible staggered conformations of the C(2)–C(3) glycerol bond and the corresponding values of torsion angles θ_3 and θ_4 are given in Figure 3. The torsion angles θ_3 and θ_4 describing the conformation of the C(2)–C(3)

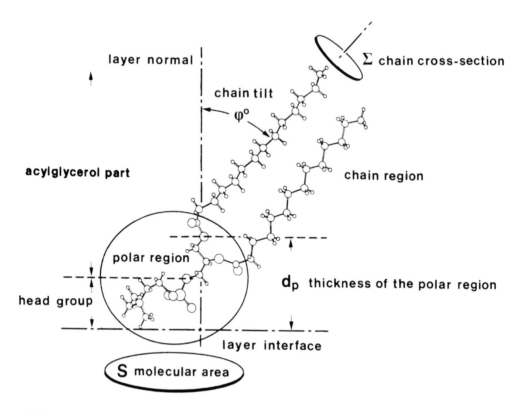

FIGURE 2.   Illustration of structural notation. A phosphatidylcholine molecule is used to define various segments of the phospholipid molecule: φ, angle of tilt between the hydrocarbon chain axis and the bilayer normal; Σ, cross-sectional area of the hydrocarbon chain projected onto a plane perpendicular to the chain axis; S, molecular area at the layer interface.[2]

glycerol bond are interrelated as shown in this figure. The torsion angle θ_4 determines the relative orientation of the two oxygen atoms O(21) and O(31) (hatched) linked to glycerol C(2) and C(3), respectively. Torsion angle θ_4 and thus the relative orientation of the two oxygens is +sc, −sc, and ap in rotamers A, B, and C, respectively (see Figure 3). Rotamer A is converted into B by a counterclockwise rotation of 120° about the C(2)–C(3) bond as shown by the arrow in Figure 3A, and rotamer B is converted into C by the same kind of rotation (see arrow in Figure 3B). In rotamers A and B, the relative orientations of the two oxygens, O(21) and O(31), on the C(2)–C(3) glycerol bond are ±sc, respectively, and hence these two rotamers will be referred to as sc or *gauche* rotamers. In rotamer C, $\theta_4 =$ ap and so is the relative orientation of the two oxygens O(21) and O(31) to which the hydrocarbon chains are attached. As rotation proceeds about the C(2)–C(3) bond and O(31) moves relative to O(21), the γ-chain moves relative to the β-chain (see Figure 3). Bonds within the γ-chain are rearranged (see Figure 3) so that the parallel alignment of the two hydrocarbon chains is warranted. Whatever the rearrangement in the γ-chain (for details see Section IV), the two hydrocarbon chains will be further apart in the ap rotamer (see Figure 3C) than in the two sc rotamers A and B.

The three staggered conformations of minimum free energy about the second glycerol C–C bond are shown in Figure 4. The conformation about the C(1)–C(2) glycerol bond is determined by torsion angle θ_1 and related to it torsion angle θ_2. The latter determines the relative orientation of oxygen O(11) attached to glycerol C(1) and oxygen O(21) attached to glycerol C(2). The torsion angle θ_2 is +sc, −sc, and ap in rotamers A, B, and C, respectively. It is clear from Figure 4, by changing torsion angle θ_2 and keeping the dia-

Rotamers about the glycerol C(2)–C(3) bond

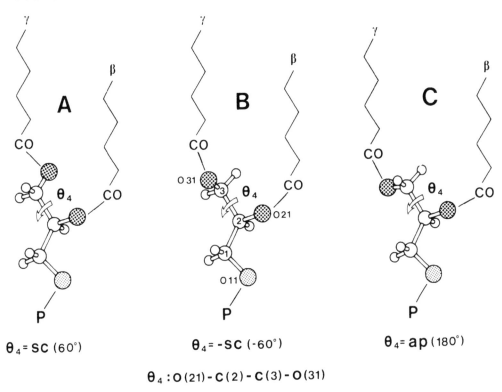

$\theta_4 = SC\,(60°)$ $\theta_4 = -SC\,(-60°)$ $\theta_4 = ap\,(180°)$

$\theta_4 : O\,(21) - C\,(2) - C\,(3) - O\,(31)$

FIGURE 3. Ball and stick models of the three staggered conformations A, B, and C of the glycerol C(2)–C(3) bond of phospholipids.[29] For atom numbering and notation of torsion angles, see Figure 1. The torsion angles θ_4 determines the relative orientation of the two ester or ether oxygens O(21) and O(31) (hatched) on glycerol C(2) and C(3), respectively. Torsion angle θ_4 is +sc, −sc, and ap in rotamers A, B, and C, respectively. The oxygen O(11) (stippled) to which the phosphate is attached is drawn downward. The arrow at torsion angle θ_4 (rotamer A) marks a counterclockwise rotation by 240° about the C(2)–C(3) bond necessary to convert rotamer A into rotamer B. Arrows at θ_4 of rotamers B and C have analogous meaning.[29]

cylglycerol part of the molecule stationary, that the orientation of the polar head group changes relative to the diacyl-C(2)–C(3) part of the molecule.

III. X-RAY SINGLE-CRYSTAL STRUCTURES

Conformations represented by single-crystal structures can be regarded as minimum free energy conformations. All single-crystal structures of glycerophospholipids available to date and some related compounds relevant to the discussion that follows are summarized in Table 3. As regards the conformation of the C(2)–C(3) glycerol bond, the existing single-crystal structures can be divided into two classes, the first one denoted by A is characterized by torsion angles θ_3/θ_4 = ap/sc consistent with rotamer A (see Figure 3A). The second class denoted by B is characterized by torsion angles θ_3/θ_4 = +sc/−sc consistent with rotamer B (Figure 3B). There are a total of 17 single-crystal structures in class I with θ_3/θ_4 = ap/ sc; torsion angle θ_3 is ap, ranging from 166 to −164°, and torsion angle θ_4 is +sc, ranging from 44 to 79° (see Table 3). There are three single-crystal structures of sphingolipids[8,13,14] and one of dilauroylphosphatidic acid[17] which all have θ_3/θ_4 = ap/sc and which are not included in Table 3. There are relatively few structures belonging to class II with θ_3 = +sc (range 45 to 78°) and θ_4 = −sc (range of −51 to −63°). In both classes of single-crystal

Rotamers about Glycerol C(1) – C(2) bond

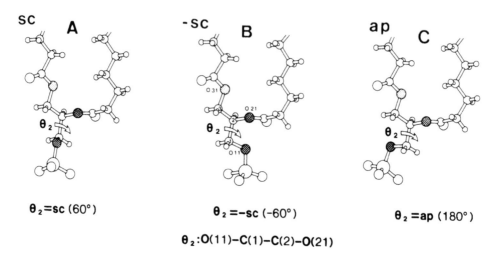

θ_2:O(11)–C(1)–C(2)–O(21)

FIGURE 4. Ball and stick models of the three staggered conformations A, B, and C of the glycerol C(1)–C(2) bond of phospholipids. For atom numbering and notation of torsion angles, see Figure 1. The torsion angle θ_2 determines the relative orientation of the ester oxygen O(11) and the ester (ether) oxygen O(21) (hatched) on glycerol C(1) and C(2), respectively. Torsion angle θ_2 is +sc, –sc, and ap in rotamers A, B, and C, respectively. The arrow at torsion angle θ_2 (rotamer A) indicates a clockwise rotation by 120° about the C(1)–C(2) bond required to convert rotamer A into rotamer B. Arrows associated with θ_2 in rotamers B and C have analogous meaning.

structures, θ_4 is either +sc or –sc. This torsion angle range apparently facilitates the parallel alignment of the two hydrocarbon chains. In contrast, the conformation with θ_4 = ap, where the two oxygen atoms on C(2) and C(3) are in an ap arrangement, is difficult to reconcile with chain stacking and intramolecular close contacts between the two hydrocarbon chains. Therefore this conformation (rotamer C, Figure 3C) is energetically unfavorable for lipids with long hydrocarbon chains.

As can be seen from Table 3, there are some single-crystal structures consistent with rotamer C, i.e., with θ_3/θ_4 = –sc/ap. However, these are single-crystal structures of constituent molecules of glycerophospholipids which lack hydrocarbon chains and hence θ_4 is not restricted by chain stacking requirements. To this group of compounds belong D-glycero-1-phosphocholine and D-glycero-1-phosphoethanolamine. On the other hand, the CdCl$_2$ complex of D-glycero-1-phosphocholine has the conformation θ_3/θ_4 = sc/–sc consistent with rotamer B. There is, however, no single-crystal structure of a long-chain lipid in which the torsion angle pair θ_3/θ_4 is –sc/ap (rotamer C, Figure 3C) and in which the normal type of parallel chain stacking occurs. Two sphingolipids, however, have been shown to crystallize as rotamer C[23,24] (see Table 3). In both cases, an unusual chain stacking mode is observed. In single crystals of glucosylphytosphingosine,[23] which corresponds structurally to a lysophospholipid, the hydrocarbon chains are packed head to tail. In this way, a fully interdigitated hydrocarbon chain stacking mode is produced and two hydrocarbon chains are accommodated per glucose residue.[23] In the single-crystal structure of N-tetracosanoylphytosphingosine,[24] the lipid molecule is V shaped with the two hydrocarbon chains pointing in opposite directions. This chain stacking mode is unique and a consequence of θ_4 = ap. Apparently, θ_4 = ap does not allow the normal type of parallel chain stacking observed with glycerophospholipids. In the single-crystal structure of N-tetracosanoylphytosphingosine,[24] the tetracosanoyl chains are arranged in one layer and the phytosphingosine chains are arranged in the opposite layer. The direction of the hydrocarbon chains in the two layers thus formed alternates in a herringbone pattern.

Table 3
TORSION ANGLES[a] OF SINGLE-CRYSTAL STRUCTURES OF MEMBRANE LIPIDS AND CONSTITUENT MOLECULES OF LIPIDS[b]

Compound[c]	Rotamer	θ_1	θ_2	θ_3	θ_4	β_1	β_2	β_3	β_4	γ_1	γ_2	γ_3	γ_4	Ref.
BrUG 1	A_γ	180	−79	174	53					164	172	−175	−178	9
BrUG 2	A_γ	172	−76	177	68					105	162	175	177	9
Deoxy HPA 1	A_γ	179		176						176	180	−178	−177	10
Deoxy HPA 2	A_γ	180		174						178	177	174	176	10
LPA^{2-}	A_γ	170	−54	177	65					−144	−176	160	173	11
PPE	A_γ	−57	70	−173	55					−170	176	164	177	4
OMPC	A_γ	−53	66	−164	79	150				−179	174	−179	−179	5
DLPE	A_γ	−52	65	−172	69	97	179	−119	65	−178	173	179	−171	6,7
DMPC 1	A_γ	58	177	−178	63	82	172	−81	45	−177	168	−173	178	12
DMPC 2	A_γ	168	−80	166	51	120	179	−134	67	102	176	180	180	12
DLG	A_β	−55	61	173	54	110	170	−159	176	91	180	65	180	15
DMPA$^-$	A_β	−54	62	−179	62	87	172	164	179	−142	180	−119	73	16
1 GPC · Cdcl₂	B	171	−72	59	−60									21
2 Deoxy LPC	B_γ	28		78						156	176	−175	178	19
3 DBrUG-pTS	B_γ	171	−61	60	−51	—			—	—	—	—	—	22
4 DLPEM₂	B_γ	176	−66	56	−60	148	173	−57	176	129	−167	166	175	18
5 DMPG−B	B_γ	71	179	45	−58	157	180	−50	−175	122	179	142	154	20
6 DMPG−A	B_β	151	−78	64	−63	159	178	177	−179	164	−170	110	−57	20
GPE	C	166	−89	−67	180									26

Table 3 (continued)
TORSION ANGLES[a] OF SINGLE-CRYSTAL STRUCTURES OF MEMBRANE LIPIDS AND CONSTITUENT MOLECULES OF LIPIDS[b]

Compound[a]	Rotamer	θ_1	θ_2	θ_3	θ_4	β_1	β_2	β_3	β_4	γ_1	γ_2	γ_3	γ_4	Ref.
GPC 1	C	172	−71	−63	<u>180</u>									25
GPC 2	C	−63	61	<u>−69</u>	<u>169</u>									25
Glc-PSp	C	75	−153	<u>−46</u>	<u>−175</u>					−173	−171	−158	180	24
24-PSp	C	−163	−51	<u>−71</u>	<u>179</u>	127	173	−147	−175	−175	57	−178	179	23

[a] The single-crystal structures presented are ordered in three groups (A, B, and C) according to their conformation about the C(2)–C(3) glycerol group (torsion angles θ_3 and θ_4). The torsion angles presented determine the conformation of the glycerol group and the parallel alignment of the hydrocarbon chains. If there are two crystallographically independent molecules present in the unit cell, they are designated by the numerals 1 and 2.

[b] Key to abbreviations:

BrUG 1, BrUG 2   3-(11-Bromoundecanoyl)-D-glycerol
DBrUG-pTS   2,3-(Di-11-bromoundecanoyl)-DL-glycero-3-(p-toluene-sulfonate)
DLG   2,3-Dilauroyl-D-glycerol
DLPE   2,3-Dilauroyl-DL-glycero-1-phosphoethanolamine
DLPEM₂   2,3-Dilauroyl-DL-glycero-1-phospho-N,N-dimethylethanolamine
DMPA⁻   Monosodium 2,3-dimyristoyl-D-glycero-1-phosphate
DMPC   2,3-Dimyristoyl-D-glycero-1-phosphocholine
DMPG⁻-A, DMPG⁻-B   2,3-Dimyristoyl-D-glycero-phospho-DL-glycerol
DeoxyHPA1, deoxyHPA2   3-Hexadecyl-deoxyglycero-1-phosphoric acid monohydrate
DeoxyLPC   3-Lauroyl-deoxyglycero-1-phosphocholine (an alternative name is 3-lauroylpropanediol-1-phosphocholine.)
Glc-PSp   Glucosylphytosphingosine[1-O-(β-D-glucopyranosyl)-D-ribo-3,4-dihydroxy-2-aminooctadecane] · HBr
GPC 1, GPC 2   D-Glycero-1-phosphocholine
GPC · CdCl₂   CdCl₂ complex of D-glycero-1-phosphocholine
GPE   D-Glycero-1-phosphoethanolamine
LPA²⁻   Disodium 3-lauroyl-DL-glycero-1-phosphate
OMPC   3-Octadecyl-2-methyl-D-glycero-1-phosphocholine monohydrate
PPE   3-Palmitoyl-DL-glycero-1-phosphoethanolamine
24-PSp   N-Tetracosanoylphytosphingosine [D-ribo-1,3,4,-trihydroxy-2-tetracosanoylamidooctadecane]

From an inspection of Table 3, it is clear that in single-crystal structures of lipids, there are not only two types of minimum free energy conformations about the C(2)–C(3) glycerol bond (represented by rotamers A and B), but each rotamer can be subdivided into two groups. These two subgroups differ in the chain stacking mode designated by β and γ. These letters are used as subscripts to capitals A and B. A_β indicates that the conformation of the C(2)–C(3) bond is that of rotamer A and that the β-chain is straight, i.e., extending in an almost perfect, continuous zigzag from the glycerol backbone. The torsion angles along this chain are close to ap. The second hydrocarbon chain is initially oriented layer-parallel and undergoes an approximately 90° bend at its second C atom. A_γ stands for the conformation of the A rotamer (see Figure 3) and for the γ-chain forming a continuous zigzag with torsion angles close to ap. What is said for A_β and A_γ regarding the hydrocarbon chain packing is also applicable to the B rotamer. In the second column of Table 3, this notation is used to classify existing single-crystal structures. Representative single-crystal structures of the two subgroups of rotamers A and B are presented in Figure 5. It can be seen that the two subgroups differ in the mode of chain stacking and also in the orientation of the glycerol group with respect to the bilayer plane. The two subgroups of rotamer A are represented by dimyristoylphosphatidylcholine[12] and dilauroylphosphatidic acid,[35] corresponding to the A_γ and A_β structure, respectively. In dimyristoylphosphatidylcholine as A_γ, the γ-chain is oriented approximately perpendicular to the bilayer plane forming a continuous zigzag with the glycerol group. The β-chain of this molecule is initially oriented layer-parallel and at the second carbon atom C(22) there is a 90° bend so that from C(22) onward this chain becomes parallel to the γ-chain (Figure 5). The torsion angles in the β-chain (β_1 to β_4) responsible for the 90° bend are marked in Table 3. (For a detailed discussion, see Hauser et al.[2]) The single-crystal structure of dimyristoylphosphatidylcholine is therefore designated A_γ to indicate that we are dealing with the A rotamer and that the γ-chain forms a straight zigzag. This packing mode is contrasted by that of the two hydrocarbon chains of dilauroylphosphatidic acid. In this case, the β-chain extends in a straight zigzag from the glycerol atom C(2). The γ-chain is initially oriented in a layer-parallel way and at C atom C(32) the γ-chain makes a 90° bend (see Figure 5, bottom left). The torsion angles in the γ-chain producing the 90° bend are γ_3 and γ_4. The structure of dilauroylphosphatidic acid is therefore designated as A_β. Dimyristoylphosphatidylcholine and dilauroylsphosphatidic acid differ in a further structural detail; in the former crystal structure, the orientation of the glycerol group is approximately perpendicular with respect to the bilayer plane while in the crystal structure of dilauroylphosphatidic acid, the glycerol group has a coplanar orientation (cf. the two structures, top and bottom on the left-hand side of Figure 5). It should be stressed that there is this difference in the orientation of the glycerol group although there is no difference in the conformation of the C(2)–C(3) glycerol bond: in both single-crystal structures, the conformation is θ_3/θ_4 = ap/sc (cf. Table 3).

The two subgroups of rotamer B are represented by the single-crystal structures of N-methyl substituted dilauroylphosphatidylethanolamine and dimyristoylphosphatidylglycerol (see Figure 5, right-hand side). In the single-crystal structure of the former, the γ-chain extends almost straight from the C(3) atom of glycerol with a minor twist about the C(3)–O(31) bond (γ_1 = 129°, cf. Table 3). The β-chain produces a 60° bend at C atom C(22), with torsion angle β_3 (defining the C(21)–C(22) bond) deviating significantly from ap: β_3 = −57°. The 60° bend ensures the parallel alignment of the two hydrocarbon chains. This single-crystal structure is therefore denoted B_γ, indicating that we are dealing with the B rotamer (θ_3/θ_4 = sc/−sc) and that the γ-chain forms a straight zigzag. In contrast, the chain stacking mode of dimyristoylphosphatidylglycerol is such that the β-chain extends straight from the glycerol backbone, while the γ-chain makes a 90° bend at C atom C(32). This is evident from a comparison of the top and bottom structure on the right-hand side of Figure 5. The single-crystal structure of dimyristoylphosphatidylglycerol is therefore denoted B_β, β indicating that the β-chain forms a straight zigzag. The structure B_β can be envisaged to

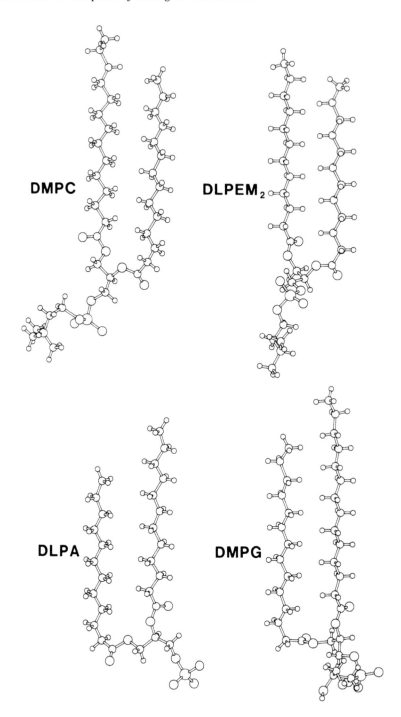

FIGURE 5.   Molecular conformation of four single-crystal structures, DMPC,[12] DLPA,[35] DLPEM$_2$,[18] and DMPG.[20] The key to the abbreviations is given in the legends to Table 3. The four selected single-crystal structures represent possible conformations about the C(2)–C(3) glycerol bond and related to it possible chain stacking modes.[29] DMPC and DLPA are representative of rotamer A; DLPEM$_2$ and DMPG are representative of rotamer B. Structural details are discussed in the text.

evolve from B_γ by a counterclockwise rotation about the C(2)–C(3) glycerol bond. By such a rotation, the C(2)–O(21) bond becomes layer-normal, while the C(3)–O(31) bond attains a layer-parallel orientation (cf. B_γ and B_β structure in Figure 5). It should be stressed that both B rotamers shown in Figure 5 have similar orientations of the glycerol group with respect to the bilayer plane: the glycerol group is inclined by about 45°. From the different single-crystal structures presented in Figure 5, it can be concluded that the orientation of the glycerol group with respect to the bilayer plane is independent of the conformation of the C(2)–C(3) bond (defined by θ_3 and θ_4). It can vary between a bilayer-normal and a bilayer-parallel orientation.

IV. THE CONFORMATION AND MOTION OF PHOSPHOLIPIDS IN THE LIQUID CRYSTALLINE FORM

Considering that lipid bilayers of intact and functional biological membranes are fully hydrated and in the liquid crystalline state, the question of the biological relevance of single-crystal structures discussed above arises. It is well known that the transition of lipid bilayers from the crystal and gel state to the liquid crystalline state is accompanied by an increase in enthalpy and entropy. The lipid bilayer takes up heat at the transition temperature and the static state of the crystal is converted into the highly dynamic state of the liquid crystal. Above the crystal-to-liquid crystal transition temperature, the phospholipid undergoes both molecular and segmental motions which have been described in some detail by spectroscopic methods. The knowledge of the structure and dynamics of phospholipids in fully hydrated, liquid crystalline bilayers is essential for an understanding of the functional role these lipids play in biological membranes. The discussion of this part of the paper is addressed to two questions. Firstly, in the highly dynamic state of fully hydrated, liquid crystalline bilayers are there one or several, coexisting preferred conformations? Secondly, if there are several coexisting conformations that are in dynamic equilibrium, is it possible to say something about the type of motions involved in conformational transitions? Although the phospholipid molecule is considered as a whole, special attention is paid to the diacylglycerol part. Information pertinent to the questions outlined above has been derived from spectroscopic techniques, above all from different NMR methods that have been applied making good use of different nuclei such as ^1H, ^{13}C, ^{31}P, and ^2H.

The question of the preferred conformation of the diacylglycerol group of phospholipids has been tackled by measuring vicinal spin-coupling constants.[27-29] For instance, the vicinal proton spin coupling constants[3] $J_{H1\ H2}$ of the H_1–C–C–H_2 bond depend on the nature of the substituents of the C–C bond and the torsion angle of this bond. It has been discussed before how conformational information can be extracted from vicinal spin-spin coupling.[28-30] One disadvantage of this approach is that the method is restricted to small aggregates such as micelles. A prerequisite for the application of this method is that well-resolved high-resolution NMR spectra must be obtained with lines narrow enough so that spin-spin coupling constants can be derived. Only small aggregate structures such as micelles or reversed micelles with diameters of ≤10 nm fulfill this condition. For instance, the resonances from small unilamellar vesicles with a diameter of ~20 nm give lines that are too broad to exhibit spin-spin interactions. The method is therefore limited to short-chain diacylphospholipids and lysophospholipids known to form small micelles in aqueous dispersions at temperatures above the critical micellar temperature, i.e., in the liquid crystalline state. The advantage of the method is that it can be applied to monomeric solutions and that the effects of changing the solvent and the experimental conditions can be readily monitored. For a detailed discussion of the assumptions involved in the derivation of fractional populations of the three staggered rotamers about a C–C bond, the reader is referred to Hauser et al.[27-29] Table 4 summarizes the results for the C(2)–C(3) glycerol bond and hence the diacylglycerol part of different

TABLE 4

The Three Staggered Conformations of Minimum Free Energy (Rotamers A to C, Figure 3) about the C(2)–C(3) Glycerol Bond of Different Phospholipids[29]

Compound	Rotamer population (%)			Experimental conditions
	A	**B**	**C**	
2,3-Dihexanoyl-*D*-glycero-1-	62	38	1	In ^2H_2O, >CMC
phosphocholine	52	42	6	In^2H_2O, <CMC
2,3-Dihexanoyl-*D*-glycero-1-	63	37	1	In ^2H_2O, pH 6.0, >CMC
phosphoethanolamine	68	32	0	In ^2H_2O, pH 9.3, >CMC
	55	38	7.5	In ^2H_2O, pH 6.0, <CMC
2,3-Di-*O*-hexyl-*D*-glycero-1-	49	44	6.5	In ^2H_2O, >CMC
phosphocholine	38—48	42—47	10—15	In^2H_2O, <CMC
2,3-Dihexanoyl-*D*-glycero-1-phospho-*L*-	62	38	1	In ^2H_2O, >CMC
serine ammonium salt	55	39	6.5	In^2H_2O, <CMC
2,3-Dipalmitoyl-DL-glycero-1-	52	40	7.5	In $C^2HCl_3/C^2H_3O^2H$, 2:1 (v/v)
phosphocholine				
2,3-Dipalmitoyl-DL-glycero-1-	51	38	11	In $C^2HCl_3/C^2H_3O^2H$, 2:1 (v/v)
phosphoethanolamine				
2,3-Dipalmitoyl-*D*-glycero-1-phospho-L-	55	38	6.5	In $C^2HCl_3/C^2H_3O^2H$, 4:3 (v/v)
serine				
Egg lysophosphatidylcholine	48	41	11	In ^2H_2O, >CMC
3-Myristoyl-*D*-glycero-1-phosphocholine	46	36	18	In ^2H_2O, >CMC
3-Lauroyl-D-glycerol-1-phosphate diso-	45	36	19	In ^2H_2O, >CMC
dium salt				
3-Lauroylpropanediol-1-phosphocholine	36	32	32	In ^2H_2O, >CMC
	33	33	33	In $C^2H_3O^2H$

phospholipids. Different short-chain diacylphospholipids and lysophospholipids were used in this study, including phosphatidylcholines, phosphatidylethanolamines, phosphatidylserines, and phosphatidic acids.[29] The results are expressed in terms of fractional populations (percent) of rotamers A, B, and C (cf. Figure 3 and Table 4). From an inspection of this table, it is clear that there are essentially two possible conformations about the C(2)–C(3) glycerol bond. The two preferred conformations are rotamer A (θ_3/θ_4 = ap/sc) and rotamer B (θ_3/θ_4 = +sc/−sc). It is interesting to note that similar to the single-crystal structures of membrane lipids (see Table 3) the dominant population is rotamer A (cf. Table 4). This is true for all diacylphospholipids studied regardless of whether the phospholipids are present as monomers or micelles. It is also seen from Table 4 that rotamer C is practically absent in micelles of diacylphospholipids indicating that this rotamer is energetically unfavorable. As pointed out in the discussion of single-crystal structures, in rotamer C the two oxygens to which the hydrocarbon chains are linked are ap and hence the parallel alignment of the two hydrocarbon chains with close intramolecular contacts is not readily accomplished. In this context it is worth noting that the coexistence of two conformations about the C(2)–C(3) bond is also consistent with minimum free energy calculations.[33] These calculations yield two conformations of about the same free energy identical to those of rotamer A and B.

The parallel alignment of the two hydrocarbon chains is preserved even in the monomeric state. Intramolecular chain stacking is energetically favorable because it probably optimizes both van der Waals' and hydrophobic interactions. Comparing the results of diacylphospholipid dispersions in H_2O below and above the critical micellar concentration, it is clear from Table 4 that in the monomeric state the populations of rotamers B and C are increased at the expense of rotamer A. However, even in the monomeric state, the population of rotamer C is still usually less than 10%.

It is surprising that rotamers A and B are also predominant in lysophospholipid micelles, though the population of rotamer C appears to be increased to about 10 to 20% (see Table

4). Lysophospholipids have a single hydrocarbon chain per molecule, usually attached to the glycerol C(3) atom, hence intramolecular chain stacking cannot come into play. Without further conformational constraints imposed on the C(2)–C(3) glycerol bond, one would expect greater flexibility about this bond. This is indeed the case for 3-lauroylpropanediol-1-phosphocholine in different solvents (see Table 4). In this case, all three staggered rotamers (A to C) are equally populated; there is apparently no preference for either of the three rotamers; instead there is probably free rotation about the two C–C bonds of propanediol. The only structural difference between lysoglycerophospholipids and 3-lauroylpropanediol-1-phosphocholine is the free OH group on C(2) of the lysophospholipids. This structural difference could account for the observed difference in behavior. The free OH-group may participate in an inter- or intramolecular hydrogen bond, thus stabilizing rotamers A and/or B.

The NMR method based on spin-spin interactions also gives dynamic information: NMR indicates that the exchange rate between different rotamers is fast on the NMR time scale. This means that in the liquid crystalline state, the phospholipid molecule switches rapidly between the possible staggered rotamers about the C(2)–C(3) bond. Therefore, the results discussed above suggest that phospholipids in the fully hydrated, liquid crystalline state switch rapidly back and forth between essentially two conformations, rotamer A (with θ_3/θ_4 = ap/sc) and rotamer B (with θ_3/θ_4 = $+$sc/$-$sc).

Comparing the NMR results with the single-crystal structures discussed in the previous section of this chapter, it is clear that in the fully hydrated, liquid crystalline state of phospholipids, there are two minimum free energy conformations about the C(2)–C(3) glycerol bond. These two conformations corresponding to rotamers A and B are the same as the two conformations prevailing in single-crystal structures of membrane lipids. As pointed out above, these are conformations in which the two ester (ether) oxygens O(21) and O(31) on glycerol C atoms C(2) and C(3), respectively, are $\pm$sc with respect to each other allowing for the parallel alignment of the two hydrocarbon chains.

It is clear from an inspection of Figure 5 that a conformational change from rotamer A to B must be coupled to conformational changes in the C–O and C–C bonds of both hydrocarbon chains in order to maintain the parallel alignment of the two hydrocarbon chains. The details of these kinds of conformational changes occurring in the liquid crystalline state of phospholipid bilayers are unknown. The single-crystal structures listed in Table 3 may be used to provide us with a clue as to these conformational changes. Figure 6 is used to read off the conformational changes involved in the two hydrocarbon chains upon transitions $A_\gamma \rightleftharpoons B_\gamma \rightleftharpoons B_\beta \rightleftharpoons A_\gamma$ (see Figure 6). It has to be borne in mind that these conformational changes do not represent real changes occurring in liquid crystalline phospholipid bilayers. These are proposed changes derived from single-crystal structures. They may be regarded as minimal changes required to maintain the parallel alignment of the hydrocarbon chains. For instance, Figure 6 may be used together with Table 3 in the following way: the conformational changes accompanying the transition $A_\gamma \rightleftharpoons B_\gamma$ are marked by small arrows inserted into rotamer A_γ (see Figure 6, top left). The transition involves primarily a change in θ_3 from ap to $+$sc and θ_4 from $+$sc to $-$sc. This change in torsion angles θ_3/θ_4 is produced by an anticlockwise rotation by 120° of the entire γ-chain about the C(2)–C(3) glycerol bond of rotamer A (see small arrow about the C(2)–C(3) bond in A_γ, Figure 6, top left). As a result of such an anticlockwise rotation about the C(2)–C(3) glycerol bond, the two hydrocarbon chains are no longer aligned. In order to realign these two chains, the following conformational changes in the two hydrocarbon chains are required. As indicated by arrows in A_γ (see Figure 6), β_1, β_3, β_4, and γ_1 undergo conformational changes. The sense of the change is also indicated by the arrow; the actual changes in torsion angles may be read from Table 3. At the same time, the orientation of the glycerol group with respect to the bilayer plane changes from an approximately perpendicular orientation in structure A_γ to one that is tilted by about 45° in structure B_γ. Changes in the orientation of the glycerol

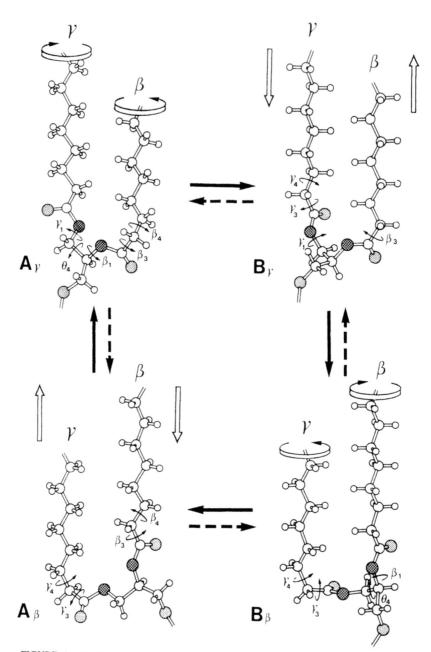

FIGURE 6.   Conformational changes involved in mutual transitions between four single-crystal structures.[29] The same four single-crystal structures as in Figure 5 are shown: DMPC,[12] DLPA,[35] DLPEM₂,[18] and DMPG.[20] (The key to abbreviations is given in the legends to Table 3.) The ester oxygens attached to the glycerol C(2)–C(3) bond are emphasized by heavy shading; all other oxygens are shaded. Reversible transitions between crystal structures are indicated by heavy arrows. The dashed arrows serve to indicate the reversible character of these transitions. Transitions indicated by horizontal, heavy arrows involve the conversion from rotamer A to B and changes in the chain stacking mode, while transitions indicated by vertical, heavy arrows involve changes in the chain stacking mode only. The small arrows associated with torsion angles β_1, β_3, β_4, and γ_1 (rotamer A_γ) indicate the torsion angles undergoing conformational changes in going from A_γ to B_γ. The light arrows on top of the two hydrocarbon chains of A_γ indicate the overall rotation of the hydrocarbon chains in going from A_γ to B_γ. The straight, light arrows at the end of the hydrocarbon chains of B_γ indicate that on going from B_γ to B_β, the chain stacking mode is changed, involving stretching of the β-chain and shortening of the γ-chain of B_γ.

group accompanying the transitions shown in Figure 6 may be identified by an inspection of Figure 6.

The light arrows on top of the two hydrocarbon chains of A_γ indicate the overall rotation of the hydrocarbon chains in going from structure A_γ to B_γ. The double arrows (heavy and dashed) indicate the reversibility of the transitions shown in Figure 6. The transitions marked by horizontal heavy/dashed arrows involve conformational changes of both the C(2)–C(3) glycerol bond as well as conformational changes in the torsion angles β_1 to β_4 and γ_1 and γ_4. In contrast, the two transitions marked by vertical, heavy/dashed arrows, i.e., $A_\gamma \rightleftharpoons A_\beta$ and $B_\gamma \rightleftharpoons B_\beta$, involve conformational changes in the two hydrocarbon chains only. These two transitions therefore primarily affect the chain stacking mode and related to it possibly the orientation of the glycerol backbone. The two transitions marked by vertical, heavy/dashed arrows involve an axial displacement of the two hydrocarbon chains by four methylene groups; this is indicated by light arrows at the end of the two hydrocarbon chains (see Figure 6, top right and bottom left). The transition $B_\gamma \rightleftharpoons B_\beta$ involves straightening of the β-chain while the γ-chains move downward making a 90° kink at C atom C(22). Such a change in the chain stacking involves significant conformational changes in torsion angles γ_1, γ_3, γ_4, and β_3 (see Figure 6, top right). Changes in these torsion angles can again be read from Table 3.

Taking the single-crystal structures (see Table 3) and NMR results discussed above together, it can be postulated that the motional average of the diacylglycerol group is the average of at least four minimum free-energy conformations presented in Figure 5 or Figure 6. We recall from the discussion of Figure 5 that the four conformations presented (A_γ, A_β, B_γ, and B_β) differ not only in the conformation about the C(2)–C(3) bond and the chain stacking mode, but also in the orientation of the glycerol group. The relative probability of structures A_γ, A_β, B_γ, and B_β can be assumed to be governed by a Boltzmann distribution. Since the minimum free energies of these structures are unknown, the relative probabilities and hence the weighting factors of these four structures are unknown. In conclusion, the motionally averaged structure of the diacylglycerol moiety of phospholipids in fully hydrated, liquid crystalline bilayers and membranes is the average of four basic structures (A_γ, A_β, B_γ, and B_β) weighted by their relative probabilities. This hypothesis was formulated by Hauser et al.[29]

It ought to be stressed that the hypothesis developed is based on spin-coupling constants analysis and X-ray crystallography. The former method is applied to highly dynamic structures such as micelles and monomers; the latter produces solid-state, static structures. These two structures can be regarded as extremes; with the structures of fully hydrated, liquid crystalline lipid bilayers, we are really interested in lying somewhere in between these two extremes. It is desirable to subject the hypothesis to experimental test using fully hydrated, liquid crystalline bilayers and methods that are sensitive to both conformational and orientational changes. Suitable candidates are deuterium NMR and IR spectroscopy. A prerequisite for the former method is the availability of selectively deuterated phospholipids containing the ^{2}H nucleus in the appropriate position.

Reviewing the existing literature on the application of ^{2}H-NMR and IR spectroscopy to the structure and dynamics of lipid bilayers would be beyond the scope of this review. It suffices to say that the interpretation of the results obtained with ^{2}H-NMR, IR, and other spectroscopic techniques are inconsistent. The following discussion is restricted to results pertinent to the question of the conformation and motion about the C(2)–C(3) bond of the diacylglycerol moiety. The interpretation of these results varies from a rigid glycerol backbone with a single conformation about the C(2)–C(3) bond to two or more conformations that are in equilibrium and exchange rapidly with frequencies $V \geq 10^5 s^{-1}$. ^{2}H-NMR results obtained with phosphatidylethanolamine and phosphatidylglycerol derived from *Escherichia coli* and selectively deuterated in the glycerol group were interpreted in terms of at least two conformations about the C(2)–C(3) glycerol bond.[30] The two deuterons on glycerol C(3) were found to be magnetically inequivalent giving rise to two separate quadrupole splittings. A twofold jump about the C(2)–C(3) bond between rotamers A and B was invoked in order to account for the observed deuterium quadrupole splittings. The model proposed here would be consistent with this interpretation. Blume et al.[31] investigated bilayers of dipalmitoylphosphatidylethanolamine selectively deuterated at glycerol C(2) above and below the crystal-to-liquid crystal transition. The crystal-type spectra were interpreted in terms of a single population of rotamer B. Upon passing through the transition temperature, the quadrupole splitting decreased by a factor of 4. This dramatic narrowing of the ^{2}H-NMR spectrum was attributed to a conformational change in the glycerol group. The interpretation given by the authors was as follows: the ^{2}H-NMR spectrum above the transition temperature is either due to a single conformation about the C(2)–C(3) bond which would have to be different from that of rotamer A and B. As an alternative interpretation, a rapid equilibrium between two or more weighted conformers about the C(2)–C(3) bond was proposed. In contrast, Strenk et al.[32] interpreted ^{2}H-NMR results obtained with liquid crystalline dimyristoylphosphatidylcholine bilayers in terms of a rigid C(2)–C(3) bond. The ^{2}H nucleus was selectively introduced into the glycerol group of the phospholipid. The rigid conformation about the C(2)–C(3) bond was concluded to be that of rotamer A. Our model is inconsistent with this interpretation which is also at variance with the interpretation of the deuterium NMR results cited above (see Gally et al.[30] and Blume et al.[31]). The interpretation of Strenk et al.[32] is also inconsistent with a recent IR study[34] using ^{13}C=O-labeled phospholipids (phosphatidylcholine, -ethanolamine, -serine, and phosphatidic acid all as dimyristoyl compound). The authors succeeded in assigning unambiguously the observed C=O bands, making good use of the vibrational isotope effect. In aqueous dispersions of phospholipids, two unresolved C=O bands are observed at 1740 and 1727 cm^{-1}. These two bands can be assigned to an anhydrous C=O group and a monohydrated C=O group, respectively. Conformational differences between the two hydrocarbon chains are negligible amounting to differences in band frequency of only 1 to 2 cm^{-1}. The main conclusion drawn from the C=O region of the IR spectra of different phospholipids is that the conformation and motion of the diacylglycerol must be such that both hydrocarbon chains become equivalent in terms of hydration of the C=O group. This implies that the motion of the diacylglycerol group in the fully hydrated, liquid crystalline state of phospholipid averages out any inequivalence of the two hydrocarbon chains which may be associated with a particular conformation of the glycerol C(2)–C(3) bond.

From the short discussion in this last part, it is clear that the problem of the conformation and motion of the diacylglycerol moiety of phospholipids in the liquid crystalline state is far from being solved. Certainly more work is needed, and it is evident from the discussion presented here that progress will depend on the successful application of a range of independent physical methods.

REFERENCES

1. **Sundaralingam, M.,** Molecular structures and conformations of the phospholipids and sphingomyelins, *Ann. N.Y. Acad. Sci.,* 195, 324, 1972.
2. **Hauser, H., Pascher, I., Pearson, R. H., and Sundell, S.,** Preferred conformation and molecular packing of phosphatidylethanolamine and phosphatidylcholine, *Biochim. Biophys. Acta,* 650, 21, 1981.
3. **Klyne, W. and Prelog, V.,** Description of steric relationships across single bonds, *Experientia,* 16, 521, 1960.
4. **Pascher, I., Sundell, S., and Hauser, H.,** Polar group interaction and molecular packing of membrane lipids. The crystal structure of lysophosphatidylethanolamine, *J. Mol. Biol.,* 153, 807, 1981.

5. **Pascher, I., Sundell, S., Eibl, H., and Harlos, K.,** The single crystal structure of octadecyl-2-methyl-glycero-phosphocholine monohydrate. A multilamellar structure with interdigitating head groups and hydrocarbon chains, *Chem. Phys. Lipids*, 39, 53, 1986.
6. **Hitchcock, P. B., Mason, R., Thomas, K. M., and Shipley, G. G.,** Structural chemistry of 1,2-dilauroyl-DL-phosphatidylethanolamine: molecular conformation and intermolecular packing of phospholipids, *Proc. Natl. Acad. Sci. U.S.A.*, 71, 3036, 1974.
7. **Elder, M., Hitchcock, P., Mason, R., and Shipley, G. G.,** A refinement analysis of the crystallography of the phospholipid, 1,2-dilauroyl-DL-phosphatidylethanolamine, and some remarks on lipid-lipid and lipid-protein interactions, *Proc. R. Soc. London Ser. A*, 354, 157, 1977.
8. **Pascher, I. and Sundell, S.,** Molecular arrangements in sphingolipids. The crystal structure of cerebroside, *Chem. Phys. Lipids*, 20, 175, 1977.
9. **Larsson, K.,** The crystal structure of the L-1 monoglyceride of 11-bromoundecanoic acid, *Acta Crystallogr.*, 21, 267, 1966.
10. **Pascher, I., Sundell, S., Eibl, H., and Harlos, K.,** Interactions and space requirement of the phosphate head group of membrane lipids: the single crystal structures of a triclinic and a monoclinic form of hexadecyl-2-deoxyglycerophosphoric acid monohydrate, *Chem. Phys. Lipids*, 35, 103, 1984.
11. **Pascher, I. and Sundell, S.,** Interactions and space requirements of the phosphate head group in membrane lipids. The crystal structure of disodium lysophosphatidate dihydrate, *Chem. Phys. Lipids*, 37, 241, 1985.
12. **Pearson, R. H. and Pascher, I.,** The molecular structure of lecithin dihydrate, *Nature (London)*, 281, 499, 1979.
13. **O'Connell, A. M. and Pascher, I.,** The crystal structure of triacetylsphingosine, *Acta Crystallogr. Sect. B*, 25, 2553, 1969.
14. **Nyholm, P.-G., Pascher, I., and Sundell, S.,** The effect of hydrogen bonds on the conformation of glycosphingolipids. Methylated and unmethylated cerebrosides studied by X-ray single-crystal analysis and model calculations, *Chem. Phys. Lipids*, in press.
15. **Pascher, I., Sundell, S., and Hauser, H.,** Glycerol conformation and molecular packing of membrane lipids: the crystal structure of 2,3-dilauroyl-D-glycerol, *J. Mol. Biol.*, 153, 791, 1981.
16. **Harlos, K., Eibl, H., Pascher, I., and Sundell, S.,** Conformation and packing properties of phosphatidic acid: the crystal structure of monosodium dimyristoylphosphatidate, *Chem. Phys. Lipids*, 34, 115, 1984.
17. **Pascher, I. and Sundell, S.,** unpublished results.
18. **Pascher, I. and Sundell, S.,** Membrane lipids: preferred conformational states and their interplay. The crystal structure of dilauroylphosphatidyl-*N,N*-dimethylethanolamine, *Biochim. Biophys. Acta*, 855, 68, 1986.
19. **Hauser, H., Pascher, I., and Sundell, S.,** Conformation of phospholipids: crystal structure of a lyso-phosphatidylcholine analogue, *J. Mol. Biol.*, 137, 249, 1980.
20. **Pascher, I., Sundell, S., Harlos, K., and Eibl, H.,** Conformation and packing properties of membrane lipids. The crystal structure of sodium dimyristoylphosphatidylglycerol, *Biochim. Biophys. Acta*, 896, 77, 1987.
21. **Sundaralingam, M. and Jensen, L. H.,** Crystal and molecular structure of a phospholipid component: L-α-glycerophosphorylcholine cadmium chloride trihydrate, *Science*, 150, 1035, 1965.
22. **Watts, P. H., Jr., Pangborn, W. A., and Hybl, A.,** X-ray structure of racemic glycerol 1,2-(di-11-bromoundecanoate)-3-(*p*-toluenesulfonate), *Science*, 175, 60, 1972.
23. **Dahlén, B. and Pascher, I.,** Molecular arrangements in sphingolipids. Crystal structure of *N*-tetracosa-noylphytosphingosine, *Acta Crystallogr. Sect. B*, 28, 2396, 1972.
24. **Abrahamsson, S., Dahlén, B., and Pascher, I.,** Molecular arrangements in glycosphingolipids: the crystal structure of glucosylphytosphingosine hydrochloride, *Acta Crystallogr. Sect. B*, 33, 2008, 1977.
25. **Abrahamsson, S. and Pascher, I.,** Crystal and molecular structure of L-α-glycerylphosphorylcholine, *Acta Crystallogr.*, 21, 79, 1966.
26. **DeTitta, G. T. and Craven, B. M.,** Conformation of *O*-(L-α-glycerylphosphoryl)-ethanolamine in the crystal structure of its monohydrate, *Nature (London) New Biol.*, 233, 118, 1971.
27. **Hauser, H., Guyer, W., Pascher, I., Skrabal, P., and Sundell, S.,** Polar group conformation of phosphatidylcholine. Effect of solvent and aggregation, *Biochemistry*, 19, 366, 1980.
28. **Hauser, H., Guyer, W., Spiess, M., Pascher, I., and Sundell, S.,** The polar group conformation of a lysophosphatidylcholine analogue in solution, *J. Mol. Biol.*, 137, 265, 1980.
29. **Hauser, H., Pascher, I., and Sundell, S.,** Preferred conformation and dynamics of the glycerol backbone in phospholipids. An NMR and X-ray single-crystal analysis, *Biochemistry*, 27, 9166, 1988.
30. **Gally, H. U., Pluschke, G., Overath, P., and Seelig, J.,** Structure of *Escherichia coli* membranes. Glycerol auxotrophs as a tool for the analysis of the phospholipid head-group region by deuterium magnetic resonance, *Biochemistry*, 20, 1826, 1981.
31. **Blume, A., Rice, D. M., Wittebort, R. J., and Griffin, R. G.,** Molecular dynamics and conformation in the gel and liquid-crystalline phases of phosphatidylethanolamine bilayers, *Biochemistry*, 24, 6220, 1982.

32. **Strenk, L. M., Westerman, P. W., and Doane, J. W.,** A model of orientational ordering in phosphatidylcholine bilayers based on conformational analysis of the glycerol backbone region, *Biophys. J.,* 48, 765, 1985.

33. **McAlister, J., Yathindra, N., and Sundaralingam, M.,** Potential energy calculations on phospholipids. Preferred conformations with intramolecular stacking and mutually tilted hydrocarbon chain planes, *Biochemistry,* 12, 1189, 1973.

34. **Blume, A., Hübner, W., and Messner, G.,** Fourier transform infrared spectroscopy of ^{13}C=O-labeled phospholipids. Hydrogen bonding to carbonyl groups, *Biochemistry,* 27, 8239, 1988.

35. **Pascher, I. and Sundell, S.,** to be published.

Chapter 1.B.3

POLARIZED ATTENUATED TOTAL REFLECTION INFRARED SPECTROSCOPY AS A TOOL TO INVESTIGATE THE CONFORMATION AND ORIENTATION OF MEMBRANE COMPONENTS

Erik Goormaghtigh and Jean-Marie Ruysschaert

TABLE OF CONTENTS

I. OVERVIEW

The determination of the conformation of biological membrane molecules by experimental means has long been challenged by the difficulties encountered in obtaining crystals of protein suitable for high-resolution X-ray crystallography and by the turbidity inherent to membrane fragments which prevents them from being analyzed by spectroscopic methods using ultraviolet (UV) or visible light. Infrared (IR) spectroscopy has long been recognized as a potentially useful method to gain information on the structure of molecules of biological interest. However, the complexity of the latter molecules, the intrinsic broadness of the absorption bands in the liquid or solid state, and the presence of water (H_2O or D_2O) whose bands overlap several interesting regions of the sample spectrum have prevented the technique from a widespread development. The recent availability of Fourier transfer infrared (FTIR) instrumentation along with computer software allowing solving to some extent the problems described above has enabled IR spectroscopy to become one of the leading techniques in the experimental search of the structure of biological molecules. Accordingly, the literature on this subject has increased greatly ever since. In some areas, IR spectroscopy has become the only technique available. Let us quote, for example, the determination on hydrated membranes of the secondary structure of membrane proteins, the determination of the orientation of some protein segments with respect to the plane of the membrane, the evaluation of the structure and orientation of the different phospholipid groups, the determination of ionization state of various chemical groups of interest, etc. Moreover, results are obtained with a relatively short time lag compared with other techniques such as nuclear magnetic resonance (NMR) of selectively deuterated molecules or X-ray crystallography. For these reasons, we think that it is a method of choice for checking or orienting conformational analysis computation. Some reviews have already been dedicated to the limited area of the domain: the secondary structure of proteins in solution in H_2O or D_2O,[1,2] lipid polymorphism,[3] or the attenuated total reflection (ATR) study of membranes.[4] The purpose of this Chapter is to present to the reader an overview of the IR spectroscopy possibilities to determine protein and other membrane components conformation and orientation in membranes. As a guideline, we have tried to make the descriptions, especially those concerning the techniques, easily accessible to the chemist or biologist, but complete enough so that the reader can grasp the meaning and the limitations of the mathematical treatments required to increase dramatically the amount of information harvested from IR spectra.

II. INTRODUCTION

Because many textbooks present excellent descriptions of the basements of IR spectroscopy (see for instance References 5 and 6), we shall limit ourselves to a few lines here.

A. VIBRATION FREQUENCIES

In its classical description, one mobile mass is linked to a fixed support by a spring characterized by a force constant k such that when the mass is displaced a distance x from its equilibrium position, the force exerted on the mass is

$$f = -kx = m \, d^2x/dt^2 \qquad (1)$$

Hence,

$$d^2x/dt^2 = -k/mx \qquad (2)$$

whose solution is

$$x = A \, 2\sin(2\pi\nu t) \qquad (3)$$

where

$$\nu = 1/2\pi \, \sqrt{(k/m)} \qquad (4)$$

which relates the frequency ν to k and m. If two masses are mobile, the same equation stands if m is replaced by the reduced mass μ:

$$\frac{1}{\mu} = \frac{1}{m_1} + \frac{1}{m^2} \qquad (5)$$

Large use is made of Equation 5 to predict the frequency of vibration upon isotopic exchange. As an example, let us consider the ν(C-H) and ν(C-D) vibration. The ratio ν (C-H)/ν(C-D) = $(\mu_{CD}/\mu_{CH})^{1/2}$ = $(13/7)^{1/2}$ = 1.363. So, for instance, the ν_s(C-H) vibration of the hydrocarbon chain of a phospholipid which occurs near 2853 cm^{-1} would be shifted upon H/D exchange to 2853/1.363 = 2094 cm^{-1}, a region of the spectrum usually devoided from other absorption bands in which the labeled molecule can be studied without interference, even in a very complex medium. Since several fatty acid chains (palmitic, myristic, and oleic) labeled or multilabeled at almost any position are now commercially available, the user has to just incorporate them in the lipid of his choice prior to start of the IR experiments. Several types of deuterium-labeled amino acids are also available. ^{18}O-labeled fatty acids, which are also commercially available, are potentially very useful for the study of the carbonyl group of phospholipids, but no work has been reported yet.

B. VIBRATIONAL BAND SHAPE

The vibrational band shape is a measure of the states of the entire population of molecules that exhibit this vibrational mode. Since vibrational periods are short relative to rotational or translational motions, their band shape represents the distribution of states by which molecules interact with their neighbors (the opposite is true in NMR, where the line shape is due to a time averaging of the molecule environments). As a consequence in IR spectroscopy, ordered aggregated states yield narrow bands in agreement with narrow distribution of molecular states. (The same conditions yield broader NMR line widths.) The band width in IR spectroscopy provides then a measure of the disorder or multiplicity of local interactions.[7] A straightforward application of this is to use low temperature (liquid nitrogen) to resolve otherwise broad and overlapped bands.

In the case of solutions, associated with each vibrational energy level are many closely spaced rotational energy levels which are unresolved in solution because of the so-called lifetime broadening effect. Vibrational transitions are therefore correspondingly broad.[5] The lifetime broadening is due the fact that the lifetime of the excited state is finite and that, as a consequence, the level of energy of the system becomes blurred by an amount δE:

$$\delta E = \hbar/\tau \tag{6}$$

where $\hbar = h/2\pi$ and τ is the lifetime of the excited state. Collisions, for instance, are responsible for modifying the system, e.g., by making them relax to their ground state. So, if collisions happen at a rate of 10^{13} per second in a solution, the corresponding δE is about 50 cm^{-1} which is a value much greater than the separation between two rotational bands. In dilute solutions, collisions become the dominant factor ruling the band broadening and the bands tend to be Gaussian. This is called "homogeneous broadening" because all molecules have an equal probability of being perturbed by collision and relax by a similar process. In an interacting solvent (polar solvents) or in solids, bands are often deviated from a pure Gaussian shape. They have been described as a convolution of a Lorentzian with a Gaussian function. This shape of the broadening function is important since an approximation of it has to be used for resolution enhancement by Fourier self-deconvolution (see Chapter 3). A more detailed analysis of the reasons determining the more Gaussian or Lorentzian character of the broadening function can be found in the study of vibrational relaxation in liquid realized by Oxtoby.[8]

C. VIBRATIONAL SPECTRA OF POLYATOMIC MOLECULES

For a molecule of N atoms, $3N - 6$ fundamental modes of vibrations (or normal modes) exist ($3N - 5$ if the molecule is linear). Even simple biological molecules such as phospholipids would therefore yield several hundreds of normal vibrations. The problem of the assignment of the bands is in practice simplified by the fact that many normal modes of vibration are localized because they involve a large displacement of just two bonded atoms with little interaction with other vibrations. They typically involve vibrations of distinct molecular groups and are present in many different molecules involving these groups. For this reason, their properties (frequency and frequency shift as a function of the conformation, hydrogen bonding, etc., as well as the orientations of their dipole moment with respect to their chemical bonds) are often used in IR spectroscopy because the information gained on their properties in one molecule is usually transferable to another. Most vibrations discussed in this paper belong to this latter category. Most of the transitions observed are transitions from the ground state to the first excited state and are called fundamental or first harmonics. The selection rules strictly allow only fundamental transitions to exist, but second harmonics or overtones are also sometimes observed. They result from the anharmonicity of the oscillator (the potential curve deviate from a parabolic shape).

III. DICHROISM

A. DETERMINATION OF MOLECULAR ORIENTATIONS

The absorbence of an IR band is proportional to

$$|\overline{E}, \partial\overline{\mu}/\partial Q|^2 = |\overline{E}|^2 \cdot |\partial\overline{\mu}/\partial Q|^2 \cdot \cos^2\Gamma \tag{7}$$

where $\overline{E}$ is the amplitude of the electric field acting on the molecule, $\partial\overline{\mu}/\partial Q$ is the transition moment, i.e., the variation of electric dipole $\overline{\mu}$ along the coordinate, Q, and Γ is the angle between $\overline{E}$ and $\partial\overline{\mu}/\partial Q$. The absorbence of a band is therefore a function of the polarization of the incident light, and polarization measurements provide information on the orientation of $\partial\overline{\mu}/\partial Q$. Indeed, the absorbence will vary from zero for $\overline{E}$ perpendicular to $\partial\overline{\mu}/\partial Q$ to a maximum for $\overline{E}$ parallel to $\partial\overline{\mu}/\partial Q$. If the orientation of $\partial\overline{\mu}/\partial Q$ with respect to a molecular axis is known and if all the molecules of the sample are oriented in the same direction, (e.g., in a membrane multilamellar system), then the orientation of the molecular axis can be calculated. The study of the dichroism of several vibrations belonging to the same molecule can yield information as to the orientation of several molecular axes and dichroism is therefore a valuable tool to determine the orientation of the molecule. We shall examine how in practice these orientations are obtained. Three types of sample can be encountered for biological samples:

1. Oriented fibers such as stretched protein fibers or polymers — Elongated molecules are sometimes embedded into a polymer matrix which is stretched. The included molecules then orient themselves with their long axis preferentially parallel to the stretching direction. All the molecular axes are therefore oriented symmetrically about the stretching direction.
2. Mono- or multilayers deposited parallel to the surface of a support transparent to the IR radiation — The spectrum is recorded by transmittance. Most biological membranes containing phospholipids spontaneously form oriented bilayers or multilayers structures upon dehydration. The different methods of preparation of such oriented arrangements are described in Chapter 5.
3. Mono- or multilayers deposited parallel to the surface of an internal multiple reflection plate — The spectrum is recorded by internal reflection spectroscopy.

The three types of samples described share common features: only one axis of symmetry exists — the stretching axis for the fiber or the normal to the plane of the membrane for the mono- or multilayer systems. This axis will be called the z-axis here. The probability of finding a molecular bond oriented along x or along y is identical. Deviation of the symmetry axis from the z-axis will also be considered. This kind of symmetry is also called uniaxial orientation.

For each of the systems described, the dichroic ratio R is defined as

$$R = \frac{A^{90°}}{A^{0°}} = \frac{(\overline{E}^{90°}, \partial\overline{\mu}/\partial Q)^2}{(\overline{E}^{0°}, \partial\overline{\mu}/\partial Q)^2} \tag{8}$$

where $\overline{E}^{90°}$ and $\overline{E}^{0°}$ are the components of the electric field of the incident radiation oriented, respectively, parallel and perpendicular to the z-symmetry-axis (for a membrane, it is, respectively, perpendicular and parallel to the plane of the membrane) and $A^{90°}$ and $A^{0°}$ are the absorbences measured for the two orthogonal polarizations of the incident radiation just described. The derivation of the expression of R which allows orientation to be measured is slightly different for each system.

1. Oriented Fibers
Three cases of increasing complexity have been distinguished.[9]

Perfect axial ordering — The symmetry axis of the molecule is parallel to the z-axis (fiber axis) which is also parallel to $\overline{E}^{90°}$, one of the two polarizations of the light. The other polarization of the light ($\overline{E}^{0°}$) is parallel to the y-axis. The beam propagates along the x-axis (Figure 1a). The oscillating dipole moment associate with the vibration of the group studied $\partial\overline{\mu}/\partial Q$ is tilted at an angle α from the molecular axis which is also the z-axis here. According to Equation 8 and to the symmetry around the z-axis, the dichroic ratio is expressed by

$$R_0 = \frac{A^{90°}}{A^{0°}} = \frac{1/2\pi \int_0^{2\pi} \cos^2\alpha \, d\Phi}{1/2\pi \int_0^{2\pi} \sin^2\alpha \sin^2\Phi \, d\Phi} \tag{9}$$

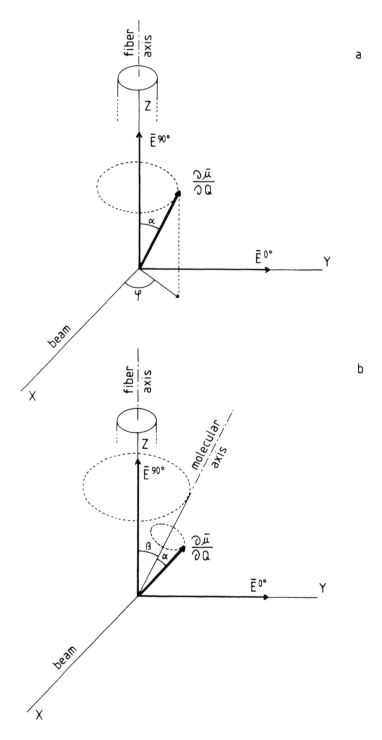

FIGURE 1. Relation between the orthogonal basis XYZ linked to the fiber and the direction of the incident IR beam, the directions of the two polarizations $\overline{E}^{90°}$ and $\overline{E}^{0°}$, and the transition moment dipole $\partial\overline{\mu}/\partial Q$. (a) The molecular axis related to the observed transition is parallel to the fiber symmetry axis Z; (b) the molecular axis is tilted at an angle β with respect to the Z-axis. α is the angle between the molecular axis and the transition dipole moment $\partial\overline{\mu}/\partial Q$.

$$R_0 = 2\cot^2\alpha \tag{10}$$

As α varies between 0 and $\pi/2$, R varies from ∞ to 0 and R = 1 for α = 54° 44′.

Partial order — In practice, it is unlikely to encounter a perfect orientation of the molecular axis parallel to the z-axis. Partial disordering can be considered from two points of view. Firstly, we may consider the sample as containing a fraction f of perfectly oriented molecules and a fraction $1 - f$ of the molecules randomly oriented. The dichroic ratio is then expressed by

$$R = \frac{2f\cos^2\alpha + 2/3(1 - f)}{f\sin^2\alpha + 2/3(1 - f)} \tag{11}$$

f is related to the degree of orientation of the molecule axis along the z-axis, i.e., along the fiber axis which is placed normal to the incident beam. It varies between 0 and 1. Secondly, alternatively, we may consider all the symmetry axes as displaced by the same angle β from the z-axis (see Figure 1b). The expression of R becomes

$$R = \frac{2\cot^2\alpha\cos^2\beta + \sin^2\beta}{\cot^2\alpha\sin^2\beta + (1 + \cos^2\beta)/2} \tag{12}$$

See Reference 9 for details of the derivation. A relation between f and an angle β has been derived by Fraser:[10]

$$f = 1 - \frac{3}{2}\sin^2\beta = (3\cos^2\beta - 1)/2 \tag{13}$$

Disordering — In practice, a distribution of the z-axes with an angle β occurs and Equation 8 must be integrated over β. It can be characterized by an orientational order parameter S defined by

$$S = (3<\cos^2\beta> - 1)/2 \tag{14}$$

where

$$<\cos^2\beta> = 2\pi \int_0^\pi C(\beta)\cos^2\beta\sin\beta d\beta \tag{15}$$

and $C(\beta)$ is an orientation density function such that the fraction of the axes between β and $\beta + d\beta$ is $C(\beta) \sin\beta\, d\beta$. An example of orientation density function is given below. For details of the derivation, the reader is referred to Fraser and MacRae.[11] By comparison with Equation 13, it can be shown that the absorption properties are equivalent to those of a specimen in which a fraction S of the z-axes is aligned parallel to the fiber axis and a fraction $(1 - S)$ is randomly distributed.[11] The dichroic ratio is now given by

$$R = \frac{2S\cos^2\alpha + 2/3(1 - S)}{S\sin^2\alpha + 2/3(1 - S)} \tag{16}$$

similar to Equation 11. It reduces to Equation 10 for a perfectly oriented system (S = 1). Since the density function $C(\beta)$ is usually not known, the value of S cannot be calculated. The evaluation of S by other means is then required for the interpretation of dichroism data. The problem of the evaluation of S is treated below and it is enough to say here that it can be greatly simplified if R is either small or large. If α is known, the S can be calculated from

$$S = \frac{(R - 1)(R_0 + 2)}{(R_0 - 1)(R + 2)} \tag{17}$$

obtained by combining Equations 16 and 10. Another potentially useful relation is the one relating the unpolarized absorbence A to the absorbences obtained with the two polarizations, $A^{90°}$ and $A^{0°}$:

$$A = 1/3(A^{90°} + 2A^{0°}) \tag{18}$$

Note that the equivalent symbols for several papers are $\overline{E}^{90°} = \overline{E}_\| = \overline{E}_v$ and $\overline{E}^{0°} = \overline{E}_\perp = \overline{E}_h$. Quite similar to the oriented fiber system are the films or stretched films in which the symmetry axis of the molecules is oriented in a single direction in the plane of the film. A clear picture of the molecular conformation elements that can be gained from this approach for poly-τ-benzyl-L-glutamate whose fibrous crystals were oriented in one direction (in the plane of the film) by rubbing the film during its formation is described by Tsuboi.[12] In this paper, the relation between R and α is expressed in a slightly different way:

$$R = \frac{2\cos^2\alpha + g}{\sin^2\alpha + g} \tag{19}$$

where

$$g = \frac{2}{3}\frac{(1 - f)}{f} \tag{20}$$

with f having the meaning defined in Equation 11, g becomes 0 for perfect ordering and infinity for random distribution.

2. Mono- or Multilayers Transmittance Spectra

Opposite to the situation encountered with fibers, no dichroism can be detected when directing the incident beam perpendicular to the film surface since the symmetry axis then lies parallel to the beam with both polarization of the light perpendicular to this symmetry axis. Dichroism, however, appears when the film is tilted at an angle θ from the incident beam.

A simple expression of R which does not take into account the disordering of the molecules has been derived by Akutsu et al.:[13]

$$R_0 = \cos^2\theta + 2\cot^2\alpha\sin^2\theta \tag{21}$$

where θ is the tilt between the film plane and the beam direction in the film and α is the angle between the oscillating transition moment $\partial\overline{\mu}/\partial Q$ and a molecular axis which is here supposed to be parallel to the Z-axis normal to the film. If the refractive index of the film is n, the incident angle θ_0 between the incident beam and the film is related to the tilt angle θ in the film by

$$n\sin\theta = \sin\theta_0 \tag{22}$$

and Equation 21 becomes

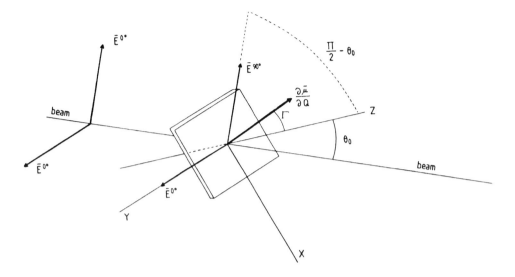

FIGURE 2. Relation between the orthogonal basis XYZ linked to the plate supporting the membrane and the direction of the incident beam, the directions of the two polarizations $\overline{E}^{90°}$ and $\overline{E}^{0°}$, and the transition moment dipole $\partial\overline{\mu}/\partial Q$. Z is normal to the plate, tilted at an angle θ_o with respect to the incident beam; Y lies in the plate plane and is normal to Z and to the incident beam. $\overline{E}^{0°}$ is parallel to Y. X, Z, and the incident beam are in the same plane. There is an angle Γ between $\overline{E}^{90°}$ and the transition dipole moment.

$$R_0 = 1 + \frac{1}{n^2} \sin^2\theta_0(2\cot^2\alpha - 1) \qquad (23)$$

This relation allows α to be determined provided that a perfect orientation of the molecular axis parallel to the Z-axis is obtained. In the simplest case, if $\partial\overline{\mu}/\partial Q$ is parallel to a chemical bond, the orientation of this chemical bond with respect to the normal to the film (= symmetry axis) is deduced immediately from Equation 21. However, a more realistic model must take into account the disordering inherent to biological membrane samples. Such a model has been developed by Rothschild and Clark[14] and was applied in the same paper to the determination of the mean orientation of α-helices of bacteriorhodopsin in oriented purple membrane. The geometry of the experimental setup is described in Figure 2.

X, Y, and Z form an orthogonal system of axes linked to the plate supporting the oriented membranes, Z is normal to the plate, and this normal is tilted at an angle θ_o with respect to the incident beam. The vectors $\overline{E}^{90°}$, $\overline{E}^{0°}$, and $\partial\overline{\mu}/\partial Q$ can be expressed as follows on the X, Y, Z axes system:

$$\overline{E}^{90°} = |\overline{E}^{90°}|(\sin(\pi/2 - \theta), 0, \cos(\pi/2 - \theta))$$

$$= |\overline{E}^{90°}|(\cos\theta, 0, \sin\theta) \qquad (24)$$

$$\overline{E}^{0°} = |\overline{E}^{0°}|(0, 1, 0) \qquad (25)$$

$$\partial\overline{\mu}/\partial Q = |\partial\overline{\mu}/\partial Q|(\sin\Gamma\cos\Phi, \sin\Gamma\sin\Phi, \cos\Gamma) \qquad (26)$$

We cannot evaluate the squared dot products of $\partial\overline{\mu}/\partial Q$ with $\overline{E}^{90°}$ and $\overline{E}^{0°}$ which are required in the expression of R (Equation 8):

$$(\overline{E}^{90°}, \partial\overline{\mu}/\partial Q)^2 = |\overline{E}^{90°}|^2 |\partial\overline{\mu}/\partial Q|^2 (\cos^2\theta\sin^2\Gamma\cos^2\Phi$$
$$+ \sin^2\theta\cos^2\Gamma + 2\sin\theta\cos\theta\sin\Gamma\cos\Gamma\cos\Phi) \qquad (27)$$

$$(\overline{E}^{0°}, \partial\overline{\mu}/\partial Q)^2 = |\overline{E}^{0°}|^2 |\partial\overline{\mu}/\partial Q|^2 \sin^2\Gamma\sin^2\Phi \tag{28}$$

Averaging Equations 27 and 28 over ϕ by

$$<\cdots>_\Phi = \frac{1}{2\pi} \int_0^{2\pi} d\Phi C(\Phi) \cdots \tag{29}$$

where . . . represents the expression to be averaged is easy since the distribution function $C(\phi) = 1$ by definition of the uniaxial property of the system. Noting that

$$\int_0^{2\pi} d\Phi\cos^2\Phi = \int_0^{2\pi} d\Phi\sin^2\Phi = \pi \tag{30}$$

$$\int_0^{2\pi} d\Phi\cos\Phi = 0 \tag{31}$$

the averaging of Equations 27 and 28 yield, respectively,

$$<(\overline{E}^{90°}, \partial\overline{\mu}/\partial Q)^2>_\Phi = |\overline{E}^{90°}|^2 |\partial\overline{\mu}/\partial Q|^2 (1/2\cos^2\theta\sin^2\Gamma + \sin^2\theta\cos^2\Gamma) \tag{32}$$

$$<(\overline{E}^{90°}, \partial\overline{\mu}/\partial Q)^2>_\Phi = |\overline{E}^{90°}|^2 |\partial\overline{\mu}/\partial Q|^2 1/2 \sin^2\Gamma \tag{32}$$

At this stage, introducing Equations 32 and 33 in Equation 8 would yield an expression identical to Equation 21 if $\Gamma = \alpha$. However, in addition to α, Γ also contains the distribution of the molecular axes about the Z-axis. Another potential contribution to Γ arises from the nonperfect parallelism between the supporting plate and the membrane planes. This is usually referred to as the mosaic spread distribution about the supporting plate normal. The different contributions to the disordering as described by Rothschild and Clark[14] appear in Figure 3. Averaging on Γ must take into account the distribution function $C(\Gamma)$ such that the average is given by

$$<\cdots\partial>_\Gamma = \int_0^\pi d\Gamma\sin\Gamma C(\Gamma) \cdots \tag{34}$$

where again . . . represents the expression to be averaged and $C(\Gamma)$ is the distribution function. $C(\Gamma)$ is assumed to be independent of ϕ, independent of a $\pm\pi$ change in θ_0 since the number of membranes facing up equals the number of membranes facing down and finally $C(\Gamma) = C(\pi - \Gamma)$. The distribution $C(\Gamma)$ can then be written as a sum of even Legendre polynomials:

$$C(\Gamma) = \sum_{n=0}^\infty \frac{4n + 1}{2} <P_{2n}(\cos\theta)> P_{2n}(\cos\theta) \tag{35}$$

where P_l is the Legendre polynomial of order l:

$$P_0 = 1$$

$$P_2 = (3\cos^2\Gamma - 1)/2$$

$$\cdot$$
$$\cdot$$

$$P_l = \frac{1}{2^l l!} \frac{d^2(\Gamma^2 - 1)^l}{d\Gamma^2} \tag{36}$$

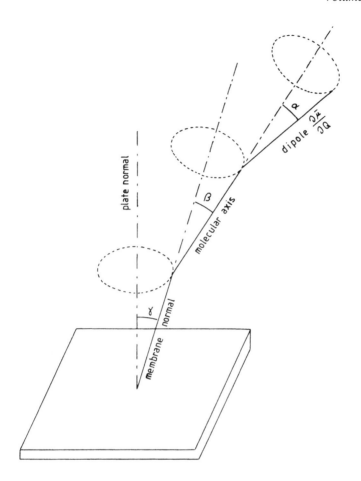

FIGURE 3. Set of nested axially symmetric distributions. The membrane normal is distributed about the plate normal (angle γ); the molecular axis is about the membrane normal (angle β); and the transition dipole moment $\partial\bar{\mu}/\partial Q$ is about the molecular axis (angle α).

and

$$<P_{21}>_{C(\Gamma)} = \int_0^\pi d\Gamma \sin\Gamma P_{21}(\cos\Gamma)C(\Gamma) \tag{37}$$

From Equation 36, $\sin^2\Gamma$ and $\cos^2\Gamma$ can be written as a function of P_0 and P_2:

$$\cos^2\Gamma = \frac{2}{3}P_2 + \frac{1}{3}P_0 \tag{38}$$

$$\sin^2\Gamma = \frac{2}{3}P_0 - \frac{2}{3}P_2 \tag{39}$$

The average of $\cos^2\Gamma$ and $\sin^2\Gamma$ have to be evaluated in order to obtain the average of Equations 32 and 33 according to Equation 34:

$$<\cos^2\Gamma>_\Gamma = \int_0^\pi d\Gamma \sin\Gamma C(\Gamma)\cos^2\Gamma \tag{40}$$

$$= \int_{-1}^{+1} d\mu C(\mu)\left(\frac{2}{3}P_2 + \frac{1}{3}P_0\right)$$

by posing $\mu = \cos\Gamma$. Introducing Equation 35 yields

$$<\cos^2\Gamma>_\Gamma = \int_{-1}^{+1} d\mu \sum_{n=0}^\infty \frac{4n+1}{2}<P_{2n}(\mu)> P_{2n}(\mu)\left(\frac{2}{3}P_2 + \frac{1}{3}P_0\right) \tag{41}$$

$$= \sum_{n=0}^\infty \frac{4n+1}{2}<P_{2n}(\mu)> \int_{-1}^{+1} d\mu P_{2n}(\mu)\left(\frac{2}{3}P_2 + \frac{1}{3}P_0\right) \tag{42}$$

$$= \sum_{n=0}^\infty \frac{4n+1}{2}<P_{2n}(\mu)> \left\{\frac{2}{3}\frac{2}{5}\delta_{n,2} + \frac{1}{3}2\delta_{n,0}\right\} \tag{43}$$

$$= \frac{2}{3}<P_2> + \frac{1}{3}<P_0> \tag{44}$$

Equation 43 being obtained by virtue of the orthogonality of the Legendre polynomials. Similarly,

$$<\sin^2\Gamma>_\Gamma = \frac{2}{3}<P_0> - \frac{2}{3}<P_2> \tag{45}$$

Averaging Equation 32 for Γ according to Equation 34 becomes

$$<(\overline{E}^{90°}, \partial\overline{\mu}/\partial Q)^2>_{\Phi,\Gamma} = |\overline{E}^{90°}|^2 |\partial\overline{\mu}/\partial Q|^2 \left\{\frac{1}{2}\cos^2\theta\left(\frac{2}{3}<P_0> - \frac{2}{3}<P_2>\right)\right.$$

$$\left. + \sin^2\theta\left(\frac{2}{3}<P_2> - \frac{1}{3}<P_0>\right)\right\} \tag{46}$$

$$= |\overline{E}^{90°}|^2 |\partial\overline{\mu}/\partial Q|^2 \left\{\frac{1}{3}<P_0> - \frac{1}{3}<P_2> + \sin^2\theta <P_2>\right\} \tag{47}$$

and Equation 33 becomes

$$<(\overline{E}^{0°}, \partial\overline{\mu}/\partial Q)^2>_{\Phi,\Gamma} = |\overline{E}^{0°}|^2 |\partial\overline{\mu}/\partial Q|^2 \frac{1}{3}\{<P_0> - <P_2>\} \tag{48}$$

The dichroic ratio is obtained by ratioing Equations 47 and 48:

$$R = 1 + 3\sin^2\theta \frac{<P_2>}{<P_0> - <P_2>} \tag{49}$$

and θ is calculated from θ_0 according to Equation 22.

It follows from the application of the addition theorem of spherical harmonics[15] that

a

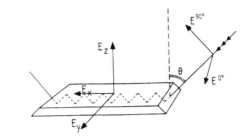

b

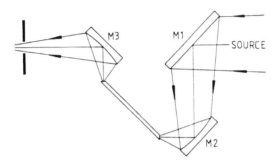

FIGURE 4. (a) Internal reflection element (IRE). The relation
between the different axes and vectors is identical to Figure 2. (b)
Experimental attenuated total reflection set-up with three mirrors,
M1, M2, and M3, which concentrate the beam into the IRE.

$$<P_2> \ = \ <P_2>_\gamma \cdot <P_2>_\beta \cdot <P_2>_\alpha \qquad (50)$$

The determination of $<P_2>_\beta$ requires therefore the knowledge of $<P_2>_\gamma$ and $<P_2>_\alpha$, $<P_2>$ being experimentally determined from R (Equation 49). We can assume $<P_2>_\alpha$ to be a δ-function so that $<P_2>_\alpha = (3\cos^2\alpha - 1)/2$. The tilt α between the symmetry axis of the molecule and $\partial\overline{\mu}/\partial Q$ can most generally be found in the literature. See, for instance, References 4, 12, and 15 or more general textbooks such as those written by Bellamy.[16,17] If the membranes are perfectly oriented parallel to the supporting plate ($\gamma = 0°$), then $<P_2>_\gamma = 1$. The quality of this approximation depends on the efficiency of the sample preparation (see Chapter 5). It is now possible to calculate the tilt β between the membrane normal and a molecular axis if we assume again that $C(\beta)$ is a γ-function. Posing $<P_2>/<P_2>_\alpha = U$, we have

$$\beta \ = \ \arccos\{(2U + 1)/3\}^{1/2} \qquad (51)$$

3. Mono- or Multilayers Attenuated Total Reflection (ATR) Spectra

The case of ATR spectroscopy performed on multilayers is very similar to the transmittance case discussed above. However, it must be stressed that a definite polarization (R <> 1) is always measured even for a completely random sample. It originates from the particular field configuration in the internal reflection element and has nothing to do with molecular ordering. It must be taken into account when interpreting ATR dichroism data. The amplitude of the different components of the electric field must now be calculated explicitly. For the geometry described in Figure 4, their expression has been derived by Harrick:[18]

$$Ey \ = \ \frac{2\cos\theta}{(1 \ - \ n_{31}^2)^{1/2}} \qquad (52)$$

$$Ex = \frac{2\cos\theta(\sin^2\theta - n_{31}^2)^{1/2}}{(1 - n_{31}^2)^{1/2}\{(1 + n_{31}^2)\sin\theta - n_{31}^2\}^{1/2}} \tag{53}$$

$$Ez = \frac{2\cos\theta n_{32}^2\sin\theta}{(1 - n_{31}^2)^{1/2}\{(1 + n_{31}^2)\sin\theta - n_{31}^2\}^{1/2}} \tag{54}$$

where $n_{21} = n_2/n_1$ and $n_{31} = n_3/n_1$, n being the refractive index, 1 being the thin film, 2 being the ATR plate, and 3 being the outside medium, usually air, so that $n_3 = 1$.

Introducing explicitly the field amplitudes Ex, Ey, and Ez in Equations 24 and 25 yields:

$$\overline{E}^{90°} = (Ex, 0, Ez) \tag{55}$$

$$\overline{E}^{0°} = (0, Ey, 0) \tag{56}$$

Using the same calculation as for the previous case (Equations 9 and 24 to 49) yields:

$$R = \frac{Ex^2}{Ey^2} + \frac{Ez^2}{Ey^2}\left(\frac{1 + 3<P_2>}{<P_0> - <P_2>}\right) \tag{57}$$

which is identical to the expression arrived at by Fringeli.[19-21] In the case of perfect alignment of the symmetry molecular axis parallel to the membrane normal, it reduces to:

$$R = \frac{Ex^2}{Ey^2} + \frac{Ez^2}{Ey^2}\frac{2\cos^2\alpha}{\sin^2\alpha} \tag{58}$$

It further reduces to Equation 23 if $Ex = Ey = Ez$. In the general case, $<P_2>_\beta$ is experimentally determined from the measurement of the dichroic ratio through Equation 51. In the case of a random distribution of the angles β, i.e., $C(\beta) = $ constant, $<P_2>_\beta = 0$ as it can be calculated from Equation 37 and R is given by

$$R = \frac{Ex^2}{Ey^2} + \frac{Ez^2}{Ey^2} \tag{59}$$

It is indeed different from unity because of the particular configuration of the field encountered in ATR. As it will be discussed later, the most practical approximation to gain information about the molecular conformation is to consider $C(\beta)$ to be a δ-function. The practical limits of this approximation will be highlighted. In the meantime, it is worth presenting numerical data obtained from Equation 57. Table 1 presents the values of the dichroic ratio as a function of α and β for three angles of incidence θ in the case of a germanium internal reflection elements (IRE) supporting a lipid film, and Table 2 presents similar results for a KRS-5 IRE. Before coming to the determination of angles, we must have a look at the orientation density function which are needed to calculate the orientation order parameters $<P_2>$ via Equation 37.

B. ORIENTATION DENSITY FUNCTIONS

Little success has yet been achieved in using model orientation density function to predict the behavior of $<P_2>_\beta$. The simplest one is described by a δ-function:

$$C(\beta) = \delta(\beta - \beta_0) \tag{60}$$

TABLE 1
Determination of Orientations by Dichroism Measurements by Attenuated Total Reflection (ATR) on Germanium Internal Reflection Elements (IRE)

$\alpha =$	90	80	70	60	50	40	30	20	10	0
$S = <P_2>_\alpha$	-0.50	-0.45	-0.32	-0.12	0.12	0.38	0.63	0.82	0.95	1.00
$\beta =$										
0	0.92	0.94	0.98	1.07	1.22	1.53	2.20	4.14	14.64	∞
10	0.93	0.94	0.98	1.07	1.22	1.50	2.08	3.50	7.73	14.64
20	0.95	0.96	1.00	1.08	1.21	1.43	1.82	2.49	3.50	4.14
30	0.98	0.99	1.03	1.09	1.19	1.34	1.55	1.82	2.08	2.20
40	1.03	1.04	1.07	1.11	1.17	1.24	1.34	1.43	1.50	1.53
50	1.10	1.10	1.11	1.13	1.15	1.17	1.19	1.21	1.22	1.22
60	1.18	1.17	1.16	1.15	1.13	1.11	1.09	1.08	1.07	1.07
70	1.26	1.25	1.21	1.16	1.11	1.07	1.03	1.00	0.98	0.98
80	1.32	1.30	1.25	1.17	1.10	1.04	0.99	0.96	0.94	0.94
90	1.35	1.32	1.26	1.18	1.10	1.03	0.98	0.95	0.93	0.92
0	0.93	0.94	0.98	1.06	1.19	1.46	2.04	3.72	12.82	∞
10	0.94	0.95	0.99	1.06	1.19	1.43	1.94	3.17	6.83	12.82
20	0.96	0.97	1.00	1.07	1.18	1.37	1.71	2.30	3.17	3.72
30	0.99	1.00	1.02	1.08	1.16	1.29	1.47	1.71	1.94	2.04
40	1.03	1.04	1.06	1.09	1.14	1.21	1.29	1.37	1.43	1.46
50	1.09	1.09	1.10	1.11	1.13	1.14	1.16	1.18	1.19	1.19
60	1.16	1.15	1.14	1.13	1.11	1.09	1.08	1.07	1.06	1.06
70	1.23	1.21	1.18	1.14	1.10	1.06	1.02	1.00	0.99	0.98
80	1.28	1.26	1.21	1.15	1.09	1.04	1.00	0.97	0.95	0.94
90	1.30	1.28	1.23	1.16	1.09	1.03	0.99	0.96	0.94	0.93
0	0.94	0.95	0.98	1.05	1.19	1.44	2.00	3.61	12.32	∞
10	0.94	0.95	0.99	1.06	1.18	1.42	1.90	3.08	6.59	12.32
20	0.96	0.97	1.00	1.06	1.17	1.36	1.68	2.24	3.08	3.61
30	0.99	1.00	1.02	1.07	1.16	1.28	1.45	1.68	1.90	2.00
40	1.03	1.03	1.05	1.09	1.14	1.20	1.28	1.36	1.42	1.44
50	1.08	1.09	1.09	1.11	1.12	1.14	1.16	1.17	1.18	1.19
60	1.15	1.15	1.14	1.12	1.11	1.09	1.07	1.06	1.06	1.05
70	1.22	1.21	1.18	1.14	1.09	1.05	1.02	1.00	0.99	0.98
80	1.27	1.25	1.21	1.15	1.09	1.03	1.00	0.97	0.95	0.95
90	1.29	1.27	1.22	1.15	1.08	1.03	0.99	0.96	0.94	0.94

Note: Values are of the dichroic ratio for different orientations of a molecular axis with respect to a normal to the plane of the membrane (angle β) as a function of the angle α between the molecular axis and the dipole moment of the transition observed and of the dichroic ratio measured. The meaning of the order parameter $<P_2>_\alpha$ can be extended to obtain an order parameter $S = f. <P_2>_\alpha$, where f is the fraction of oriented structures and $1 - f$ is the fraction of randomly oriented ones. For example, if $\alpha = 20°$ and $f = 1$, the table must be entered with $S = <P_2>_\alpha = 0.82$ (column 8); if $f = 46\%$, then $S = 0.82, 46\% = 0.38$, and the table must be entered with a value of 0.38 (column 6). The refractive indices used in the computation are $n_1 = 4.00$, $n_2 = 1.55$, and $n_3 = 1.00$. In the upper part of the table, an incidence angle $\theta = 30°$ was considered. The resulting amplitudes of the electric field Ex, Ey, and Ez are, respectively, 1.72, 1.789, and 0.826; $E_\perp = 1.789$, $E_\parallel = 1.907$, and $R^{random} = 1.14$. In the middle part of the table, an angle of incidence $\theta = 45°$ was considered. The resulting amplitudes of the electric field Ex, Ey, and Ez are, respectively, 1.41, 1.461, and 0.628; $E_\perp = 1.461$, $E_\parallel = 1.544$, and $R^{random} = 1.13$. In the lower part of the table, an angle of incidence $\theta = 60°$ was considered. The resulting amplitudes of the electric field Ex, Ey, and Ez are, respectively, 1.00, 1.033, and 0.434; $E_\perp = 1.033$, $E_\parallel = 1.090$, and $R^{random} = 1.11$.

TABLE 2
Determination of Orientations by Dichroism Measurements by Attenuated Total Reflection (ATR) on KRS-5 Internal Reflection Elements (IRE)

α =	90	80	70	60	50	40	30	20	10	0
$S = \langle P_2 \rangle_\alpha$	−0.50	−0.45	−0.32	−0.12	0.12	0.38	0.63	0.82	0.95	1.00
β =										
0	0.60	0.63	0.70	0.86	1.14	1.68	2.88	6.33	25.00	∞
10	0.62	0.64	0.71	0.86	1.13	1.63	2.67	5.19	12.71	25.00
20	0.65	0.67	0.74	0.88	1.11	1.50	2.19	3.40	5.19	6.33
30	0.71	0.73	0.79	0.90	1.07	1.34	1.71	2.19	2.67	2.88
40	0.80	0.82	0.86	0.93	1.04	1.18	1.34	1.50	1.63	1.68
50	0.92	0.92	0.94	0.97	1.00	1.04	1.07	1.11	1.13	1.14
60	1.06	1.05	1.03	1.00	0.97	0.93	0.90	0.88	0.86	0.86
70	1.20	1.18	1.12	1.03	0.94	0.86	0.79	0.74	0.71	0.70
80	1.32	1.28	1.18	1.05	0.92	0.82	0.73	0.67	0.64	0.63
90	1.36	1.32	1.20	1.06	0.92	0.80	0.71	0.65	0.62	0.60
0	0.78	0.79	0.83	0.92	1.08	1.38	2.05	3.97	14.39	∞
10	0.79	0.80	0.84	0.92	1.07	1.35	1.93	3.34	7.53	14.39
20	0.81	0.82	0.86	0.93	1.06	1.28	1.67	2.34	3.34	3.97
30	0.84	0.85	0.88	0.94	1.04	1.19	1.40	1.67	1.93	2.05
40	0.89	0.90	0.92	0.96	1.02	1.10	1.19	1.28	1.35	1.38
50	0.95	0.96	0.97	0.98	1.00	1.02	1.04	1.06	1.07	1.08
60	1.03	1.03	1.02	1.00	0.98	0.96	0.94	0.93	0.92	0.92
70	1.11	1.10	1.07	1.02	0.97	0.92	0.88	0.86	0.84	0.83
80	1.18	1.16	1.10	1.03	0.96	0.90	0.85	0.82	0.80	0.79
90	1.20	1.18	1.11	1.03	0.95	0.89	0.84	0.81	0.79	0.78
0	0.81	0.82	0.86	0.93	1.07	1.33	1.91	3.59	12.67	∞
10	0.81	0.82	0.86	0.93	1.06	1.31	1.81	3.04	6.69	12.67
20	0.83	0.84	0.87	0.94	1.05	1.24	1.58	2.17	3.04	3.59
30	0.86	0.87	0.90	0.95	1.04	1.16	1.35	1.58	1.81	1.91
40	0.90	0.91	0.93	0.97	1.02	1.09	1.16	1.24	1.31	1.33
50	0.96	0.96	0.97	0.98	1.00	1.02	1.04	1.05	1.06	1.01
60	1.03	1.03	1.02	1.00	0.98	0.97	0.95	0.94	0.93	0.93
70	1.10	1.09	1.06	1.02	0.97	0.93	0.90	0.87	0.86	0.86
80	1.15	1.14	1.09	1.03	0.96	0.91	0.87	0.84	0.82	0.82
90	1.18	1.15	1.10	1.03	0.96	0.90	0.86	0.83	0.81	0.81

Maximum Resolution Requested: 1 cm⁻¹ (r = 1 cm)

σ_1	2.5	5.0	7.5	10.0	12.5	15.0	17.5	20.0
f								
1.000	0.74	1.05	1.29	1.49	1.66	1.82	1.96	2.10
0.900	0.79	1.09	1.33	1.53	1.70	1.86	2.01	2.14
0.800	0.81	1.11	1.35	1.55	1.72	1.88	2.03	2.16
0.700	0.83	1.13	1.37	1.57	1.74	1.90	2.05	2.18
0.600	0.84	1.15	1.38	1.58	1.76	1.92	2.06	2.20
0.500	0.86	1.17	1.40	1.60	1.77	1.93	2.08	2.21
0.400	0.88	1.18	1.42	1.62	1.79	1.95	2.10	2.23
0.300	0.90	1.21	1.44	1.64	1.81	1.97	2.12	2.25
0.200	0.93	1.23	1.47	1.66	1.84	2.00	2.14	2.28
0.100	0.97	1.27	1.50	1.70	1.87	2.03	2.18	2.31
0.090	0.98	1.28	1.51	1.71	1.88	2.04	2.18	2.32
0.080	0.98	1.28	1.51	1.71	1.88	2.04	2.19	2.32
0.070	0.99	1.29	1.52	1.72	1.89	2.05	2.19	2.33
0.060	1.00	1.30	1.53	1.72	1.90	2.05	2.20	2.33

TABLE 2 (continued)
Determination of Orientations by Dichroism Measurements by Attenuated Total
Reflection (ATR) on KRS-5 Internal Reflection Elements (IRE)

Maximum Resolution Requested: 1 cm^{-1} (r = 1 cm)

σ_1	2.5	5.0	7.5	10.0	12.5	15.0	17.5	20.0
0.050	1.01	1.30	1.54	1.73	1.91	2.06	2.21	2.34
0.040	1.02	1.31	1.55	1.74	1.92	2.07	2.22	2.35
0.030	1.03	1.33	1.56	1.75	1.93	2.08	2.23	2.36
0.020	1.05	1.34	1.57	1.77	1.94	2.10	2.24	2.38
0.010	1.08	1.37	1.60	1.80	1.97	2.13	2.27	2.40
0.005	1.11	1.40	1.63	1.82	1.99	2.15	2.29	2.43
0.002	1.13	1.42	1.65	1.84	2.02	2.17	2.32	2.45
0.001	1.16	1.45	1.67	1.87	2.04	2.19	2.34	2.47

Maximum Resolution Requested: 2 cm^{-1} (r = 0.5 cm)

σ_1	2.5	5.0	7.5	10.0	12.5	15.0	17.5	20.0
f								
1.000	1.05	1.49	1.82	2.10	2.35	2.57	2.78	2.97
0.900	1.14	1.57	1.91	2.19	2.44	2.66	2.87	3.06
0.800	1.18	1.62	1.95	2.23	2.48	2.70	2.91	3.10
0.700	1.22	1.65	1.98	2.26	2.51	2.74	2.94	3.13
0.600	1.26	1.69	2.02	2.30	2.55	2.77	2.97	3.17
0.500	1.29	1.72	2.05	2.33	2.58	2.80	3.01	3.20
0.400	1.33	1.76	2.09	2.37	2.62	2.84	3.04	3.24
0.300	1.38	1.80	2.13	2.41	2.66	2.88	3.08	3.28
0.200	1.44	1.86	2.19	2.46	2.71	2.93	3.14	3.33
0.100	1.53	1.94	2.27	2.54	2.78	3.01	3.21	3.40
0.090	1.54	1.95	2.28	2.55	2.80	3.02	3.22	3.41
0.080	1.55	1.97	2.29	2.56	2.81	3.03	3.23	3.42
0.070	1.57	1.98	2.30	2.58	2.82	3.04	3.24	3.43
0.060	1.59	1.99	2.32	2.59	2.83	3.06	3.26	3.45
0.050	1.60	2.01	2.33	2.61	2.85	3.07	3.28	3.46
0.040	1.63	2.04	2.36	2.63	2.87	3.09	3.29	3.48
0.030	1.66	2.06	2.38	2.65	2.90	3.12	3.32	3.51
0.020	1.70	2.10	2.42	2.69	2.93	3.15	3.35	3.54
0.010	1.76	2.16	2.47	2.74	2.99	3.20	3.41	3.59
0.005	1.82	2.22	2.53	2.80	3.04	3.25	3.46	3.64
0.002	1.88	2.27	2.58	2.85	3.09	3.30	3.50	3.69
0.001	1.94	2.32	2.63	2.89	3.13	3.35	3.55	3.73

Note: This table is similar to Table 1, but computed for a KRS-5 IRE. The refractive indices used in the computation are $n_1 = 2.35$, $n_2 = 1.55$, and $n_3 = 1.00$. In the upper part of the table, an incidence angle $\theta = 30°$ was considered. The resulting amplitudes of the electric field Ex, Ey, and Ez are, respectively, 1.49, 1.94, and 1.179; $E_\perp = 1.914$, $E_\parallel = 1.898$, and $R^{random} = 0.99$. In the middle part of the table, an angle of incidence $\theta = 45°$ was considered. The resulting amplitudes of the electric field Ex, Ey, and Ez are, respectively, 1.380, 1.563, and 0.719; $E_\perp = 1.563$, $E_\parallel = 1.555$, and $R^{random} = 0.99$. In the lower part of the table, an angle of incidence $\theta = 60°$ was considered. The resulting amplitudes of the electric field Ex, Ey, and Ez are, respectively, 0.99, 1.105, and 0.474; $E_\perp = 1.105$, $E_\parallel = 1.100$, and $R^{random} = 0.99$.

which defines a perfect orientation with respect to the z-axis. This type of distribution is not realistic for most membranes. More realistic is the Kratky density function. It has already been used for polymers, fibers, and membranes. It describes the orientation distribution of rodlets embedded in a matrix upon stretching the matrix. The stretching ratio v (length after stretching/length before stretching) enters as a parameter in the density function:

$$C(\beta) = \frac{v^3}{4\pi(1 + (v^3 - 1)\sin^2\beta)^{3/2}} \qquad (61)$$

For $v = 1$ (no stretching), the rodlets are randomly oriented. $C(\beta)$ is plotted as a function of β for different values of v in Figure 5. Integration yields:

$$\langle\cos^2\beta\rangle = \frac{v^3}{v^3 - 1}\left\{1 - \frac{\tan^{-1}(v^3 - 1)^{1/2}}{(v^3 - 1)^{1/2}}\right\} \qquad (62)$$

The relation between $\langle P_2\rangle_\beta$ and v is plotted in Figure 6.

The Kratky distribution function has been used by Fringeli et al.[19] to evaluate v and $\langle P_2\rangle_\beta$ from ATR measurements carried out on a liquid crystal made out of one part of 4-(4'-n-propylbenzylidene amino)-benzonitrile and two parts of 4(4'-n-hexylbenzylidene amino)-benzonitrile. Orientation was obtained under the influence of an electric field. Depending on the vibration considered, v varied from 1 to 2.2 and their related order parameter varied between 0 and 0.48.

Another simple distribution density function model is a uniform distribution of the z-axes in the range $0 < \beta < \beta_0$. In this case, we have

$$\langle\cos^2\beta\rangle = 1/3(1 + \cos\beta_0 + \cos^2\beta_0) \qquad (63)$$

$$\langle P_2\rangle_\beta = 1/2\cos\beta_0(1 + \cos\beta_0) \qquad (64)$$

A new approach to the problem of the determination of $C(\beta)$ could come from conformational and statistical analysis. IR dichroism measurements would provide a tool to check the theoretical data provided that a good estimate of the mean orientation can be obtained by other means.

It appears from the experimental point of view that it is very difficult to assess the quality of a model of density distribution function. The lack of accuracy on the values of R indeed prevents different models to be distinguished. We will now focus on these experimental problems and on the approximations which are legitimate.

C. USING POLARIZATION DATA TO OBTAIN ORIENTATIONS

Table 1 and 2 report the value of the dichroic ratio for different angles β (angle between a molecular axis and the normal to the membrane) as a function of an order parameter S. In the case of perfect ordering, $S = \langle P_2\rangle_\alpha$. A perfect ordering of the molecular axes has been considered to calculate the values of β_0 from $\langle P_2\rangle_\beta = (3\cos^2\beta_0 - 1)/2$. If a distribution of the angles β occurs about β_0, we must now introduce the order parameter f for this distribution in S as explained in the tables. The wider the distribution, the smaller is f and consequently the smaller is S. Unless the distribution function $C(\beta)$ is precisely known (a few examples are given in the previous paragraph), little can be done to obtain the mean value of β. At first glance, it seems to be a rough approximation to consider that the distribution of the angles β is a δ-function (i.e., $f = 1$). However, it allows one to set a limit to the angle β. Indeed, for a given mean value of $\beta = \beta_0$, the absolute value of $\langle P_2\rangle_\beta$ is maximum if $C(\beta) = \delta(\beta - \beta_0)$ ($f = 1$) and tends to 0 when $C(\beta)$ tends to an isotropic distribution. The limiting value so set to β is particularly useful in two situations. These are encountered when R is either sufficiently larger or sufficiently smaller than the value found for an isotropic system. Let us take here a hypothetical example: the orientation of a peptidic α-helix embedded in a bilayer is measured by ATR. (Conditions for IR spectroscopy are those of the legend of Table 1.) The dichroic ratio for amide I whose dipole moment $\partial\bar{\mu}/\partial Q$ lies approximately parallel (say that parallel is $\alpha = 0$ for the sake of this example)

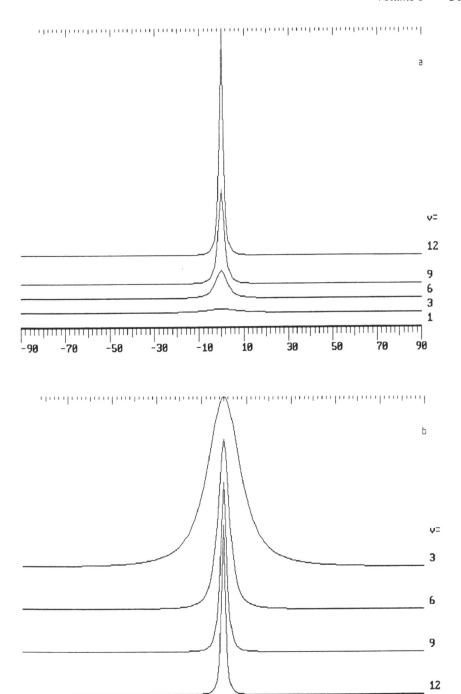

FIGURE 5.   (a) Kratky orientation distribution function (Equation 61) for five values of the extension ratio v. The curves are on the same scale, but are offset for the clarity of the figure; (b) same curves as in (a), but rescaled and offset so that the width of the distributions can be compared.

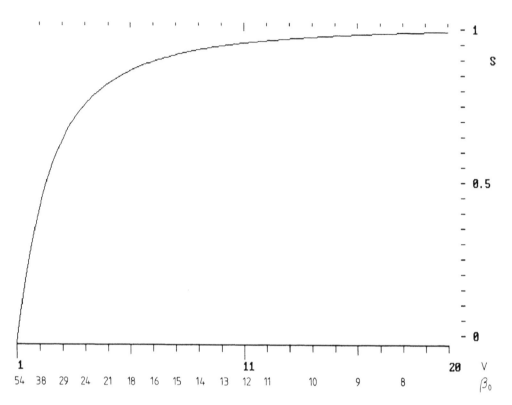

FIGURE 6.   Order parameter S = $<P_2>_\beta$ for a Kratky distribution function of the angles β as a function of the extension factor v. The shape of the distribution function is reported in Figure 5 for five values of v. The second abscissa scale reports the angle β_o calculated from S for a density distribution function C(β) = δ(β − β_o) so that β_o = $(\arccos((2 S + 1)/3))^{1/2}$.

to the long helix axis is measured to be 3.6. Looking at Table 1 (germanium IRE, θ = 45°), it can be seen that the dichroic ratio is sufficiently large to rule out any value of β larger than 23° which clearly means that the helix is a transmembrane helix. Note that this result comes without any prior knowledge on C(β). The same reasoning holds for small values of R, although with somewhat less accuracy. For example, if R had been equal to 0.98, Table 1 indicates that the helix is now tilted between 90 and 70° with respect to the membrane normal, i.e., is tilted at almost 20° with respect to the membrane plane. In the latter case, the problem of the accuracy on R is crucial (see Table 1) and should be examined carefully. One way to enlarge the range of R for which C(β) is clearly distinguished from a random or close to random situation is to decrease the angle of incidence θ or to improve the index matching between the sample and the IRE. The striking difference between Table 1 calculated for a germanium IRE with θ = 45° and Table 2 calculated for a KRS-5 IRE with θ = 30° is due to both effects. In the latter case, an orientation of the helix axis parallel to the membrane would yield a dichroic ratio close to 0.6 (provided that the distribution function C(β) is sufficiently narrow), easily distinguishable from a random distribution (R = 0.99). In the former case, the same molecular orientation leads to a dichroic ratio close to 0.93 which is difficult to distinguish from a random distribution (R = 1.13). However, as explained in Chapter 4, some particular optical properties of the internal reflection spectroscopy limit the use of small angles of incidence simultaneous to good index matching.

For intermediate values of R, no sufficient information is brought along as to the limit values of $<P_2>_\beta$ and the range of possible angles is too wide to be really useful. However, it is still legitimate to use the following trick. Another vibration (whose dipole is preferentially perpendicular to the first one) of the same (or rigidly linked) chemical group is looked for.

If the dichroic ratio of that band is itself either much larger or smaller than the random value, it means that the ordering at the level of that particular group is high and that in the first approximation Table 1 or 2 can be entered as it. This trick was used, for instance, to determine the orientation of the long and short quinone axis of the adriamycin bound onto cardiolipin bilayers.[22]

A special case for which the uncertainty can be removed arisesia band is known to contain a single dichroic contribution and a random contribution, e.g., the amide I band of a membrane protein is known to have a membrane helix and a disordered conformation in its part protruding outside the membrane. The nondichroic contribution tends to push the global value of R toward its random value, yielding wider ranges of permitted values for β. If a fraction f of the band is due to the dichroic contribution and a fraction $1 - f$ is due to isotropic contributions, adapting the relation developed by Rothschild et al.[30,31] to ATR allows Equation 57 to be rewritten as

$$R = \frac{Ex^2}{Ey^2} + \frac{Ez^2}{Ey^2} \left(\frac{1 + 3f<P_2>}{<P_0> - f<P_2>} \right) \qquad (65)$$

which is identical in form to considering an additional order parameter whose meaning has been introduced with Equation 11. Introducing f as explained in Tables 1 or 2 obviously further limits the range of permitted angles β.

Now, if no convincing information about the ordering for a given vibration can be gained out of the polarized IR spectra, it is still possible to resort to other techniques. The quality of the orientation of the membranes with respect to the support can be checked by light-polarized microscopy. It is worth mentioning here the electron microscopy approach developed by Clark et al.[32] Working on a facsimile of freeze-fracture of purple membranes oriented by the isopotential spin dry centrifugation (see Chapter 5), they were able to calculate the distribution of the normal of the membrane fragments about the mean. Even though orientation was better close to the surface supporting the film, up to $1 - \mu m$ depth, the membrane order parameter $<P_2>_\gamma$ was slightly higher than 0.9. Now the quality of the orientation of the molecule bonds studied within the membrane has to be estimated by other methods such as optical measurements, X-ray and neutron diffraction, and NMR. To be useful, previous studies must relate as nearly as possible to the same molecules under the same experimental conditions and the spectroscopist evaluates whether a value of $<P_2>_\beta$ can be transferred to his own experiment. It is, for instance, widely accepted that hydrocarbon chains of phospholipid membrane have an order parameter close to 1 below their phase transition.[4,23]

D. PRACTICAL PROBLEMS
1. Experimental Evaluation of the Dichroic Ratio R

From its definition (Equation 8), R is the ratio of the integrated absorbence of a band recorded with the incident light polarized at 90 and at 0°. The requirement of area determination raises the acute problem of baseline determination. Three cases can be envisaged.

1. The band considered is well separated from other bands. The choice of the baseline is straightforward (Figure 7). In the example given in Figure 7, two synthetic Lorentzians were summed; the surface of the low-frequency one in spectrum b was set to one half of its value in spectrum a. When the baselines are chosen as depicted in Figure 7, the dichroic ratios were, respectively, 0.97 and 2.1 for the high- and low-frequency Lorentzians instead of their real values of 1 and 2.

2. The width of the band considered is very different from the width of the bands superimposing the former. It can then be tentatively assumed that in first approximation

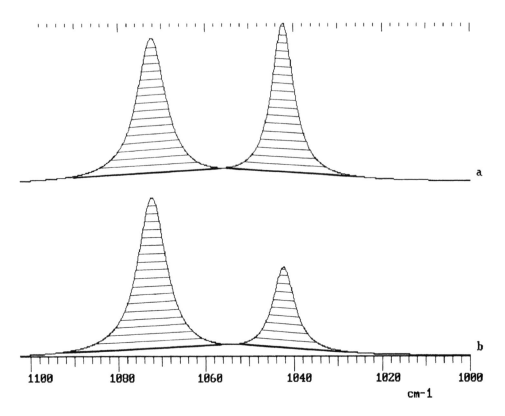

FIGURE 7.   Sum of two Lorentzians of areas 1 and 0.8 for spectrum (a) and 1 and 0.4 for spectrum (b). The half width at half height σ is 4 and 3 cm^{-1} for the high- and low-frequency Lorentzians and separation is 30 cm^{-1}. The spectrum contains 1024 points. The hatched area represents the surface calculated by drawing a straight baseline between the minima of the spectrum.

the baseline can be drawn as depicted in Figure 8. To check the validity of this assumption, we have simulated this situation in Figure 8 by superimposing two Gaussian lines: a broad one with a width of 20 cm^{-1} and a narrow band with a width of 4 cm^{-1} whose intensity was doubled from each spectrum b to spectrum a in order to simulate a dichroic ratio R = 2. The bands were then integrated with the baselines shown in Figure 8. The calculated dichroic ratio after integration of the low-frequency Lorentzians were, respectively, 2.4, 2.6, and 2.6 for spectra 1, 2, and 3 of Figure 8, i.e., significantly too large. More realistic values are expected if the band widths are even more different. For instance, if the width of the low-frequency band in the cases of spectra 3 of Figure 8 is 2 cm^{-1} instead of 4 cm^{-1}, the calculated value of R becomes 2.2 instead of the value of 2.6 found before (data not shown), closer to the real value of 2. The $j_w(CH_2)$ of the phospholipid hydrocarbon chains ranges in this category.

3.   The band is superimposed by other bands of similar width. The only practical solution is to separate the different components of the envelope by a curve-fitting procedure. Fourier self-deconvolution may be necessary prior to curve fitting if the envelope components cannot be clearly distinguished. This procedure is described in Chapter 3. Many bands associated with different protein conformations fall in this category and it will be elaborated upon later in this chapter.

2. Orientation of $\partial\bar{\mu}/\partial Q$ With Respect to the Chemical Bonds

As far as the vibrations of phospholipids and proteins are concerned, data about the relation between the orientation of $\partial\bar{\mu}/\partial Q$ and the chemical bonds of the molecule exist in

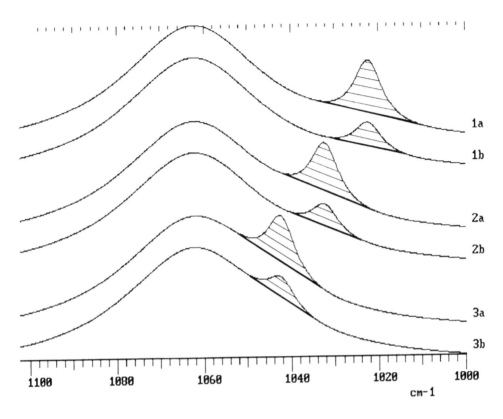

FIGURE 8. Sum of two Lorentzians of areas 1 and 0.1 for spectra (a) and 1 and 0.05 for spectra (b). The half width at half height σ is 20 and 4 cm^{-1} for the high- and low-frequency Lorentzians and separation is 40 cm^{-1} for spectrum 1, 30 cm^{-1} for spectrum 2, and 20 cm^{-1} for spectrum 3. Each spectrum contains 1024 points. The hatched area represents the surfaces discussed in the text.

the literature and are given in the sections treating these vibrations. Most of these orientations were determined by normal coordinate analysis, but some of them were experimentally checked. Let us quote the orientations of the transition dipoles of 1,4- and 1,8-dihydroxyanthraquinone[24,25] which were very useful to determine the orientation of adriamycin with respect to cardiolipin membrane[22] and the orientation of the transition dipoles of anthracene, phenazine, and acridine.[26] In the former cases (anthraquinone derivatives), polarized spectra were recorded from crystals in which the molecule orientation was known with respect to the crystal axis, while in the latter case, they were obtained from stretched polyethylene sheets, a method available to orient planar molecules.[27]

3. Miscellaneous

Refractive indices — The values of the refractive indices in the IR region are still subject to discussion. A value of 1.50 to 1.55 is generally used for phospholipids[4] and a value of 1.7 is used for proteins,[14,28] even though a value as low as 1.5 has been discussed in the case of photosynthetic proteins.[29]

Buffers and salts — Buffers and salts can be used in ATR provided that no absorption bands show up in the spectral region to be studied. However, the weight of the buffering molecules and salt ions per volume unit should not exceed the weight of the membrane molecules in the same volume unit if the multilayers are prepared by the solvent evaporation technique (see Chapter 5). Indeed, excess of salt mechanically disrupts the flat orientation of the multilayers and prevents good contact between the IRE and the sample. Dramatically weak signal and poor orientation result from excess of buffer and salt. Best results are obtained when the membranes are dispersed in pure water.

Precipitates — Because the intensity of the spectrum is very dependent on the quality of the contact between the sample and the IRE, some precipitates which poorly stick to the IRE require much more material to obtain good-quality spectra. In a mixture, the contribution of a precipitate component can be totally absent from the spectrum.

IRE surface — It is obvious that poorly polished IRE or scratched plates will not be able to perfectly orient the membranes and dichroism will be low. The hydrophobic/hydrophilic quality of the surface depends on the nature of the IRE chosen and on the cleaning process. Germanium IRE are most useful because of the hardness of their surface. A simple cleaning with a detergent, then with methanol, and finally with chloroform is sufficient for membrane applications. The surface obtained after this treatment is clean but hydrophobic. Plasma cleaning is required if aqueous solutions are to be spread on the plate since it yields a more hydrophilic surface.

Efficiency of the experimental setup — The efficiency of the experimental setup to measure polarization is decreased by at least two reasons: (1) the polarizer always lets a percentage of the light with unwanted polarization direction through (the quality of the polarizer used is here crucial) and (2) the convergence of the beam (see Figure 4b) results in a loss of parallelism in the incident light and therefore in a disordering of the $\bar{E}^{90°}$ and $\bar{E}^{0°}$ vectors with respect to the plate surface.

Other sources of problems — Other sources of problems include contamination of the sample with dirty glassware. Since very small amounts of materials are sometimes handled (a few micrograms), traces of contaminant can be problematic. In our hands, new glass tubes are definitively not suitable for use without prior sulfochromic acid cleaning. Thorough purging of the spectrophotometer with dry air or nitrogen is also absolutely required. Fourier deconvolution (see Chapter 3) indeed strongly enhances the narrow bands arising from the presence of H_2O vapor.

IV. DATA MANIPULATION

A. SPECTROPHOTOMETERS AND DATA ACQUISITION

Any kind of data manipulation by a computer requires that the spectra are digitally encoded. This requirement is filled for most of the spectrophotometers available today since they are usually working under computer control. Two classes of apparatus are available: the dispersive instrument which uses a monochromator to scan the sample with the different light components and the so-called Fourier transform spectrophotometers based on the Michelson interferometer. In the latter case, the interferograms are Fourier transformed into the frequency IR spectra. The advantage of the Fourier transform spectrophotometer over dispersive instruments can be summarized by an increase of the signal-to-noise ratio and by the possibility to record a complete spectrum in a matter of seconds. Moreover, most of the Fourier transform instruments can be equipped with mercury cadmium telluride (MCT) fast detectors which allow the study of low-transmitting samples such as dilute aqueous solutions or samples recorded by ATR. More details concerning the advantage of the Fourier transform spectrophotometers are discussed elsewhere.[33,34] It is only fair to say that a high signal-to-noise ratio can also be obtained with dispersive instruments in a reasonable amount of time if the user is interested only by a small domain of the IR spectra. In the latter case, the user should consider that for most applications, it is not required to record the spectra with too high a resolution since the signal to noise ratio is proportional to the voltage at the amplifier input, itself proportional to the square of the slit width (resolution). Resolutions better than 2 cm^{-1} are not necessary for biological samples in the liquid or solid states since the intrinsic broadness of the bands is much larger than 2 cm^{-1} (see Chapter 1). On the other hand, since the voltage corresponding to the noise at the amplifier input is proportional to the square root of the time constant of the amplificator t_o, the time constant is related to the width of the slit w as follows:

$$t = t_0(w_0/w)^4 \tag{66}$$

i.e., for a slit twice smaller (resolution twice better), a time constant 16 times higher is to be used in order to keep the signal to noise ratio at the same level. Moreover, the maximum scanning rate permissible varies as the fifth power of the slit.[35] Additional spectra recorded successively is another way to decrease the signal to noise ratio. The latter decreases as $\sqrt{N}$, where N is the number of spectra added.

B. FOURIER SELF-DECONVOLUTION

The mathematical technique of spectrum self-deconvolution useful for biological sample spectra has been essentially developed by Kauppinen et al.[36-39] and by Yang and Griffiths.[40-42] The goal of the technique is to enhance the spectral resolution so that the different components of a complex band can be resolved and eventually submitted to a curve fitting procedure for quantitative analysis. The principle of self-deconvolution consists of considering that in the liquid or solid state the vibrational absorption bands are intrinsically broadened (or convolved) by a function. The self-deconvolution uses this function to ''unbroaden'' (or deconvolve) the spectrum. This deconvolution is most conveniently achieved by the use of the Fourier transforms, even though other methods can also be used.[35,43]

The procedure encounters a major theoretical problem which is the knowledge of the shape of the convoluting function. As we have seen in Chapter 1, this function is thought to be essentially Lorentzian, but its exact shape is still to be defined. However, a pure Lorentzian shape has been successfully assumed by many investigations for self-deconvolution of spectra of lipids and proteins. The width FWHH (full width at half height) of the Lorentzian has still to be chosen. The correct value can only be found by trial and error. If FWHH is too small, little narrowing is obtained. If it is too large, negative side lobes appear. This is illustrated in Figures 9 to 11. A synthetic spectrum is made out of two Lorentzian line shapes separated by half of their FWHH (see Figure 9). Only a slight asymmetry is visible in the sum spectrum, but it is impossible to determine the number and the frequency of the components of the band envelope. When the Fourier self-deconvolution is correctly applied (see Figure 10), the narrowing of these components results in a much higher-resolution spectrum and the determination of the number and position of the components is obvious. As it will be discussed below, the K factor reports correctly the resolution increase (i.e., the factor by which the FWHH of each component is decreased). Figure 11 reports the result of a deconvolution where the FWHH was overestimated by a factor of 2. Clearly, resolution enhancement is poor and negative side lobes appear. The presence of such negative side lobes in deconvolved real spectra indicates overdeconvolution. Usually, it is not possible to determine a single value for the FWHH of several absorption bands of different origins and each peak has to be treated separately. This is, however, not a real constraint when studying the structure of proteins since the same amide I band is then analyzed over and over for different proteins and different conditions. From the practical point of view, the Fourier self-deconvolution is limited by three instrumental factors:

1. The instrumental resolution used when the spectrum is recorded limits the information available and obviously the resolution after Fourier self-deconvolution cannot be improved beyond that point. (There is not information in the interferogram past a point $x = 1$ per instrument resolution.)
2. The space between two digitally encoded points must be at the most equal to the nominal resolution of the spectrophotometer, otherwise information is lost.

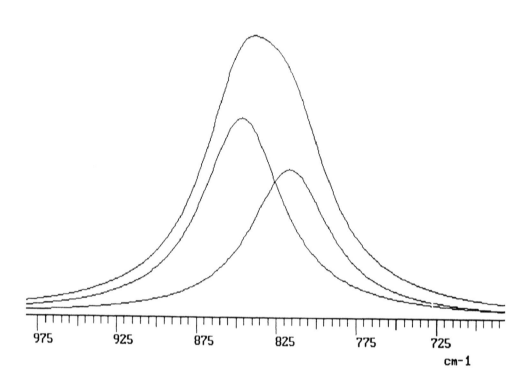

FIGURE 9.   Two Lorentzians of half width at half height σ = 30 cm^{-1} each separated by 30 cm^{-1} and their sum.

3.   The noise is experimentally the most constraining source of information loss and its dramatic effect on the deconvolved spectrum is illustrated in Figure 12. The high-frequency noise whose amplitude does not exceed 0.1% of the total spectrum amplitude (it is barely visible on the undeconvolved spectrum) tremendously increases for K > 3. As a rule of thumb, the maximum K value applied should not exceed 2 if the noise maximum amplitude is 1% or 3 if the noise maximum amplitude is 0.1%.

C. RESOLUTION ENHANCEMENT FACTOR

A resolution enhancement factor K is defined as the ratio of the line width before self-deconvolution to that after.[37] If the spectrum is deconvoluted with a Lorentzian line,

$$L_0(\nu) = \frac{\sigma_1/\pi}{\sigma_1^2 + \nu^2} \tag{67}$$

where σ_1 is one half of the FWHH of the Lorentzian, then the interferogram of the spectrum has to be divided by the Fourier transform of $L_0(\nu)$ which is given by

$$F\{L_0(\nu)\} = \int_{-\infty}^{+\infty} L_0(\nu)\exp(-i2\pi\nu x)d\nu \tag{68}$$

$$= \exp(-2\pi\sigma_1|x|) \tag{69}$$

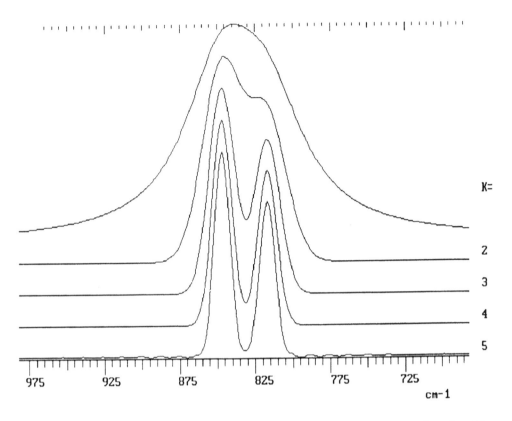

FIGURE 10. Fourier self-deconvolution of the spectrum of Figure 9 resulting from the sum of two Lorentzians as a function of the resolution enhancement factor K. Deconvolution was performed with a Lorentzian function ($\sigma = 30$ cm^{-1}) and a Gaussian apodization adjusted to obtain the desired value of K.

In order to prevent the high-frequency noise from being unnecessarily amplified, an apodization is also applied, i.e., the spectrum is convoluted by a smoothing function. A Gaussian line has been used in major works concerning protein secondary structure and will be taken as an example here. If the spectrum is to be convoluted with a Gaussian line,

$$G_0(\nu) = \frac{\ln 2}{\sqrt{\pi}\sigma_g} \exp(-\ln 2\nu^2/\sigma_g^2) \tag{70}$$

where σ_g is one half of the FWHH of the Gaussian. The interferogram of the deconvoluted spectrum then has to be multiplied by the Fourier transform of $G_0(\nu)$ which is given by

$$F\{G_0(\nu)\} = \sqrt{\ln 2} \exp - \pi^2 x^2 \sigma_g^2/\ln 2 \tag{71}$$

note that $\sigma_g = 1/2L$ of references.[36-39]

The resolution enhancement factor K defined as the ratio of the width of the deconvoluting Lorentzian by the width of the convoluting Gaussian correctly describes the ratio of the IR band width before by the band width after the mathematical treatment provided that the Lorentzian band width to be used is precisely known. The process can then indeed be seen as the convolution of a δ-function resulting from the correct deconvolution of a Lorentzian by itself by a Gaussian, the result being the convoluting Gaussian itself. If σ_l is underestimated, the factor K has no physical meaning anymore.

The interferogram of the spectrum is multiplied by the deconvolution-apodization function DA(x):

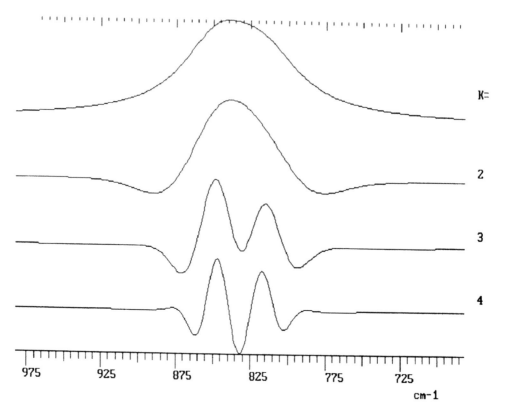

FIGURE 11.   Fourier self-deconvolution of the spectrum of Figure 9 resulting from the sum of two Lorentzians as a function of the resolution enhancement factor K. Deconvolution was performed with a Lorentzian function ($\sigma = 60$ cm^{-1}) and a Gaussian apodization adjusted to obtain the desired value of K.

$$DA(x) = \sqrt{\ln 2}\ \exp\{2\pi\sigma_1|x| - \pi^2\sigma_g^2 x^2/\ln 2\} \tag{72}$$

The computation is performed as follows. For a frequency spectrum of N points encoded every k cm^{-1}, $x_{max} = 1/k$ cm, the interval in x is dx $= 1/(N{\cdot}k)$. The real and the imaginary part of the Fourier transformed spectrum, A(x) and B(x), respectively, are multiplied by DA(x):

$$A(i \cdot dx) = A(i \cdot dx) \cdot DA(i \cdot dx) \tag{73}$$

$$B(i \cdot dx) = B(i \cdot dx) \cdot DA(i \cdot dx) \tag{74}$$

for i = 0 to N/2 and i·dx = x. Because of the symmetry properties of the Fourier transform,

$$A((N + 1 - i) \cdot dx) = A(i \cdot dx) \tag{75}$$

$$B((N + 1 - i) \cdot dx) = -B(i \cdot dx) \tag{76}$$

for i = 1 to N/2 −1. If σ_1 is ill-defined, the resolution enhancement factor K loses its meaning as has already been exemplified in Figure 11. Moreover, the same K factor can yield different shapes of the function DA(x) according to the value of σ_1 chosen. The shape of DA(x) for K = 2 for $\sigma_1 = 8$, 12, and 16 cm^{-1} is reported in Figure 13.

It is worth studying the properties of DA(x) so that the user can predict in the general case which frequencies will be most enhanced and how a given cut off of the high-frequency

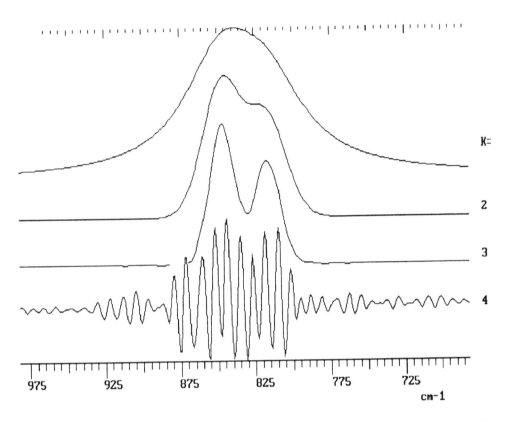

FIGURE 12.   Fourier self-deconvolution of the spectrum resulting from the sum of two Lorentzians presented in Figure 8. Conditions are identical to those of Figure 9, but 0.01% of the high-frequency noise has been added to the original spectrum.

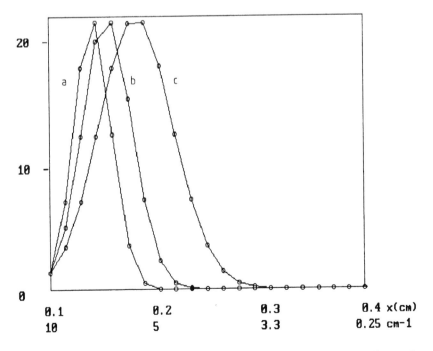

FIGURE 13.   Shape of the DA(x) function for a resolution enhancement factor K = 2 for different values of σ_1; a, $\sigma_1 = 16$ cm^{-1}; b, $\sigma_1 = 12$ cm^{-1}; c, $\sigma_1 = 8$ cm^{-1}.

noise can be obtained. Because of the symmetry of the Fourier transform around $x = 0$, only positive values of x will be considered hereafter. From the derivatization of Equation 72, the DA(x) function has one maximum x_{max} given by

$$x_{max} = \frac{\ln 2}{\pi} \frac{\sigma_1}{\sigma_g^2} \tag{77}$$

The function falls to its value in $x = 0$, $(DA(0) = \sqrt{\ln 2})$, again when $x = 2x_{max}$. The frequency which is most enhanced is adjusted for a given value of σ_1 by changing σ_g.

It is important to realize here that if a noise is random before applying self-deconvolution, it is no longer random after self-deconvolution with the DA(x) function since some frequencies are specifically enhanced. The noise appears then as usual IR absorption bands and is very easily confused with real signal. Only a preliminary check of the noise level or a close watch of the region of the spectrum free of any real signal can prevent the confusion of real signal with noise. Upon data accumulation, the noise should decrease, but not the real signal.

From another point of view, it is useful to be able to determine for a given σ_1 which value of σ_g is going to yield a cut off at a position $x = r \approx 1$ per maximum resolution desired, f being a fraction of the maximum of the function, i.e.,

$$DA(r) = f\sqrt{\ln 2} \; \exp\{\ln 2(\sigma_1^2/\sigma_g^2)\} \tag{78}$$

The value of σ_g is then given by

$$\sigma_g = \{(2\pi\sigma_1 r - \ln f + (\ln^2 f - 4\pi\sigma_1 r \ln f)^{1/2})/(2\pi^2 r^2/\ln 2)\}^{1/2} \quad 0 < f \leqslant 1 \tag{79}$$

Tables 3 and 4 report the value of σ_g as a function of the "maximum resolution" $1/r$ at which DA(x) falls to a fraction f of its maximum as a function of f and σ_1 for four values of $1/r$.

V. MATERIALS USED IN ATTENUATED TOTAL REFLECTION (ATR) AND THEIR OPTICAL PROPERTIES

Internal reflection spectroscopy is greatly dependent on the optical properties of the internal reflection element and on the incidence angle. The laws governing internal reflection spectroscopy have been described by Harrick.[18] It is useful here to summarize the properties of some usual internal reflection elements when working with lipid or protein films and polarized light. We shall consider only the case of "thin films" which are much thinner than the penetration depth.

A. PENETRATION DEPTH

It has been demonstrated from Maxwell's equations that an electromagnetic disturbance exists in the medium beyond the reflecting interface. It is an evanescent wave whose electric field amplitude E_0 falls off exponentially with distance z from the surface, i.e.,

$$E = E_0 e^{-z/dp} \tag{80}$$

The electric field amplitude E falls at $1/e$ at the penetration depth dp which is related to the wavelength λ and to the angle of incidence with respect to a normal to the IRE θ by

$$d_p = \frac{\lambda/n_1}{2\pi(\sin^2\theta - n_{21}^2)^{1/2}} \tag{81}$$

TABLE 3

Evaluation of Fourier Self-Deconvolution Parameters as a Function of the Maximum Resolution Required for Typical Values of σ_1 and σ_g

Maximum Resolution Requested: 4 cm^{-1} (r = 0.250 cm)

σ_1	2.5	5.0	7.5	10.0	12.5	15.0	17.5	20.0
f								
1.000	1.49	2.10	2.57	2.97	3.32	3.64	3.93	4.20
0.900	1.67	2.28	2.75	3.15	3.50	3.81	4.11	4.38
0.800	1.76	2.37	2.84	3.23	3.58	3.90	4.19	4.46
0.700	1.84	2.44	2.91	3.30	3.65	3.97	4.26	4.53
0.600	1.91	2.51	2.98	3.37	3.72	4.04	4.33	4.60
0.500	1.99	2.59	3.05	3.44	3.79	4.11	4.40	4.67
0.400	2.08	2.67	3.13	3.52	3.87	4.18	4.47	4.74
0.300	2.18	2.76	3.22	3.61	3.95	4.27	4.55	4.82
0.200	2.30	2.88	3.33	3.72	4.06	4.37	4.66	4.93
0.100	2.49	3.05	3.50	3.88	4.22	4.53	4.82	5.08
0.090	2.52	3.08	3.52	3.90	4.24	4.55	4.84	5.10
0.080	2.55	3.11	3.55	3.93	4.27	4.58	4.86	5.13
0.070	2.58	3.14	3.58	3.96	4.30	4.60	4.89	5.15
0.060	2.62	3.17	3.61	3.99	4.33	4.63	4.92	5.18
0.050	2.66	3.21	3.65	4.03	4.36	4.67	4.95	5.22
0.040	2.71	3.26	3.69	4.07	4.41	4.71	4.99	5.26
0.030	2.78	3.32	3.75	4.12	4.46	4.76	5.05	5.31
0.020	2.87	3.40	3.83	4.20	4.53	4.83	5.12	5.38
0.010	3.01	3.53	3.95	4.32	4.65	4.95	5.23	5.49
0.005	3.14	3.65	4.07	4.43	4.76	5.06	5.33	5.59
0.002	3.27	3.77	4.18	4.54	4.86	5.16	5.44	5.69
0.001	3.39	3.88	4.29	4.64	4.96	5.26	5.53	5.79

Maximum Resolution Requested: 8 cm^{-1} (r = 0.125 cm)

σ_1	2.5	5.0	7.5	10.0	12.5	15.0	17.5	20.0
f								
1.000	2.10	2.97	3.64	4.20	4.70	5.15	5.56	5.94
0.900	2.47	3.33	4.00	4.56	5.05	5.50	5.91	6.30
0.800	2.66	3.51	4.17	4.73	5.22	5.67	6.08	6.46
0.700	2.83	3.67	4.33	4.88	5.37	5.82	6.23	6.61
0.600	2.99	3.82	4.47	5.03	5.52	5.96	6.37	6.75
0.500	3.16	3.98	4.63	5.18	5.66	6.10	6.51	6.89
0.400	3.35	4.15	4.79	5.34	5.82	6.26	6.66	7.04
0.300	3.56	4.35	4.98	5.52	6.00	6.44	6.84	7.22
0.200	3.84	4.61	5.22	5.76	6.23	6.66	7.06	7.44
0.100	4.25	4.99	5.59	6.11	6.57	7.00	7.39	7.76
0.090	4.31	5.04	5.64	6.16	6.62	7.05	7.44	7.81
0.080	4.38	5.10	5.69	6.21	6.67	7.10	7.49	7.86
0.070	4.45	5.17	5.76	6.27	6.73	7.16	7.55	7.92
0.060	4.53	5.24	5.83	6.34	6.80	7.22	7.61	7.98
0.050	4.62	5.33	5.91	6.42	6.88	7.30	7.69	8.05
0.040	4.74	5.43	6.01	6.51	6.97	7.39	7.78	8.14
0.030	4.88	5.56	6.13	6.63	7.08	7.50	7.89	8.25
0.020	5.06	5.73	6.30	6.79	7.24	7.65	8.04	8.40
0.010	5.37	6.02	6.57	7.05	7.49	7.90	8.28	8.64
0.005	5.66	6.28	6.82	7.30	7.73	8.13	8.51	8.86
0.002	5.93	6.54	7.06	7.53	7.96	8.36	8.73	9.08
0.001	6.19	6.78	7.30	7.76	8.18	8.57	8.94	9.28

TABLE 3 (continued)
Evaluation of Fourier Self-Deconvolution Parameters as a Function of the Maximum Resolution Required for Typical Values of σ_1 and σ_g

Note: Half width at half height σ_g of the apodization Gaussian as a function of 1°; half width at half height σ_1 of the deconvoluting Lorentzian function and 2° as a function of f; the value of the deconvolution-apodization function expressed as a fraction of its maximum value at a position r on the interferogram corresponding to the maximum resolution requested.

where n_1 is the internal reflection element refractive index, n_2 is the index of the sample in contact with the reflection element, and $n_{21} = n_2/n_1$. Hence, d_p increases with the wavelength and when $n_{21} \rightarrow 1$ (better index matching). For a lipid film ($n_2 = 1.55$) and a KRS plate ($n_1 = 2.35$) at an angle of incidence of 45°, $d_p = 1\lambda$ ($= 5 \ \mu m$ at 2000 cm^{-1}). If a germanium plate ($n_1 = 4$) is used with a 45° incidence angle, $d_p = 0.11\lambda$, and for a 30°C incidence angle, $d_p = 0.40\lambda$.

If we consider a surface occupied per molecule at 60 Å^2 and a mean molecular weight of 750 for a phospholipid, then 1 cm^2 of a single bilayer weighs 0.4 μg. If the bilayer thickness is 100 Å including the interbilayer space in a multilayer system, then 100 of them can be stacked in 1 μm and the lipid weight is now 40 μg/cm^2. For 50 × 20 × 2 mm IRE, about 5 cm^2 is usable on one side. Those numbers will have to be taken into account to determine the approximate mean thickness of the sample.

B. ABSORBENCE VS. REFLECTION SPECTRA

It must be noted that in the general case, the reflection spectrum can be different from an absorption spectrum. For a reflection spectrum, the absorption parameter a is defined as the reflection loss per reflection:

$$a = (100 - R)\% \tag{82}$$

where R is the reflectivity of the surface which represents the reflected power. For an absorption spectrum, the transmittance I/I_0 is defined by the absorption coefficient α and the sample thickness d:

$$\frac{I}{I_0} = \exp(-\alpha d) \approx 1 - \alpha d \ \text{for low absorption} \tag{83}$$

For one internal reflection, an effective thickness d_e can be defined as

$$d_e = a/\alpha \tag{84}$$

so that

$$R = 1 - \alpha d_e \tag{85}$$

d_e is therefore a measure of the strength of coupling to the sample. It represents the actual thickness of film that would be required to obtain the same absorption in transmission measurements.

For multiple reflections, the reflected power is given by

$$R_N = (1 - \alpha d_e)^N \approx 1 - N\alpha d_e \ \text{ for } \ \alpha d_e \ll 1 \tag{86}$$

where N is the number of reflections. It is therefore possible to increase the sensitivity of

TABLE 4
Optical and Physical Constants of the Most Usual Materials Used to Build Internal Reflection Elements (IRE)

Materials	Refractive index n_1	θ_{cs} (°)	θ_{ca} (°)	Hardness (Knoop)	$de_\perp$	$de_\parallel$	$Nde_\perp$	$Nde_\parallel$	N	Aperture	Remark
Ge											
30°	4.0	15	23	550	1.43	1.63	62.0	70.5	43	4.0	
45°					1.17	1.31	29.2	32.7	25	2.8	
60°					0.83	0.92	11.9	13.3	14	2.3	
Si											
30°	3.42	17	27	1150	1.72	1.92	74.3	81.1	43	4.0	
45°					1.40	1.54	35.0	38.4	25	2.8	
60°					1.00	1.08	14.3	15.6	14	2.3	
ZnS											
30°	2.42	24	40	355	2.68	2.69	115.9	116.5	43	4.0	$\theta > \theta_{ca}$
45°					2.18	2.19	54.6	54.8	25	2.8	
60°					1.55	1.55	22.3	22.4	14	2.3	
KRS-5											
30°	2.35	25	41	40	2.79	2.74	120.8	118.7	43	4.0	$\theta > \theta_{ca}$
45°					2.28	2.26	57.0	56.0	25	2.8	
30°					1.61	1.60	23.3	23.1	14	2.3	

Note: The optical properties of IRE reported have been calculated for use with thin phospholipid films ($n_2 = 1.55$) in contact with air ($n_3 = 1$). $de_\perp$ and $de_\parallel$ were calculated according to Equations 90 and 91, respectively; N was calculated according to Equation 92 and the aperture was calculated according to Equations 93 to 94; $\theta_{cs} = \sin^{-1} n_{21}$ and $\theta_{ca} = \sin^{-1} n_{31}$. The refractive index of other materials, e.g., ZnSe ($n_1 = 2.24$, hardness = 150) or CdTe ($n_1 = 2.65$, hardness = 45), are close enough to those already used in the Table, so that their other properties can be estimated by comparison with the other materials.

the method by increasing d_e and N. For very thin films (d $\ll$ dp), the electric field can be assumed to be constant over the film thickness and the effective thickness is then given by

$$d_e = n_{21}E_0^2d/\cos\theta \tag{87}$$

where d is the actual thickness of the film.

The electric field amplitude in the film is given by

$$E_\perp = \frac{2\cos\theta}{(1 - n_{31}^2)^{1/2}} \tag{88}$$

$$E_\parallel = \frac{2\cos\theta\{(1 + n_{32}^4)\sin^2\theta - _{31}^2\}^{1/2}}{(1 - n_{31}^2)\{(1 + n_{31}^2)\sin\theta^2 - n_{31}^2\}^{1/2}} \tag{89}$$

where medium 1 is the IRE, medium 2 is the thin film, and medium 3 is the medium beyond the thin film. The effective thicknesses for perpendicular and parallel polarization are, respectively,

$$de_\perp = \frac{4n_{21}d\cos\theta}{(1 - n_{31}^2)} \tag{90}$$

$$de_\parallel = \frac{4n_{21}d\cos\theta\{(1 + n_{32}^4)\sin^2\theta - n_{31}^2\}}{(1 - n_{31}^2)\{(1 + n_{31}^2)\sin^2\theta - n_{31}^2\}} \tag{91}$$

These equations are good to a few percent when d $<0.1/2\pi\cdot\lambda/n_1$, e.g., when at 1000 cm^{-1}, d <40 nm for germanium and d <70 nm for KRS-5. For $\theta = 45°$ in these conditions, the absorption coefficient should not exceed 10^5. While for bulk materials, the lower limit of the working angle is governed by the IRE/sample interface, $\theta_c = \sin^{-1} n_{21}$; for thin films, the lower limit of the working angle is only limited by the IRE/medium 3 interface, $\theta_{ca} = \sin^{-1}n_{31}$. For $\theta <\theta_{cs}$, the total reflection occurs at the 1-2 interface, but for $\theta_{ca} <\theta <\theta_{cs}$, the light is partially reflected by the sample/medium 3 interface and these values of θ can be used if the outer surface of the film is uniform and parallel to the IRE surface. Optical constants can be derived from measurements at these angles.[44] In practice, it is wise to use values of $\theta <\theta_{ca}$ when working with biological samples. Finally, it must be noted that spectra can be much distorted if good physical contact between the IRE and the sample is not obtained.

To summarize the factors affecting the sensitivity of a measurement, the absorbence of a band increases:

1. With the number N of internal reflection — If l is the length of the IRE and t is its thickness, we have

$$N = \frac{1}{t}\cot\theta \tag{92}$$

    N must be the integer and odd for the geometry described in Figure 4.
2. When the incidence angle θ becomes smaller and tends to θ_{cs} — However, at small incidence angles, the aperture A decreases, letting less light into the IRE:

$$A = t\csc\theta \tag{93}$$

$$A = 2t\sin\theta \quad \text{for} \quad \theta < 45° \tag{94}$$

It must be taken into account as a limiting experimental factor at small angles. Highly sensitive MCT detectors available can probably overcome this problem to a certain extent.

3. When the index matching is better between the sample and the IRE ($n_{21} \rightarrow 1$) — However, this reduces in turn the range of incidence angles θ available for measurements.

C. PROPERTIES OF VARIOUS INTERNAL REFLECTION ELEMENTS (IRE)

From the practical point of view, an important property of the IRE is its hardness. Indeed, it determines how quickly the surface is going to be damaged. Since scattering follows a law in λ^{-4}, intensity losses at high wave numbers becomes quickly considerable. In our hands, polishing the IRE with the help of a polishing kit requires a lot of skilled work and never yields high-quality surfaces. The properties of the most usual IRE are summarized in Table 4.

VI. SAMPLE PREPARATION: OBTENTION OF ORIENTED MEMBRANES

When the orientation of various molecular axes is measured with respect to a normal to the plate supporting the membrane by dichroism measurements (see Chapter 2), it is required that the membranes themselves orient parallel to the supporting plate. A perfect orientation of the membranes has been described by an order parameter, $<P_2>_\gamma = 1$ (Equation 50). Two questions arise for the preparation of oriented membranes: (1) what technique is available and what degree of orientation can be achieved and (2) can we make sure that the procedure does not modify the conformation to be studied? Several procedures will be quickly overviewed.

A. THE LANGMUIR-BLODGETT TECHNIQUE

A multilayer assembly is obtained by transferring a monolayer spread at the air-water interface by a cycle of dipping and withdrawal of the supporting plate through the monolayer. The surface pressure of the monolayer is kept constant during the process by moving a barrier on the surface. The barrier displacement allows control of the amount of material transferred on the plate. The details of the technique are described elsewhere.[45,46] This procedure allows the study of single monolayer or bilayer or multilayer arrangements. Single monolayers of DPPC transferred on a germanium IRE at low pressure (20 mN/m) or high pressure (40 mN/m) results, respectively, in ordered and disordered states of the DPPC molecules similar to those observed in liposomes below and above the phase transition. However, when the number of layers transferred (z-type) is increased, the ordered form is always found, suggesting a rearrangement of the layers so that a closer packing of the molecules is obtained.[47] Similar rearrangements of the DPPC molecules to form islands of well-packed molecules in monolayers transferred at low pressure have been suggested by Okamura et al.[48] Other evidence of reorganization has been brought by Fringeli.[4,49,50] As far as the diffusion rate of the molecules in the monolayer is concerned, experiments of fluorescence recovery after photobleaching indicate that the lipid diffusion rate reflects the fluidity of the film at the air-water interface before deposit.[51] Transition temperatures are also observed in multilayer arrangements.[51] As a conclusion, it appears that the layer system transferred on the solid support is able to evolve toward a more stable situation when the initial molecular situation is experimentally forced to be unstable. However, this final more stable situation is probably closer to that prevailing in real membrane systems. The hydration of the molecules seems to preserve the conformation of the molecules existing in solution.

The role of this hydration on DMPC, DPPC, and DSPC and their phase transition have been recently studied.[53] As an example of determination of conformational parameters obtained on such multilayers of DPPE by dichroism measurements, the reader is referred to the work of Akutsu et al.[13]

B. THE SOLVENT EVAPORATION TECHNIQUE

Because of the often poor attachment of the layers encountered while building up multilayer arrangements by the previous technique, most workers have resorted to the simple and efficient solvent evaporation technique. It consists of drying on the supporting plate a solution or suspension of the membranes in either organic or aqueous solvent. While evaporating, the capilarity forces flatten the membrane which spontaneously forms multilayers arrangements.[4] Hydration of the molecules can take place subsequently by flushing the sample-containing chamber with nitrogen saturated with H_2O or D_2O.[22,52] The technique is very convenient to study proteins inserted into lipid films since usual reconstitution techniques can be used. Orientation of protein secondary structures can then be studied by dichrism.[52,55] Addition of sugars such as trehalose to the membrane sample can prevent the destabilizing effects of dehydration on the bilayers[56-59] and on proteins.[60] Removal of defects in the structure of oriented multilayers can be achieved by different methods such as annealing[61] or compression-dilatation.[62] The procedure described in the next paragraph is another way to improve the ordering of the multilayers.

C. ISOPOTENTIAL SPIN-DRY CENTRIFUGATION

In this technique, drying occurs during centrifugation at high g. It takes advantage of the initial layer-by-layer deposition of centrifugation to form parallel arrays. The surface of the support is designed to be isopotential during the centrifugation. Solvent evaporation can take place into the evacuated spin chamber through a small hole. Centrifugation alone can achieve a pressure of 10^6 dyn/cm^2 which is, however, not enough to eliminate thermal membrane curvature fluctuations. Solvent evaporation exerts, via capillary suction, much larger compaction pressures sufficient to eliminate the space between the layers. A theory about the membrane orientation during the isopotential spin-dry centrifugation is described elsewhere.[30-32] For another example, the reader is referred to the work of Bazzi and Woody[63] on the orientation of the α-helices of cytochrome c oxidase.

VII. CONFORMATIONAL INFORMATION CONTAINED IN INFRARED (IR) SPECTRA

In the study of membrane phospholipids and proteins, IR spectroscopy brings two types of information:

1.   An orientational information — This can be obtained provided that oriented membranes can be prepared. Orientation of various chemical bonds or chemical groups can then be determined by studying the polarization of their specific absorption bands. Chapter 2 was dedicated to this aspect, the methods used, and their limitation.
2.   A purely conformational information — It comes from normal mode analysis computation and from the empirical observation that the frequency of a group is, sometimes strongly, dependent on the molecular conformation. For this reason, a simple observation of a IR spectrum can provide us with valuable details on the molecular conformation. This aspect of IR spectroscopy applied to membranes deserves an entire paper, but we shall limit ourselves here to a brief overview of the kind of information that can be gained.

A. PHOSPHOLIPID MOLECULES

The different regions of the phospholipid molecule will be examined successively. The assignments of the bands as well as the orientation of the transition dipole moment with respect to molecular axes have been reviewed.[4] Only the main characteristics of the bands frequently used in the literature are listed.

The hydrocarbon chain region — The symmetric and antisymmetric C–H (CH$_2$) stretching bands around 2850 and 2925 cm^{-1} have their dipole oriented ∥ (parallel) and ⊥ (perpendicular) to the H–C–H bisector, respectively. These modes of vibration are uncoupled from the rest of the molecule and are therefore independent on the nature of the lipid polar head group. Their frequency reflects the number of *gauche* conformers in the acyl chain (allows estimation of the *trans/gauche* ratio) and the band width increases with the acyl chain mobility.[64,65] Both can be used to monitor lamellar gel structure transition to a lamellar liquid-crystalline phase as well as a transition to the hexagonal H$_{ii}$ phase.[65] Since the amplitude of the frequency shift observed during the phase transition does not exceed 2 to 3 cm^{-1}, special algorithms are required to obtain the accuracy required.[66] The effect of cholesterol[67] and proteins[68,69] has been studied at this level. Using deuterium-labeled acyl chains allows performance of the measurements for a specific lipid in a complex environment such as natural membranes.[70,71] The CH$_2$ bending mode is located near 1472 cm^{-1} for an all-*trans* conformation of the acyl chains and falls to about 1466 cm^{-1} above the phase transition.[4,64] Splitting occurs in some types of packing.[72] The dipole is directed along the H–C–H bisector. The CH$_2$ wagging band progression between 1180 and 1345 cm^{-1} appears only when the acyl chains are in the all-*trans* conformation.[4,73,74] The integration of one of these bands (usually the band near 1200 cm^{-1} is the most convenient to use) can be used to quantify the proportion of acyl chains in the all-*trans* conformation.[23,75] The dipole of this transition is oriented parallel to the all-*trans* chain axis and is often used for determination of chain orientation.[4] The CH$_2$ rocking near 720 cm^{-1} is sensitive to chain packing in crystals.[76,77] The band width reflects chain mobility. It sharpens, for instance, in the presence of mellitin.[78]

The glycerol backbone region — The C=O stretching near 1730 cm^{-1} contains the contribution of both sn-1 and sn-2 acyl chains which usually adopt different conformations. The high-frequency component is assigned to the sn-1 straight chain in PC and the low-frequency component is assigned to the bent sn-2 chain.[4] Hydrogen bonding is known to decrease the frequency of the band.[79] Difference in the hydration between sn-1 and sn-2 chains might explain part of their difference of position on the IR spectrum. Results obtained by Wong and Mantsch indicate that no hydration of the sn-1 C=O group occurs in DMPC, DPPC, DPPE, and DHPC. The sn-2 is located at somewhat lower frequency. This frequency is further decreased upon hydration.[80] In general, a broad contour results from the overlapping of sn-1 and sn-2 chains, but different components can be resolved by Fourier self-deconvolution.[80,81] These results can be checked for some of the phospholipids for which an X-ray diffraction structure is known.[82] Addition of cholesterol perturbs specifically the sn-2 chain.[83] Effects of Li$^+$ and Ca^{2+} on the conformation and hydration of PS have been reported by Casal et al.[84,85] The most thorough investigation of the carbonyl stretching frequency has been carried out by Blume et al.[86] They prepared synthetic phospholipid (DMPC, DMPE, DMPG, and DMPA) in which one of the two ^{12}C=O group was labeled with a ^{13}C=O. The shift of about 40 cm^{-1} of the labeled acyl chain allowed monitoring of the carbonyl stretching frequency for each chain without interference of the other. The C–O single bond stretching is clearly resolved for the sn-1 chain (1180 cm^{-1}) for which the C–CO–O–C group is planar and for the sn-2 chain (1165 cm^{-1}) for which the C–CO–O–C group is *gauche*.[4] The dipole is about perpendicular to the C=O double bond. A shift from one conformation to the other may be observed by monitoring these two frequencies.

The phosphate group region — The symmetric and antisymmetric (PO$_2^-$) stretchings are sensitive to hydration, e.g., upon dehydration following Ca^{2+} binding, the antisymmetric

(PO_2^-) stretching is shifted from 1221 to 1238 cm^{-1} (dehydrated), indicating that phosphate, but not the carboxyl group of PS, is responsible for Ca^{2+} binding.[84,85] Splitting may occur upon crystallization. The frequency of the symmetric and antisymmetric O–P–O vibration and of the PO_2 wagging are of direct diagnostic interest for the conformation (antiplanar-antiplanar, antiplanar-*gauche*, *gauche-gauche*) of the R–O–PO_2–O–R' group.[85] More information about the phosphate group frequencies for the solid or solution state of PE[87] compared for different phospholipids[88,89] can be found in the literature.

The terminal head group region — The terminal head group region gives rise to numerous bands according to the nature of the phospholipid. Let us quote here the antisymmetric (CH_3) bending of the choline group whose dipole is directed along the symmetry axis of the choline group and the symmetric C–N–$(CH_3)_3^+$ stretching which has the same dipole orientation and which is found at 920 to 930 cm^{-1} for the *trans* conformation of the O–C–C–N frame and at 875 to 895 cm^{-1} for the *gauche* conformation.[4] For PS, the C=O stretching of the carboxylic group is located near 1736 cm^{-1} for the –COOH form and near 1623 cm^{-1} for the –COO$^-$ form (1640 cm^{-1} if hydrated).

B. PROTEINS AND PEPTIDES

It has been known for a long time that protein IR spectra are sensitive to secondary structure. The amide I band (amide carbonyl stretching) is the most useful band to study since it is the most conformationally sensitive and since it falls between 1600 and 1700 cm^{-1}, a region with little lipid absorption (except for PS). However, it was only in 1986 that a systematic quantitative estimation of protein secondary structure was obtained after Fourier self-deconvolution and subsequent curve fitting of the amide I' band;[90,91] (the prime (') means that a H/D exchange has been realized). The sensitivity of the shape of amide I' on the protein secondary structure appears in Figure 14 where the ATR spectra of three membrane proteins in a bilayer environment are presented. Porin is very rich in β-sheet structure, bacteriorhodopsin is rich in α-helices, and glycophorin contains both. Assignment of the different frequencies found in amide I' to the different recognized secondary structures was made on an empirical basis as well as on theoretical grounds.[92] The way the quantitative determination of the secondary structures and orientation were determined for membrane proteins from ATR spectra is developed in References 52 and 93. This is illustrated in Figure 15 for papain, a protein which contains an equal amount of α-helix and β-sheet structure. The number and the approximate frequency of the different components are obtained after Fourier self-deconvolution (here K = 2.4). A curve fitting with Lorentzian lines is then realized. The results of the curve fitting reported in Figure 15a are then used as input parameters for a second curve fitting performed on the original spectrum. This procedure avoids some of the drawbacks of the curve fitting techniques[94,95] and prevents artifacts possibly introduced by the deconvolution to interfere with the quantitative analysis. The areas of the components assigned to a same structure are added and the percentage of that structure in the protein is taken to be that resulting area divided by the total amide I' area. This supposes that the extinction coefficient is identical for all the secondary structures. When this procedure was extended to a series of well-characterized proteins, the mean difference between the values so obtained and the X-ray values amounted to no more than 2% (SD 8%) for all the proteins and all the structures when using a quite automatic procedure which requires no human decision between the recording of the spectra and the obtention of the secondary structure (unpublished results). A similar approach is used by several other investigators.[1,96-101] Both conformational and orientational parameters can be studied simultaneously. Figure 16 reports the ATR polarized spectra of bacteriorhodopsin incorporated into DMPC multilayers. Polarization appears more clearly on the difference spectrum 90 to 0°. The lipid C=O stretching at 1730 to 1740 cm^{-1} is very weakly polarized, probably because it is composed of several contributions with various orientations. The frequency of the peptidic C=O stretching (amide I) at 1600 cm^{-1} indicates a largely α-helix structure of

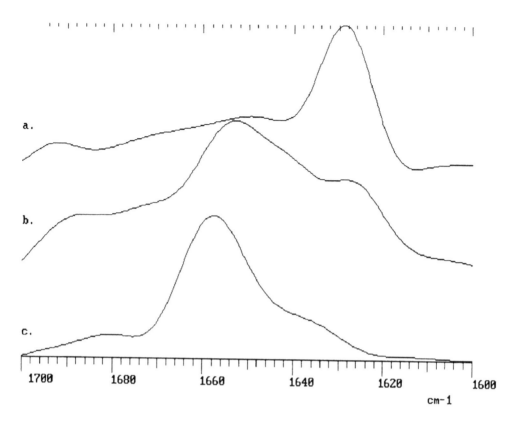

FIGURE 14.   IR spectrum in the amide I region of three membrane proteins reconstituted into liposomes and then prepared for ATR by the solvent evaporation technique. (a) Porin; (b) glycophorin A; (c) bacteriorhodopsin.

the protein. The Fourier self-deconvolution/curve fitting analysis (not shown) determines a content of 51% for the α-helix and 14% for the β-sheet structures. The amide I band is strongly polarized at 90°, particularly on its high-frequency side, indicating a transmembrane orientation of the helices. The orientation of the lipid hydrocarbon chains perpendicular to the membrane plane is assessed by (1) the 90° polarization of the CH_2 wagging at 1200 cm^{-1} (dipole parallel to the all-*trans* chain axis) and (2) by the 0° polarization of the CH_2 bending at 1470 cm^{-1} (dipole parallel to the H–C–H bisector, i.e., perpendicular to the chain axis).

VIII. CONCLUSIONS

The data presented in this Chapter indicate some possible applications of IR spectroscopy in the determination of conformational and orientational parameters of biological membrane molecules. Even though these data precisely define some conformational features of the molecules studied as well as the orientation of several molecular bonds with respect to the membrane, they are not sufficient to provide a clear molecular model of complex assemblies. We suggest here that the information gained by IR spectroscopy can be allied to conformational analysis in two ways:

1.   The introduction in the molecular structure as fixed values of the conformational parameters prior to minimization would dramatically reduce the number of degrees of freedom and therefore reduce the time required to realize the minimization computation. Orientational parameters would be useful at the level of the computation of the association of the membrane molecules in monolayers.

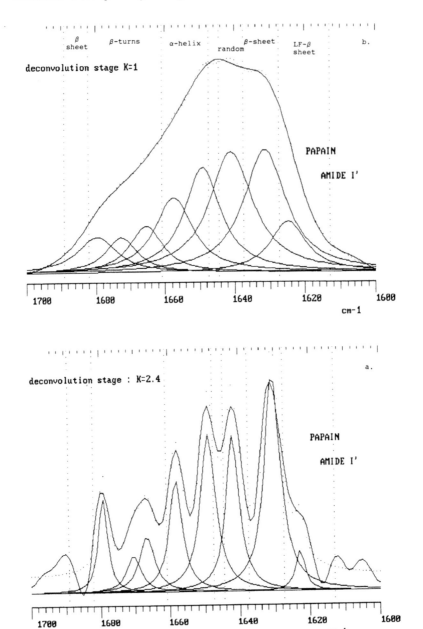

FIGURE 15.   Fourier self-deconvolution and curve fitting realized on the amide I′ band of papain. (See text for details of the procedure.) K is the resolution enhancement factor. The vertical dotted lines indicate the frequency limits in which each secondary structure is found.

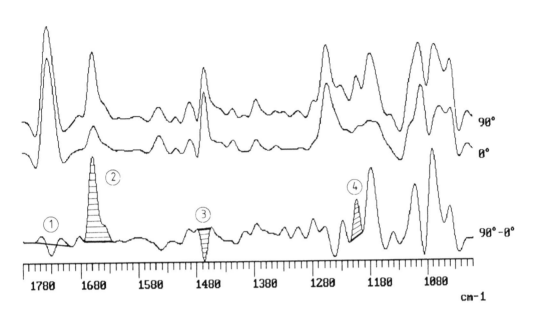

FIGURE 16.   Polarized IR spectra of bacteriorhodopsin reconstituted in DMPC liposomes. Multilayers were formed by the solvent evaporation technique on a germanium IRE at 45°. Spectra were recorded by ATR. The difference spectrum 90 to 0° is rescaled. A positive deviation indicates that the dipole is oriented preferentially perpendicular to the membrane plane and a negative deviation suggests an orientation parallel to the membrane plane: 1, lipid acyl chain carbonyl stretching; 2, peptidic carbonyl stretching (amide I); 3, lipid hydrocarbon chain CH_2 bending; 4, lipid hydrocarbon chain CH_2 wagging.

2.   If the conformational analysis were performed *ab initio* without constraints, the IR data would be useful to check the validity of some of the features of the model arrived at by conformational analysis.

Finally, we mentioned in Chapter 2 a possible interaction between conformational and statistical analysis with the computation of the order parameters.

ACKNOWLEDGMENTS

We are indebted to Dr. Schomblond for reminding us of the basements of the Legendre polynomials. E. G. is an Action de Recherche Concertée fellow. We thank the "Banque Nationale de Belgique" and the "Caisse Générale d'Epargne et de Retraite — Fonds Cancérologique" for financial support.

REFERENCES

1. **Surewicz, W. K. and Mantsch, H. H.,** New insight into protein secondary structure from resolution-enhanced infrared spectra, *Biochim. Biophys. Acta*, 952, 115, 1980.
2. **Susi, H. and Byler, D. M.,** Resolution-enhanced Fourier transform infrared spectroscopy of enzymes, *Methods Enzymol.*, 130, 290, 1986.
3. **Casal, H. L. and Hantsch, H. H.,** Polymorphic phase behaviour of phospholipid membranes studied by infrared spectroscopy, *Biochim. Biophys. Acta*, 779, 381, 1984.
4. **Fringeli, U. P. and Günthard, H. H.,** Infrared membrane spectroscopy, in *Molecular Biology, Biochemistry and Biophysics*, Vol. 31, Grell, E., Ed., Springer-Verlag, Berlin, 1981, 270.
5. **Campbell, I. D. and Dwek, R. A.,** in *Biological Spectroscopy*, Benjamin Cummings, Menlo Park, CA, 1984.
6. **Brey, W. S.,** *Physical Chemistry and Its Biological Applications*, Academic Press, New York, 1978.
7. **Alben, J. O. and Fiamingo, F. G.,** Fourier transform infrared spectroscopy, in *Optical Techniques in Biological Research*, Rousseau, D. L., Ed., Academic Press, New York, 1984, 133.
8. **Oxtoby, D. W.,** Vibrational relaxation in liquids, *Annu. Rev. Phys. Chem.*, 32, 77, 1981.
9. **Fraser, R. D. B.,** The interpretation of infrared dichroism in fibrous protein structures, *J. Chem. Phys.*, 21, 1511, 1953.
10. **Fraser, R. D. B.,** Interpretation of infrared dichroism in fibrous proteins — the 2μ region, *J. Chem. Phys.*, 24, 89, 1956.
11. **Fraser, R. D. B. and MacRae, T. P.,** in *Conformation in Fibrous Proteins and Related Synthetic Polypeptides*, Academic Press, New York, 1973, chap. 5.
12. **Tsuboi, M.,** Infrared dichroism and molecular conformation of α-form poly-τ-benzyl-L-glutamate, *J. Polym. Sci.*, 59, 139, 1962.
13. **Akutsu, H., Kyogoku, Y., Nakahara, H., and Fukuda, K.,** Conformational analysis of phosphatidylethanolamine in multilayers by infrared spectroscopy, *Chem. Phys. Lipids*, 15, 222, 1975.
14. **Rothschild, K. J. and Clark, N. A.,** Polarized infrared spectroscopy of oriented purple membranes, *Biophys. J.*, 25, 493, 1979.
15. **Morse, P. M. and Feshbach,** *Methods of Theoretical Physics*, McGraw-Hill, New York, 1953.
16. **Bellamy, L. J.,** *The Infrared Spectra of Complex Molecules*, Vol. 1, 3rd ed., Chapman and Hall, London, 1977.
17. **Bellamy, L. J.,** *The Infrared Spectra of Complex Molecules, Advances in Group Frequencies*, Vol. 2, 2nd ed., Chapmann and Hall, London, 1980.
18. **Harrick, N. J.,** *Internal Reflection Spectroscopy*, Interscience, New York, 1967.
19. **Fringeli, U. P., Schadt, M., Rihak, P., and Günthard, H. N.,** Hydrocarbon chain ordering in liquid crystals investigated by means of infrared attenuated total reflection (IR-ATR) spectroscopy, *Z. Naturforsch, Teil A*, 31, 1098, 1976.
20. **Fringeli, U. P., Müldner, H. G., Günthard, H. H., Gasche, W., and Leuzinger, W.,** The structure of lipids and proteins studied by attenuated total reflection (ATR) infrared spectroscopy. I. Oriented layers of tripalmitin, *Z. Naturforsch, Teil B*, 27, 780, 1972.
21. **Fringeli, U. P.,** The structure of lipids and proteins studied by attenuated total reflection (ATR) infrared spectroscopy. II. Oriented layers of a homologous series: phosphatidylethanolamine to phosphatidylcholine, *Z. Naturforsch, Teil C*, 32, 20, 1977.
22. **Goormaghtigh, E., Brasseur, R., Huart, P., and Ruysschaert, J. M.,** Study of the adriamycin-cardiolipin complex structure using attenuated total reflection infrared spectroscopy, *Biochemistry*, 26, 1789, 1987.
23. **Fringeli, U. P.,** A new crystalline phase of L-α-dipalmitoylphosphatidylcholine monohydrate, *Biophys. J.*, 34, 173, 1981.
24. **Smulevich, G., Angeloni, L., Giovannardi, S., and Marzocchi, M. P.,** Resonance Raman and polarized light infrared spectra of 1,4-dihydroxyanthraquinone. Vibrational studies of the ground and excited electronic states, *Chem. Phys.*, 65, 313, 1982.
25. **Smulevich, G. and Marzocchi, M. P.,** Single crystal and polarized infrared spectra of two forms of 1,8-dihydroxyanthraquinone. Vibrational assignment and crystals structures, *Chem. Phys.*, 94, 99, 1985.
26. **Radziszewski, J. G. and Michl, J.,** Symmetry assignment of vibrations in anthracene, phenazine, and acridine from infrared dichroism in stretched polyethylene, *J. Chem. Phys.*, 82, 3527, 1985.
27. **Thulstrup, E. W.,** *Aspects of the LD and MCD of Planar Organic Molecules*, Springer-Verlag, Heidelberg, 1980.
28. **Hennicker, C. J.,** Infrared refractive indices of some oriented polymers, *Macromolecules*, 6, 514, 1973.
29. **Nabedryk, E. and Breton, J.,** Orientation of intrinsic proteins in phosphosynthetic membranes. Polarized infrared spectroscopy of chloroplasts and chromatophores, *Biochim. Biophys. Acta*, 635, 515, 1981.
30. **Rothschild, K. J., Sanches, R., and Clark, N. A.,** Infrared absorption of photoreceptor and purple membranes, *Methods Enzymol.*, 88, 696, 1982.

31. **Rothschild, K. J., Sanches, R., Hsiao, T. L., and Clark, N. A.,** A spectroscopic study of rhodopsin alpha-helix orientation, *Biophys. J.,* 31, 53, 1980.
32. **Clark, N. A., Rothschild, K. J., Luippold, D. A., and Simon, B. A.,** Surface-induced lamellar orientation of multilayer membrane arrays. Theoretical analysis and a new method with application to purple membrane fragments, *Biophys. J.,* 31, 65, 1980.
33. **Griffith, P. R., Ed.,** in *Transform Techniques in Chemistry,* Plenum Press, New York, 1978.
34. **Ferraro, J. R. and Basile, L. S., Eds.,** *Fourier Transform Infrared Spectroscopy,* Vols. 1 to 3, Academic Press, New York, 1978 to 1987.
35. **Blass, W. E. and Halsey, G. W.,** *Deconvolution of Absorption Spectra,* Academic Press, New York, 1981.
36. **Kauppinen, J. K., Moffat, D. J., Mantsch, H. H., and Cameron, D. G.,** Fourier self-deconvolution: a method for resolving intrinsically overlapped bands, *Appl. Spectrosc.,* 35, 271, 1981.
37. **Kauppinen, J. K., Moffat, D. J., Mantsch, H. H., and Cameron, D. G.,** Fourier transforms in the computation of self-deconvoluted and first-order derivatives spectra of overlapped band contours, *Anal. Chem.,* 53, 1454, 1981.
38. **Kauppinen, J. K., Moffat, D. J., and Mantsch, H. H.,** Noise in Fourier self-deconvolution, *Appl. Opt.,* 20, 1866, 1981.
39. **Kauppinen, K. J., Moffat, D. J., Mantsch, H. H., and Cameron, D. G.,** Smoothing of spectral data in the Fourier domain, *Appl. Opt.,* 21, 1866, 1982.
40. **Yang, W. S. and Griffiths, P. R.,** Optimization of parameters for Fourier self-deconvolution. I. Minimization of noise and side-lobes without apodization, *Comput. Enhanced Spectrosc.,* 1, 157, 1983.
41. **Yang, W. S. and Griffiths, P. R.,** Optimization of parameters for Fourier self-deconvolution. II. Band multiplits, *Comput. Enhanced Spectrosc.,* 2, 69, 1984.
42. **Griffiths, P. R.,** Fourier transform infrared spectroscopy, *Science,* 222, 297, 1983.
43. **Nikolov, S. and Kantchev, K.,** Deconvolution of Lorentzian broadened spectra. I. Direct deconvolution, *Nucl. Instrum. Methods Phys. Res.,* A256, 161.
44. **Crawford, B., Golpen, J. T., and Swanson, D.,** The measurement of optical constants in the infrared by attenuated total reflection, in *Advances in Infrared and Raman Spectroscopy,* Clark, R. J. H. and Hester, R. E., Eds., Heyden, London.
45. **Blodgett, K. B. and Langmuir, I.,** Built up films of barium stearate and their optical properties, *Phys. Rev.,* 51, 964, 1937.
46. **Khun, H., Möbius, B., and Bücher, H.,** Spectroscopy of monolayer assemblies, in *Techniques of Chemistry,* Vol. 1, Part III 6, Weinberger, A. and Rossiter, B., Eds., John Wiley & Sons, New York, 19, 577.
47. **Lotta, T. I., Laakkonen, L. J., Virtanen, J. A., and Kinnunen, P. K. J.,** Characterization of Langmuir-Blodgett films of 1,2-dipalmitoyl-sn-glycero-3-phosphatidylcholine and 1-palmitoyl-2-(10-pyren-1-yl)decanoyl)-sn-glycero-3-phosphatidylcholine by FTIR-ATR.
48. **Okamura, E., Umumera, J., and Takenaka, T.,** Fourier transform infrared-attenuated total reflection spectra of dipalmitoylphosphatidylcholine monomolecular films, *Biochim. Biophys. Acta,* 812, 139, 1985.
49. **Kopp, F., Fringeli, U. P., Mühlethaler, K., and Günthard, H. H.,** Instability of Langmuir-Blodgett layers of barium stearate, cadmium arachidate and tripalmitin, studied by means of electron microscopy and infrared spectroscopy, *Biophys. Struct. Mech.,* 1, 75, 1975.
50. **Kopp, F., Fringeli, U. P., Mühlethaler, K., and Günthard, H. H.,** Spontaneous rearrangement in Langmuir-Blodgett layers of tripalmitin studied by means of ATR infrared spectroscopy and electron microscopy, *Z. Naturforsch. Teil C,* 30, 711, 1975.
51. **Tiede, D. M.,** Incorporation of membrane proteins into interfacial films: model membranes for electrical and structural characterization, *Biochim. Biophys. Acta,* 811, 357, 1985.
52. **Cabiaux, V., Brasseur, R., Wattiez, R., Falmagne, P., Ruysschaert, J. M., and Goormaghtigh, E.,** Secondary structure of diphtheria toxin and its fragments interacting with acidic liposomes studied by polarized infrared spectroscopy, *J. Biol. Chem.,* 264, 4928, 1989.
53. **Mellier, A. and Diaf, A.,** Infrared study of phospholipid hydration. Main phase transition of saturated phosphatidylcholine/water multilamellar samples, *Chem. Phys. Lipids,* 46, 51, 1988.
54. **Yang, P. W., Stewart, L. C., and Mantsch, H. H.,** Polarized attenuated total reflectance spectra of oriented purple membranes, *Biochem. Biophys. Res. Commun.,* 145, 298, 1987
55. **Okamura, E., Umumera, J., and Takenaka, T.,** Orientation gramicidin D incorporated into phospholipid bilayers: a Fourier transform infrared-attenuated total reflection spectroscopy study.
56. **Crowe, L. M., Womersley, C., Crowe, J. H., Reid, D., Appel, L., and Rudolph, A.,** Prevention of fusion leakage in freeze-dried liposomes by carbohydrates, *Biochim. Biophys. Acta,* 861, 131, 1986.
57. **Hauser, H. and Strauss, G.,** Stabilization of small unilamellar phospholipid vesicles during spray-drying, *Biochim. Biophys. Acta,* 897, 331, 1987.
58. **Crowe, J. H., Spargo, B. J., and Crowe, L. M.,** Preservation of dry liposomes does not require retention of residual water, *Proc. Natl. Acad. Sci. U.S.A.,* 84, 1537, 1987.

59. **Crowe, J. H. and Crowe, L. M.,** Factors affecting the stability of dry liposomes, *Biochim. Biophys. Acta,* 939, 327, 1988.

60. **Goormaghtigh, E., Ruysschaert, J. M., and Scarborough, G. A.,** High yield incorporation of the *Neurospora* plasma membrane H$^+$ATPase into proteoliposomes: lipid requirement and secondary structure of the enzyme by IR spectroscopy, in *The Ions Pumps: Structure, Function and Regulation,* Stein, W. D., Ed., Alan R. Liss, New York, 51.

61. **Powers, L. and Pershan, P. S.,** Monodomain samples of dipalmitoylphosphatidylcholine with varying concentration of water and other ingredients, *Biophys. J.,* 20, 137, 1977.

62. **Asher, S. A. and Pershan, P. S.,** Alignment defect structures in oriented phosphatidylcholine multilayers, *Biophys. J.,* 27, 393, 1979.

63. **Bazzi, M. D. and Woody, R. W.,** Oriented secondary structure in integral membrane proteins. I. Circular dichroism and infrared spectroscopy of cytochrome oxidase in multilamellar films.

64. **Mantsch, H. H., Madec, C., Lewis, R. N. A. H., and McElhaney, R. N.,** Thermotropic phase behavior of model membranes composed of phosphatidylcholines containing iso-branched fatty acids. II. Infrared and ^{31}P NMR spectroscopic studies, *Biochemistry,* 24, 2440, 1985.

65. **Casal, H. L. and Mantsch, H. H.,** Polymorphic phase behaviour of phospholipid membranes studied by infrared spectroscopy, *Biochim. Biophys. Acta,* 779, 381, 1984.

66. **Cameron, D. G., Kauppinen, J. K., Moffat, D. J., and Mantsch, H. H.,** Precision in condensed phase vibrational spectroscopy, *Appl. Spectrosc.,* 36, 245, 1982.

67. **Umumera, J., Cameron, D. G., and Mantsch, H. H.,** A Fourier transform infrared spectroscopic study of the molecular interaction of cholesterol with 1,2-dipalmitoyl-sn-glycero-3-phosphocholine, *Biochim. Biophys. Acta,* 602, 32, 1980.

68. **Dluhy, R. A., Mendelsohn, R., Casal, H. L., and Mantsch, H. H.,** Interaction of dipalmitoylphosphatidylcholine and dimyristoylphosphatidylcholine-d$_{54}$ mixtures with glycophorine. A Fourier transform infrared investigation, *Biochemistry,* 22, 1170, 1983.

69. **Anderle, G. and Mendelsohn, R.,** Fourier transform infrared studies of CaATPase/phospholipid interaction: survey of lipid classes, *Biochemistry,* 25, 2174, 1986.

70. **Casal, H. L., Cameron, D. G., Smith, I. C. P., and Mantsch, H. H.,** *Acholeplasma laidlawii* membranes: a Fourier transform infrared study of the influence of protein on lipid organization and dynamics, *Biochemistry,* 19, 444, 1980.

71. **Cameron, D. G., Casal, D. G., and Mantsch, H. H.,** The application of Fourier transform infrared transmission spectroscopy to the study of model and natural membranes, *J. Biochem. Biophys. Methods,* 1, 21, 1979.

72. **Dluhy, R. A. D., Chowdhry, B. Z., and Cameron, D. G.,** Infrared characterization of conformational differences in the lamellar phases of 1,3-dipalmitoyl-sn-glycero-2-phosphocholine, *Biochim. Biophys. Acta,* 821, 437, 1985.

73. **Chapman, D.,** Infrared spectra and the polymorphysm of glycerides. III. Palmitodistearins and dipalmitostearins, *J. Am. Chem. Soc.,* 56, 2715, 1956.

74. **Chapman, D.,** Infrared spectroscopy of lipids, *J. Am. Oil Chem. Soc.,* 42, 353, 1965.

75. **Fringeli, U. P. and Fringeli, M.,** Pore formation in lipid membranes by alamethicin, *Proc. Natl. Acad. Sci. U.S.A.,* 76, 3852, 1979.

76. **Chapman, D.,** The 720 cm^{-1} band in the infrared spectra of crystalline long-chain compounds, *J. Am. Chem. Soc.,* 57, 4489, 1957.

77. **Snyder, R. G.,** Vibrational correlation splitting and chain packing for the crystalline *n*-alkanes, *J. Chem. Phys.,* 71, 3229, 1979.

78. **Verma, S. P., Wallach, H. D. F., and Smith, I. C. P.,** The action of melittin on phosphatide multibilayers as studied by infrared dichroism and spin labeling. A model approach to lipid-protein interactions.

79. **Mushayakarara, E. C., Wong, P. T. T., and Mantsch, H. H.,** Detection by high pressure spectroscopy of hydrogen bonding between water and triacetyl glycerol, *Biochem. Biophys. Res. Commun.,* 134, 140, 1986.

80. **Wong, P. T. T. and Mantsch, H. H.,** High pressure infrared spectroscopic evidence of water binding sites in 1,2-diacyl phospholipids, *Chem. Phys. Lipids,* 46, 213, 1988.

81. **Lotta, T. I., Virtanen, J. A., and Kinnunen, P. K. J.,** Fourier transform infrared study on the thermotropic behaviour of fully hydrated 1-palmitoyl-2-(-10-(pyren-1-y)decanoyl)-sn-glycero-3-phosphatidylcholine, *Chem. Phys. Lipids,* 46, 13, 1988.

82. **Boggs, J. M.,** Lipid intermolecular hydrogen bonding: influence on structural organization and membrane function, *Biochim. Biophys. Acta,* 906, 353, 1987.

83. **Bush, S. F., Levin, H., and Levin, I. W.,** Cholesterol-lipid interactions: an infrared and Raman spectroscopic study of the carbonyl stretching mode region of 1,2-dipalmitoyl phosphatidylcholine bilayers, *Chem. Phys. Lipids,* 27, 101, 1980.

84. **Casal, H. L., Martin, A., and Mantsch, H. H.,** Infrared studies of fully hydrated unsaturated phosphatidylserine bilayers. Effect of Li$^+$ and Ca^{++}, *Biochemistry,* 26, 7395, 1987.

85. **Casal, H. L., Mantsch, H. H., Paltauf, F., and Hauser, H. H.,** Infrared and ^{31}P NMR studies of the effects of Li$^+$ and Ca^{++} on phosphatidylserines, *Biochim. Biophys. Acta,* 919, 275, 1987.

86. **Blume, A., Hübner, W., and Messner, G.,** Fourier transform infrared spectroscopy of ^{13}C=O labeled phospholipids. Hydrogen bonding to carbonyl groups, *Biochemistry,* 27, 8239, 1988.

87. **Akutsu, H. and Kyogoku, Y.,** Infrared and Raman spectra of phosphatidylethanolamine and related compounds, *Chem. Phys. Lipids,* 14, 113, 1975.

88. **Goni, F. M. and Arrondo, L. R.,** A study of phospholipid phosphate groups in model membranes by Fourier transform infrared spectroscopy, *Faraday Discuss. Chem. Soc.,* 81, 117, 1986.

89. **Fookson, J. E. and Wallach, D. F. H.,** Structural differences among phosphatidylcholine, phosphatidylethanolamine, and mixed phosphatidylcholine/phosphatidylethanolamine multilayers: an infrared absorption study, *Arch. Biochem. Biophys.,* 189, 195, 1978.

90. **Byler, D. M. and Susi, H.,** Examination of the secondary structure of proteins by deconvolved FTIR spectra, *Biopolymers,* 25, 469, 1986.

91. **Susi, H. and Byler, D. M.,** Resolution-enhanced Fourier transform infrared spectroscopy of enzymes, *Methods Enzymol.,* 130, 290, 1986.

92. **Krimm, S. and Bandekar, J.,** Vibrational spectroscopy and conformation of peptides, polypeptides, and proteins, *Adv. Protein Chem.,* 38, 181, 1986.

93. **Cabiaux, V., Goormaghtigh, E., Wattiez, R., Falmagne, P., and Ruysschaert, J. M.,** *Biochimie,* 71, 153, 1989.

94. **Maddams, W. F.,** The scope and limitations of curve fitting, *Appl. Spectrosc.,* 34, 245, 1980.

95. **Fraser, R. D. B. and Suzuki, E.,** The use of least square in data analysis, in Molecular Biology, Part C, Physical Principles and Techniques of Protein Chemistry, Leach, S. J., Ed., Academic Press, New York, 1973, 301.

96. **Surewicz, W. K., Moscarello, M. A., and Mantsch, H. H.,** Secondary structure of the hydrophobic myelin protein in a lipid environment as determined by Fourier-transform infrared spectrometry, *J. Biol. Chem.,* 262, 8598, 1987.

97. **Surewicz, W. K., Moscarello, M. A., and Mantsch, H. H.,** Fourier transform infrared spectroscopic investigation of the interaction between myelin basic protein in dimyristoylphosphatidylglycerol bilayers, *Biochemistry,* 26, 3881, 1987.

98. **Yang, P. W., Mantsch, H. H., Arrondo, J. L. R., Saint-Girons, I., Guillou, Y., Cohen, G. N., and Bârzu, O.,** Fourier transform infrared investigation of the *Escherichia coli* methionine aporepressor, *Biochemistry,* 26, 2706, 1987.

99. **Surewicz, W. K., Mantsch, H. H., Stahl, G. L., and Epand, R. M.,** Infrared spectroscopic evidence of conformational transitions of an atrial natriuretic peptide, *Proc. Natl. Acad. Sci. U.S.A.,* 84, 7028, 1987.

100. **Surewicz, W. K. and Mantsch, H. H.,** Solution and membrane structure of enkephalins as studied by infrared spectroscopy, *Biochem. Biophys. Res. Commun.,* 150, 245, 1988.

101. **Arrondo, J. L. R., Young, N. M., and Mantsch, H. H.,** The solution structure of concanavalin A probed by FTIR spectroscopy, *Biochim. Biophys. Acta,* 952, 261, 1988.

Index

INDEX

A

Absorbence vs. reflection in ATR materials, 316—319

Acyl chain orientational order, 23—26, 66—72

Amphipathic nature of lipids, 124

Amphiphilic structures, 211

B

Bead friction constant, 175

Bilayer
chain packing, see Chain packing
condensed-phase cooperative phenomena, 41—43
formation steps, 215
lateral diffusion coefficients, 161—164
membrane thermodynamics, 154—161
lipid domain and interfacial region formation, 30—36
nonequilibrium properties at main transition, 30—41
sheet interactions, 28
static properties near main transition, 20—30

Biological membrane simulation
conclusions, 167—168
lateral diffusion, 161—164
modeling and computer simulation models, 152—154
protein distribution as measured by perturbing probes, 164—167
thermodynamics of bilayer membranes, 154—161

Boltzmann probability distribution, 10—12

Brownian dynamics
algorithms and errors, 175—177
chain conformation simulations, 172—196
hydrodynamics, 173—175
inertial effects, 177—178
selected results of chain conformation simulations, 188—195
simulation-based model
building in chain tilt, 187—188
fits to NMR relaxation data, 184—187
potential of mean force, 180—184

Buffers and salts in infrared spectroscopy, 307—308

C

Chain analysis of monolayer core
interacting chains, 92—103
isolated chains, 97—98

Chain distributions in Brownian model, 191—192

Chain packing, 213—215
in bilayers and micelles, 124—127, 132—137
molecular dynamics studies, 145—146
Monte Carlo analysis, 137—145

Chain stacking, 266—274

Chain tilt, 128—130, 187—188

Chemical bonds in molecular orientation, 306—307

Cholesterol X-ray diffraction analysis, 257—260

Cholesterol-containing lipid bilayers, 62—71

Cluster formation and cluster statistics in lipid monolayer, 46—47

Continuum models
of biological membranes, 160—161
of lipid aggregates, 129—132

Cooperative conformational model of lipid monolayer interactions, 95—103

Cooperative phenomena in lipid membranes, see Lipid membranes

Correlation function of lipid monolayer core, 114

Crankshaft model compared with Brownian, 192

Cross-sectional area, 25, 64—66

Crystalline variables, 38

Crystallization
bilayer, 38—41
monolayer, 47—50

D

Decoupling in static-phase lipid monolayer, 47—50

Density distribution of monolayer core, 114

Diacylglycerols
phospholipids in liquid crystalline form, 277—282
structural and conformational notation, 266—271
X-ray single-crystal structures, 271—277

Differential scanning calorimetry, 26

Dihexaecylphosphatidylethanolamine, 41

Dimyristolphosphatidic acid, 43, 57

Dimyristoylphosphatidylcholine, 65—66, 72—73

Dipalmitolyphosphatidylethanolimine, 41

DMPE, 43, 52

Domain size, 34

E

Energy field TAMMO model, 204—206

Fluctuation-dissipation theorem, 11

Fourier transform spectrometry, 308—309

Fractal pattern formation in lipid monolayer, 54—62

Free energy, 21—22, 99—100, 114
minimum about C(2)–C(3) glycerol bond, 278
per chain of lipid monolayer core, 115

Friction constant estimation, 173—175

G

Ganglioside GM1 X-ray diffraction analysis, 260

Glycerol backbone region, 41—42, 321

Gramidicin, 233—241

H

Hydrocarbon chain region of phospholipids, 127—132, 321

Hydrodynamic interaction, 176

Hydrophobic core of lipid monolayer
interacting chains, 92—102